Diabetic Eye Disease - From Therapeutic Pipeline to the Real World

Edited by Giuseppe Lo Giudice

Published in London, United Kingdom

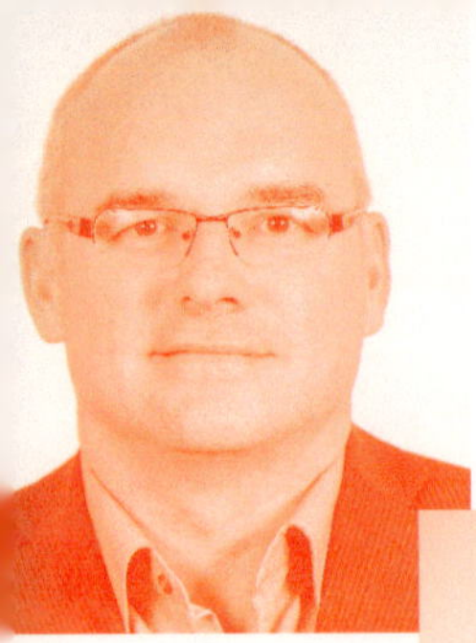
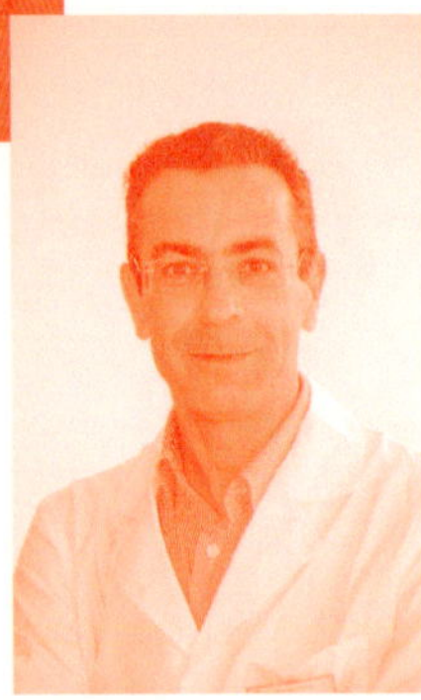
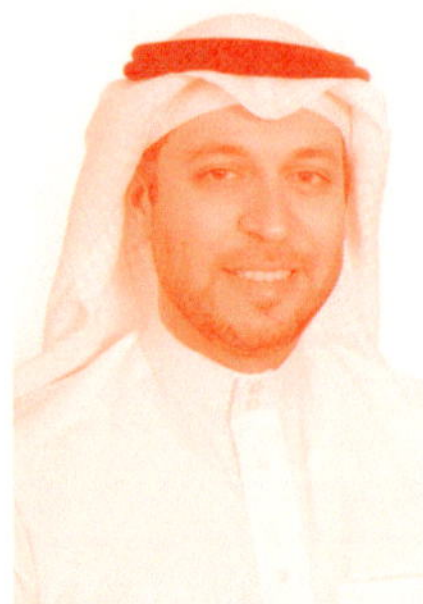
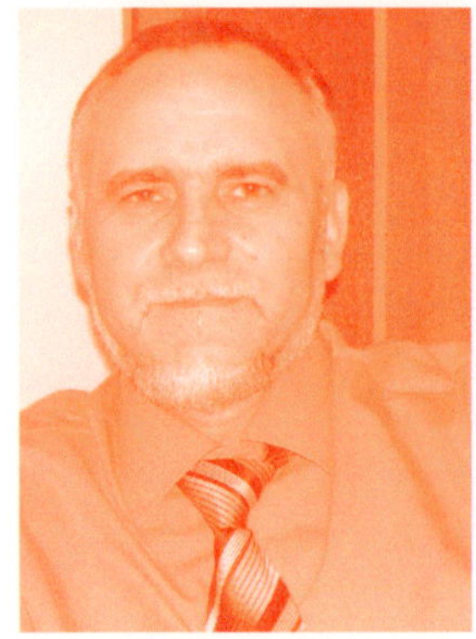
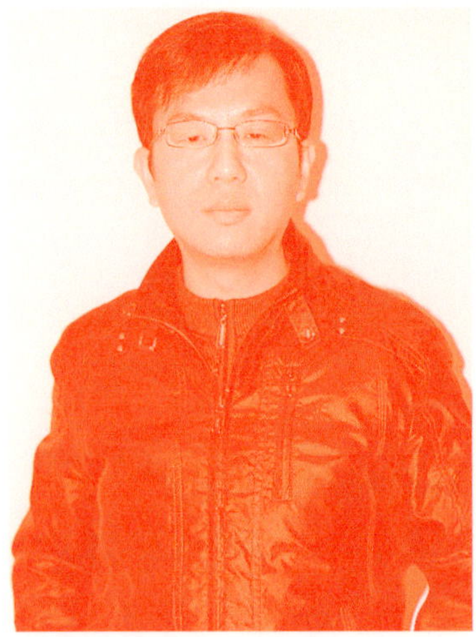
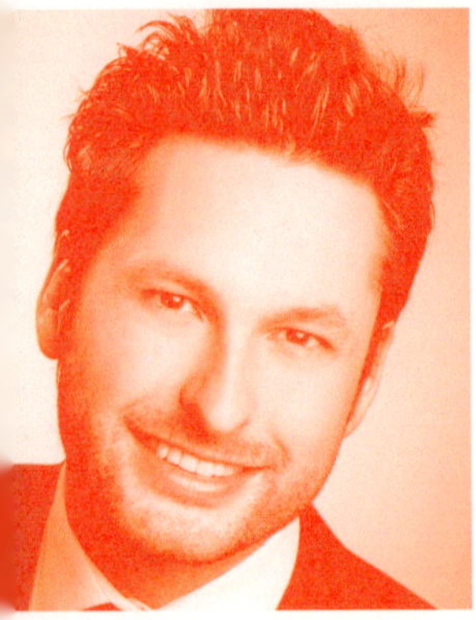
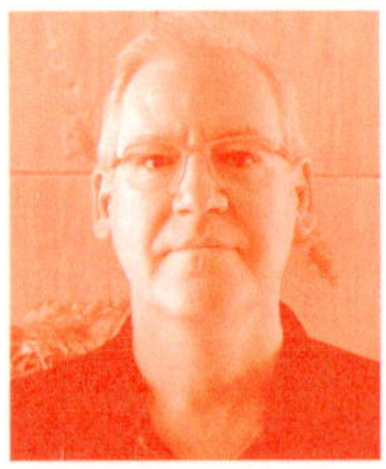

IntechOpen

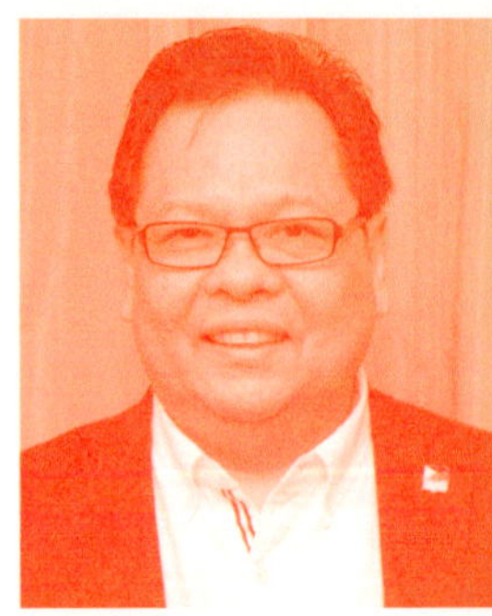
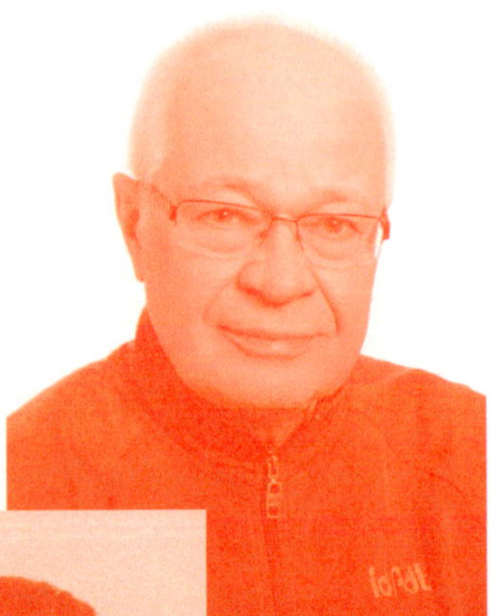
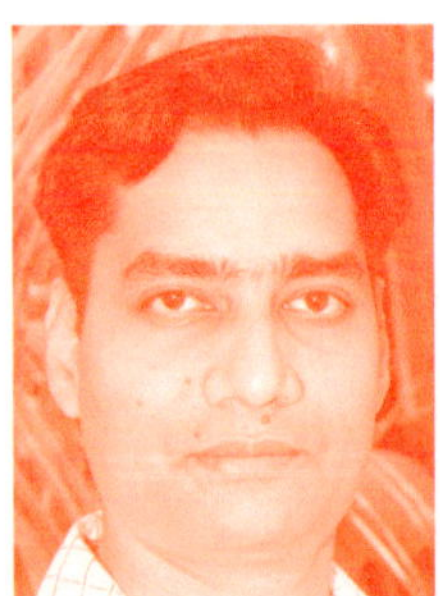
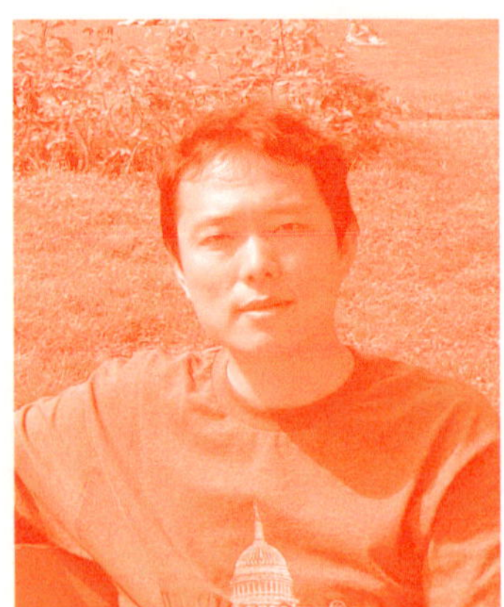
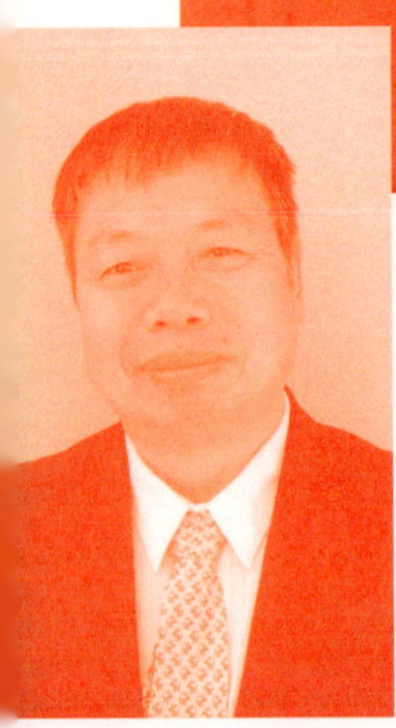
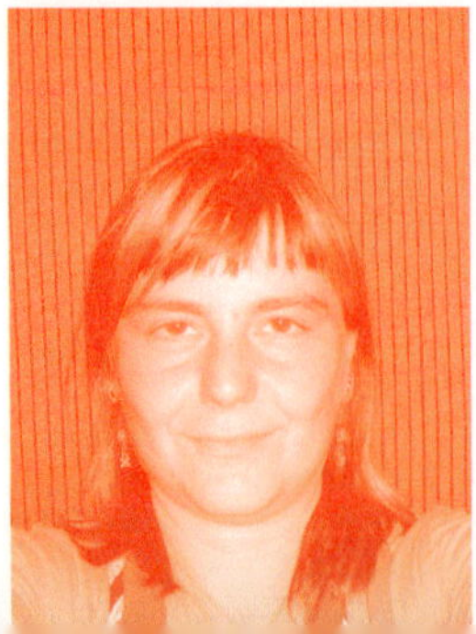

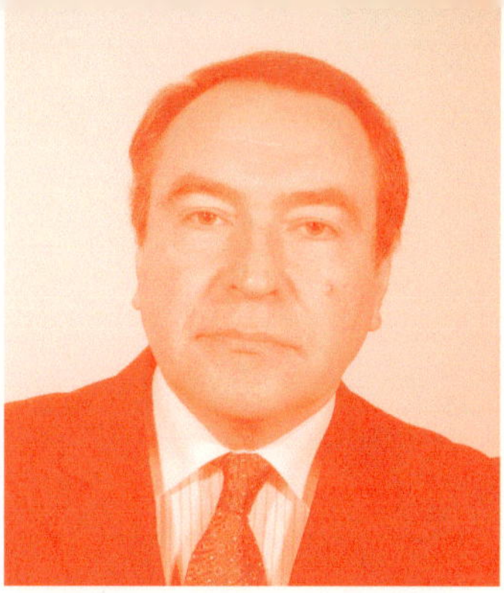
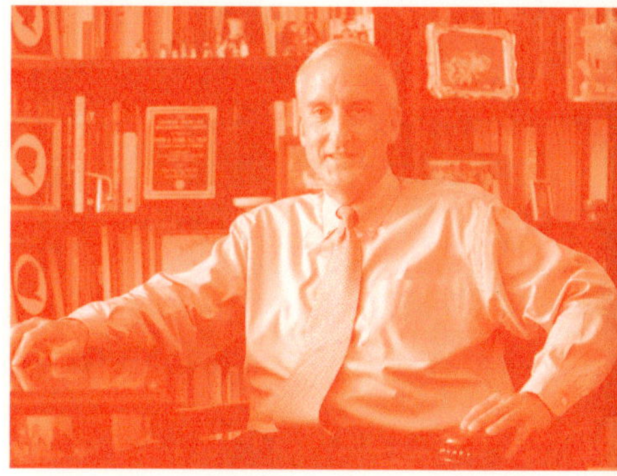
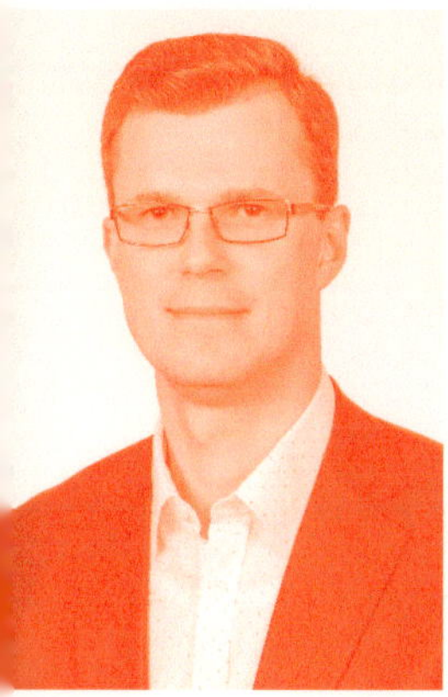
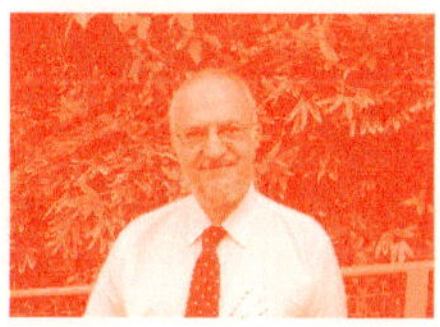
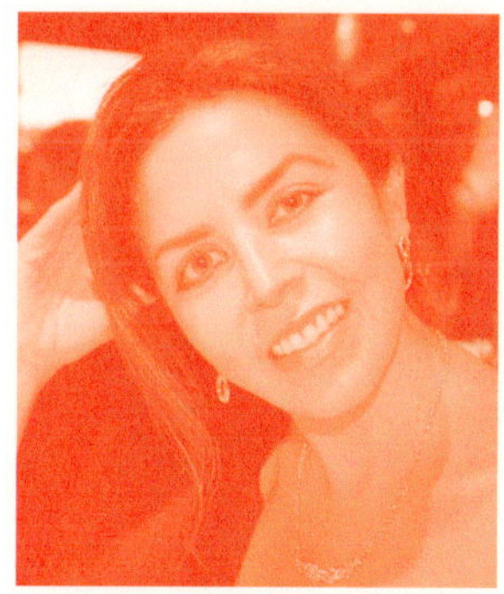

Supporting open minds since 2005

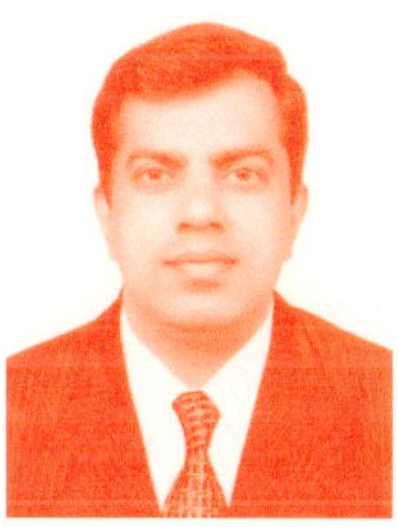
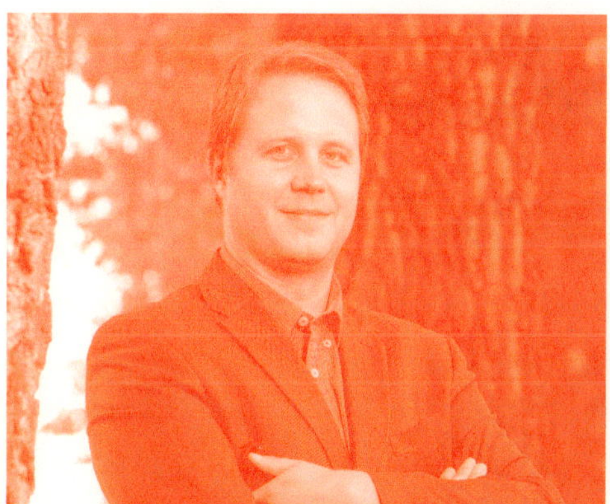
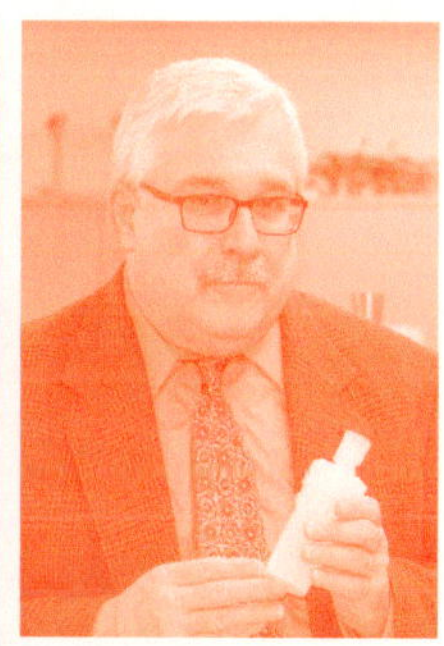
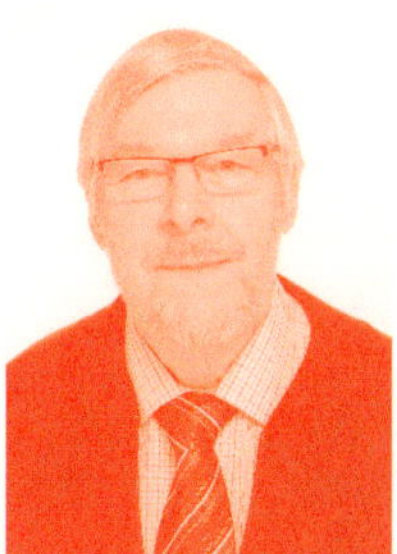
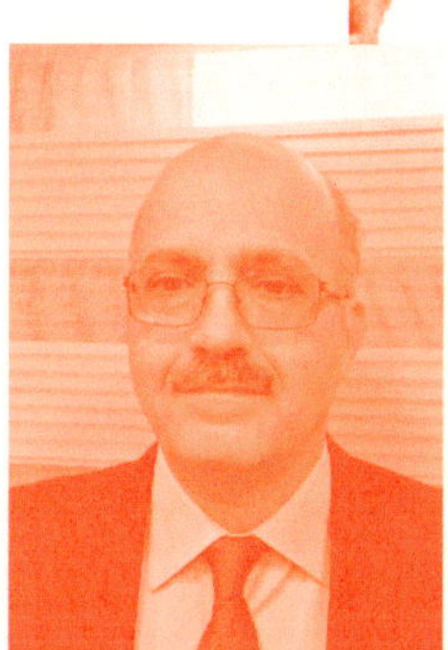
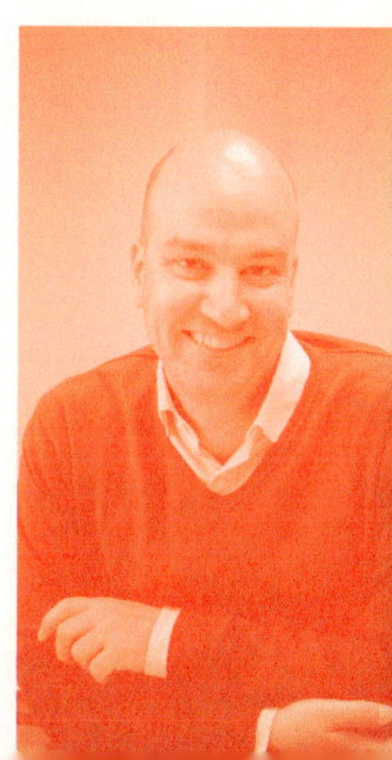
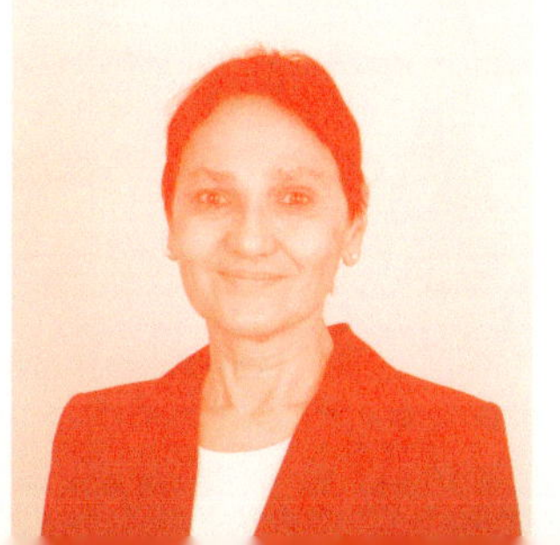

Diabetic Eye Disease - From Therapeutic Pipeline to the Real World
http://dx.doi.org/10.5772/intechopen.95737
Edited by Giuseppe Lo Giudice

Contributors
Anuj Sharma, Deepesh Arora, Surabhi Ruia, Koushik Tripathy, Maya G. Pandova, Natalia Kislitsyna, Sergei Novikov, Jesus Hernan H Gonzalez-Cortes, Jesus Emiliano Gonzalez-Cantu, Aditya Sudhalkar, Sergio Eustolio Hernandez-Da Mota, Jesus Mohamed-Hamsho, Javier Alan Garza-Chavarria, Alper Bilgic, Payal Naresh Shah, Mahesh P. Shanmugam, Divyansh K. Mishra, Florian Baltă, Irina Elena Cristescu, Ioana Teodora Tofolean, Natalia Lobanovskaya, Rehan M. Hussain, Lauren M. Ciulla, Nimesh A. Patel, Nicolas A. Yannuzzi, Ioana Damian, Simona-Delia Nicoara, Sevil - Kestane, Ogugua Ndubuisi Okonkwo, Toyin Akanbi, Chineze Thelma Agweye, Lakshmi Kanta Mondal, Subhasish Pramanik, Subhankar Chowdhury, Chiranjit Bose, Debgopal Bera, Koena Bhattacharjee

First published in London, United Kingdom, 2022 by IntechOpen
IntechOpen is the global imprint of INTECHOPEN LIMITED, registered in England and Wales, registration number: 11086078, 5 Princes Gate Court, London, SW7 2QJ, United Kingdom
Printed in Croatia

British Library Cataloguing-in-Publication Data
A catalogue record for this book is available from the British Library

Additional hard and PDF copies can be obtained from orders@intechopen.com

Diabetic Eye Disease - From Therapeutic Pipeline to the Real World
Edited by Giuseppe Lo Giudice
p. cm.
Print ISBN 978-1-83969-764-7
Online ISBN 978-1-83969-765-4
eBook (PDF) ISBN 978-1-83969-766-1

For EU product safety concerns:
IN TECH d.o.o., Prolaz Marije Krucifikse Kozulić 3, 51000 Rijeka, Croatia, info@intechopen.com or visit our website at intechopen.com.

Meet the editor

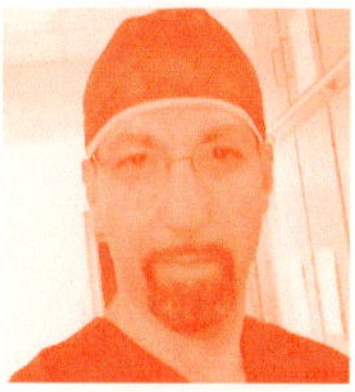

Giuseppe Lo Giudice obtained an MD from the University of Messina, Italy. He completed his ophthalmological residency at the Department of Ophthalmology, University of Padua, Italy. He was a fellow in the Ophthalmology Department, Gironcoli Ophthalmic Center, from 2002 to 2004. He was an assistant in ophthalmology at Conegliano Hospital Conegliano, Treviso, Italy, from 2004 to 2007. Since 2007, Dr. Giudice has been a surgeon and vice-director at San Antonio Hospital, University of Padua. His fields of interest include treatments for retinal diseases (proliferative retinopathies, age-related macular degeneration, and diabetic retinopathy) and vitreoretinal surgery. He has more than twenty-five years of experience in clinical research as well as in clinical trials and laboratory research. He performed more than 10,000 anterior segment surgeries (cataract surgery, glaucoma surgery, corneal transplantation) in the last five years. He has also performed more than 700 vitreo-retinal surgeries in the last two years at San Antonio Hospital.

Contents

Preface

Diabetic retinopathy (DR) is a disease characterized mainly by damage to the blood vessels in the retina. A large body of evidence supports the role of both inflammation and neurodegeneration in the development and progression of DR. Treatments for DR and diabetic macular edema (DME) have made tremendous advances in recent decades, but modalities with better efficacy and longer durability are still needed. Many ongoing trials are aiming to validate new treatment options. These range from new drugs to advances in dosing or administration of established pharmaceuticals to entirely new modalities. This book begins with a description of the mechanisms of development and progression of DME and with the characterization of the early stages of DR. Inflammation appears to be a key player in the pathogenesis of this condition. It has been noted that levels of inflammatory mediators like hypoxia-inducible factor, TNF-α, IL-6, and IL-1B, among others, are elevated in the diabetic's vitreous gel. Furthermore, oxidative stress-mediated lipid and protein-derived biomolecules not only add important mediators in the pathogenesis of DR, but also accelerate the progression and severity of microangiopathy.

Multimodal imaging represents a new diagnostic tool in the field of ophthalmology. Imaging tools such as optical coherence tomography and optical coherence tomography angiography are used for screening this pathology, but a new diagnostic advantage derived from the possibility of obtaining high-resolution retinal images of photoreceptors and retinal vessels by adaptive optics faces new perspectives in retinal physiology and pathophysiology.

This book also discusses standards and novel approaches, as well as current surgical options and treatment techniques. Anti-VEGF therapies such as ranibizumab, aflibercept, and off-label bevacizumab have become a first-line treatment for DME, however new therapeutic approaches are becoming more interesting as alternative pathways, such as the Tie-2 angiopoietin pathway, that may address unmet needs, with potential for greater efficacy or durability when compared to monotherapy or combination treatment. The book concludes with chapters on the latest concepts of vitreoretinal surgical approaches for both the DME with and/or without internal limiting membrane peeling and for proliferative DR.

Giuseppe Lo Giudice
San Antonio Hospital,
University of Padua,
Padua, Italy

Section 1

Clinical Presentation of Diabetic Retinopathy and Pathogenesis

Chapter 1

Pathophysiology of Diabetic Retinopathy

Natalia Lobanovskaya

Abstract

Diabetic retinopathy is a prototypical microvascular disorder. Hyperglycemia causes a multiple pathological changes in the retinal vasculature. It has been suggested that apoptosis of pericytes due to high glucose levels plays a key role in the development of the earliest events during diabetic retinopathy. Advancement of the disease resulted in a progressive vessel leakage leading to edematous distortion of macula and increase in hypoxia inducing development of neovascularization with sight threatening complications. Four basis hypotheses explaining the hyperglycemia harmful effects were suggested: (1) increased glucose flux through the aldose reductase pathway, (2) overproduction of advanced glycation end products, (3) activation of protein kinase C isoforms, and (4) increased glucose flux via the hexosamine pathway. It was admitted as well that apoptosis of neurons and glial cell activation occur even earlier than vascular damage. Disturbance in glial cell functions leads to increase in metabolic abnormalities such as glutamate accumulation, promotion of inflammation, and oxidative stress resulting in neuron apoptosis and deterioration of vascular disorders. Clarification of significant biochemical mechanisms involving in the development of diabetic retinopathy can help to create new effective ways in diabetic retinopathy treatment.

Keywords: diabetic retinopathy, diabetic maculopathy, microvascular changes, metabolic pathways

1. Introduction

Diabetic retinopathy (DR) is a common complication of diabetes. Elevated blood glucose levels induce alterations in a number of metabolic pathways that trigger microvascular lesions. It can cause significant vision deterioration due to development of macular edema or proliferative DR leading to intravitreal hemorrhages and tractional retinal detachment. Elaboration of effective methods in the treatment of DR is based on understanding of pathogenesis of this disease.

2. Blood flow changes

A hallmark of diabetes is a high blood glucose levels. It was shown in nondiabetic animals that infusion of glucose causes a rapid increase of retinal blood flow [1]. Patients with mild or no DR demonstrated significantly increased retinal blood volume flow compared with nondiabetic participants [2, 3]. Apparently, blood flow abnormalities contribute to the pathogenesis of DR and precede the earliest visible signs of diabetic retinal complications. Blood flow in the retina is controlled mostly by metabolic autoregulation. Metabolic autoregulation is an adaptation of the diameter of vessels to the metabolic demands in the tissues. Oxygen saturation is a principal metabolic stimulus for blood flow changes in the retina. Impaired metabolic autoregulation in patients with DR may be due to changes in the retinal metabolism. It was founded that glucose flux through the polyol pathway in DR disrupts balance between pyruvate and lactate levels that resulted in pseudohypoxia and increased blood flow [4]. Probably, this is a direct mechanism of glucose-induced hyperperfusion in DR [5]. It was shown that increased blood flow induces increase in shear stress followed by a damage of the endothelial cell lining and basement membrane thickening [6]. Production of the vasoconstrictor endothelin-1 (ET-1) by endothelial cells is changed depending on the level and duration of the shear stress [7]. At the same time increased shear stress stimulates production of vasodilators, namely prostacyclin (PGI_2) and nitric oxide (NO) followed by additional increase in blood flow [8, 9]. Hyperglycemia by its direct deleterious effect on pericytes inhibits contraction of small vessels, impairing autoregulation [10]. The dilatation of retinal vessels during the early stages of DR is accompanied with impaired pressure autoregulation. Pressure autoregulation is a capacity of the resistance vessels to adjust diameter to maintain stable microcirculation during changes in the arterial blood pressure. Thereby, in DR the systemic blood pressure more easily conveys to the capillary bed, increasing tangential stress on the capillary wall where it contributes to the formation of microaneurysms, hemorrhages, and breakdown of the blood-retina barrier (BRB) [6, 11]. The fact that hyperperfusion is essential in the development of DR is confirmed by conditions that are associated with its progression and characterized by increased blood flow. Hypertension is an important risk factor for the incidence and progression of DR [12–14]. Pregnancy in patients with diabetes is often associated with a deterioration in DR [15].

3. Microvascular changes

DR initially is a disorder of retinal capillaries that later propagates to the larger vessels. In the early stages of DR, microvascular lesions are characterized by development of microaneurysms, capillary leakage resulting in intraretinal hemorrhages, hard exudates, retinal edema, and also capillary occlusion resulting in ischemia and cotton wool spots formation. More advanced stages of DR are associated with vascular changes such as vein beading, loop formation, intraretinal microvascular abnormalities (IRMA). DR progression leads to neovascularization, intravitreal hemorrhages, expanding of fibrous tissue, causing retinal traction and detachment. Exudative or ischemic forms of the sight threatening diabetic maculopathy may develop in any stage of DR [16].

Long before any clinically visible alterations occur, histological and pathophysiological changes in the wall of the vessels develop, involving thickening of the basement membrane, loss of pericytes, disturbance of endothelial cell functions. A crucial role in the progress of the disease is played by pericytes, developmentally originating from mesoderm. Pericytes are located along the endothelial cell tube, embracing with their cytoplasmic processes endothelial cells and providing mechanical support for the capillary wall [17, 18]. Pericytes are known as specialized contractile cells and function in the capillaries such as smooth muscle cells in the larger vessels, controlling vascular tone, and perfusion pressure [18, 19]. Pericytes are encased in a basement membrane (BM) that is continued with the endothelial BM (**Figure 1A**). The pericyte-endothelial cell interface is mainly divided by the BM. However, it was demonstrated that pericyte and endothelial cell plasma membranes contact across the BM fenestra [20]. There are different types of contacts described between endothelial cells and pericytes:

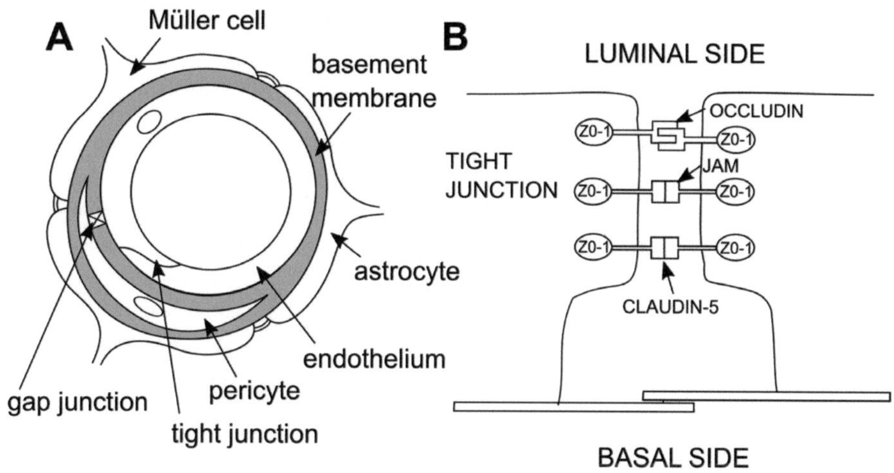

Figure 1.
Blood-retina barrier. (A) Schematic transverse section of capillary showing the endothelium, basement membrane, pericyte, and gap junction. (B) Schematic drawing of the proteins linked with tight junctions between endothelial cells. JAMs – junction adhesion molecules, ZO-1 – zonula occludens-1. (Modified from Ueno [29]).

peg-and-socket junctions, adhesion plaques, and gap junctions. In peg-and-socket contacts, cytoplasmic fingers of the pericytes interposed into the deep endothelial cell invaginations and, as assumed, support anchorage [21]. Adhesion plaques at the pericyte and endothelial cell plasma membrane serve as a mechanical binding among two cells, which allows the contraction or relaxation of the pericyte to be conveyed to the endothelial cell and thereby to affect capillary diameter [22]. Gap junctions are supposed to permit a direct connections between the cytoplasm of pericyte and endothelial cell [23]. It was proposed that ionic currents, the passage of small molecules and nucleotides, occur between endothelial cells and pericytes through the gap junctions [23, 24]. Moreover, it was shown that pericytes suppress capillary endothelial cell proliferation when cells are co-cultured in physical contact with each other, probably via gap junctions [25]. Interactions between endothelium and pericytes are also regulated by cell adhesion molecules, produced by both cell types, imbalance of which may cause leakage of the BRB during the early stages of DR [26]. Thereby, pericytes in the capillaries are closely associated with endothelial cells and regulate each other functions. Total cytoplasmic areas of the pericytes enveloping capillary and the cytoplasmic areas of the endothelial cells covering these capillaries comprise an average 1:1 ratio in human, which is much higher than that in other tissues [27, 28]. The cause for this high ratio is the necessity for an exceedingly high barrier function in the retina itself in order to prevent an extra fluid accumulation that could result in vision impairment. It seems that pericyte coverage in capillaries correlates positively with endothelial barrier characteristics in different tissues, and greater pericytes density apparently provides better integrity for the vasculature [27]. The BRB comprises the inner BRB (iBRB) and the outer BRB (oBRB). The iBRB is formed by the continuous lining of endothelial cells, tight junctions (zonula occludens) between adjacent endothelial cells and interconnecting pericytes. Tight junction proteins between apical regions of retinal pigment epithelial cells are structural components of the oBRB [29, 30]. The tight junctions are composed of integral membrane proteins, namely: claudin, occludin, junction adhesion molecules, and a number of accessory proteins such as zonula occludens –1 (ZO-1), ZO-2, ZO-3 (**Figure 1B**) [29, 31]. Pericytes are supposed to maintain the integrity of the iBRB by induction of expression of occludin and other junction proteins [30]. The early feature of DR is loss of pericytes, induced by high glucose levels that has been shown in a row of experiments. Naruse and colleagues demonstrated that high concentration of glucose inhibited proliferation of retinal capillary pericytes in the culture [32]. In particular, fluctuating glucose levels increased pericyte apoptosis in vitro [33]. Since pericytes are important compound of the capillary wall and maintain a capillary structure, loss of them results in localized outpouching of the microvessel wall. This process is linked with microaneurysms development, which is the earliest clinical sign of DR. Progressive pericyte apoptosis in complex with hypoxia causes dilation of the capillaries, venous caliber abnormalities such as venous beading and venous loops. Microaneurysms and dilated capillaries are usually incompetent and leaky [16]. Pericyte loss is accompanied by dysfunction and apoptosis of endothelial cells as well. Endothelial cells play an important role in the regulation of capillary permeability and tone. These cells are responsible for metabolism of BM, coagulation balance, migration, and adhesion of leucocytes to the vessel wall, production of ET-1 [34]. It was demonstrated in vitro that endothelium in high glucose conditions secreted more BM material such as collagen and fibronectin IV, and overexpression of these products remained detectable even after endothelial cells were returned to normal glucose exposure [35, 36]. Thickening of BM in the early phase of DR may prevent endothelium-pericytes contacts that increases pericyte apoptosis due to deprivation of nourishment, while endothelium, losing control of proliferation from pericyte is involved in the formation of new vessels in later stages of retinopathy. Thickened BM reduces a diameter of affected vessels and facilitates capillary obliteration. Dolgov and colleagues demonstrated weakening of endothelial intercellular gap junctions in the vessels during DR [37]. It was shown an increased apoptosis in cultured endothelial cells exposed by high glucose levels [38]. Furthermore, high glucose affects functions of endothelium indirectly by increased production of vasoactive agents and growth factors in other cells [39]. Thereby, DR progression leads to pericyte and endothelium pronounced disappearance, thickening of BM, and formation of acellular capillaries (tubes formed by basement membrane only), capillary occlusion, and ischemia. Non-perfusion in some capillaries induces hypoxia, dilatation, and increased intracapillary pressure in others. Thereby, loss of pericytes impaired functions and later apoptosis of endothelium resulted in progressive retinal ischemia and BRB breakdown. BRB disintegration may occur at the level of both the iBRB and oBRB, causing accumulation of intraretinal fluid and plasma proteins first of all in the inner and outer plexiform layers of the retina, which is visible ophthalmoscopically as intraretinal hemorrhages, retinal edema, and hard exudates. Fluid accumulation in the macular region can cause a macular edema leading to neuronal distortion and visual impairment [16]. Diabetic macular edema may be focal or diffuse. Focal edema is mainly caused by leakage from microaneurysms, whereas diffuse macular edema is a result of generalized leakage from dilated capillaries throughout the posterior pole, which is coupled with occlusion of capillaries. Diabetic maculopathy can associate with ischemia as well, due to mostly capillary obliteration, which is the main cause of visual impairment in this case. Progressive vessel occlusion increases retinal hypoxia and leads to the formation of significant non-perfusion areas in the retina, cotton wool spots, or soft exudates and intraretinal microvascular abnormalities (IRMA). Cotton wool spots develop in cases of retinal arteriole occlusion and focal ischemia, which courses blockage of axoplasmic current and accumulation of large spheroidal axon swellings ("cystoid bodies") and intra-axonal organelles in the retinal nerve-fiber layer [40]. IRMA is a tortuous collateral vessel located midway between arteries and veins. It is hypothesized that IRMAs are either dilated preexisting capillaries or newly formed vessels developing due to obliteration of capillaries and ischemia. IRMAs practically have no leakage and usually do not cross major large vessels [41]. In response to tissue hypoxia, vascular endothelial growth factor (VEGF) is released and stimulates angiogenesis. New vessels usually emerge from venous part of the retinal vasculature and grow uncontrolled [42]. If these vessels break the inner limiting membrane, they are defined as retinal neovascularization. New vessels penetrate through the inner limiting membrane, proliferate along the posterior hyaloid. They are fragile and may tear leaking blood into the retina and vitreous. Subsequently, a fibrovascular scar tissue grows from the retinal surface into the vitreous cavity. Fibrous tissue retraction may course tractional retinal detachment and vision loss [43, 44].

4. Metabolic pathways implicated in hyperglycemia-induced lesion of vasculature

The Diabetes Control and Complications Trial (DCCT) clinical trial confirmed that chronic hyperglycemia is detrimental in the development and progression of DR, though the exact mechanisms of microvascular lesions due to hyperglycemia are not yet fully understood [45]. A lot of interconnecting biochemical pathways are involved in hyperglycemia-induced vascular pathologies. Four major mechanisms explaining how hyperglycemia causes diabetic complications include: (1) increased glucose flux through the polyol pathway, (2) increased formation of advanced glycation end products (AGE), (3) activation of the protein kinase C (PKC) pathway, and (4) a fourth mechanism has been suggested recently: increased glucose metabolism through the hexosamine pathway [46].

4.1 Increased polyol pathway flux

Excessive glucose in diabetes is metabolized through the polyol pathway. In the polyol pathway, aldose reductase (AR) reduces glucose to sorbitol (polyol), using nicotinamide adenine dinucleotide phosphate (NADPH) as a cofactor. Subsequently, sorbitol is slowly metabolized into fructose by sorbitol dehydrogenase (SDH) with NAD^+ reduced to NADH. Sorbitol is a sugar alcohol and strongly hydrophilic; therefore sorbitol cannot diffuse easily across the cell membrane. It was demonstrated that excessive intracellular storage of sorbitol results in hyperosmotic cellular damage [47]. Increased polyol pathway flux is considered to have several negative effects on retinal cells. Concomitant decrease of NADPH results in less NADPH availability for use by glutathione reductase, which uses NADPH as a cofactor to regenerate intracellular glutathione. Glutathione protects cells by neutralizing reactive oxygen species (ROS). Thereby, reduced NADPH in a hyperglycemic environment could course or exacerbate intracellular oxidative stress. Fructose produced by the polyol pathway is metabolized consequently to fructose-3-phosphate or 3-deoxyglucosone, which are potent glycating substances and can lead to generation of AGEs [48]. The presence of AR was shown in the ganglion retinal cells, Müller cell processes, retinal pigment epithelium, and the pericytes and endothelial cells of retinal capillaries in diabetic models in animals. These studies also pointed out increased apoptosis of pericytes due to AR activity [49, 50]. It was demonstrated in other work, however, the presence of AR in the cytoplasm of pericytes but not in endothelial cells in experimental diabetes [51]. Sato and colleagues observed accumulation of sugar alcohols in pericytes in contrast with similar cultured endothelial cells [52]. It was shown that AR was localized in human retinal pericytes but not in the endothelial cells [53, 54]. This data suggested that a selective degeneration and loss of retinal pericytes may be due to AR activity. Some studies showed that aldose reductase inhibitors (ARIs) were able to reduce the incidence and severity of diabetic retinal lesions occurring in the galactose-fed animals. The administration of ARIs to animal model of diabetes indicated that

ARIs can prevent pericyte loss, formation of microaneurysms, hemorrhages, and abnormal growth of endothelial cells in areas of pericytes loss [55, 56]. Thickening of basement membrane in the retinal capillaries was significantly inhibited by administration of ARI in animal diabetic model [57]. It was shown in human genetic studies that certain polymorphisms of the AR gene are associated with elevated tissue levels of AR and higher risk of diabetic complications [58]. However, sorbinil retinopathy clinical trial, where ARI sorbinil was administred for 2–3 years to adults with insulin-dependent diabetes, had no clinically important effect on DR [59]. Probably, it is important to develop more effective ARIs.

4.2 Increased formation of advanced glycation end products (AGE)

AGEs are built up at a permanent but slow rate starting at the embryonic development, accumulate through entire life, and linked with aging. However, AGEs formation is markedly accelerated in diabetes because of hyperglycemic environment [60]. AGEs are formed from the non-enzymatic reaction of sugars, such as glucose and fructose with free amino groups of proteins, lipids, and nucleic acids. The initial products of this reaction, such as Schiff bases, which spontaneously reform themselves into Amadori products, are reversible. Further reactions and molecular rearrangements result in the formation of irreversible crossed-linked derivatives termed AGEs, which are composed of a heterogeneous class of molecules that are yellow brown pigments, fluoresce. AGEs capable of forming cross-links with other structures and interact with cells via specific cell-surface AGE-binding receptors (RAGE), triggering inflammatory events, production of growth factors, generation of reactive oxygen intermediates induce oxidative stress [61, 62]. AGEs are toxic because they can modify intracellular proteins, including those involved in the regulation of gene transcription, or transfigure the extracellular matrix proteins, leading to reduction of the cell-to-cell interaction and vascular dysfunction, and also can modify circulating blood proteins. It demonstrated free radical generation by glycation products in vitro [63, 64]. The interaction of AGEs with RAGE has been involved in the development of DR. It was demonstrated that retinal endothelial cells, pericytes, and ganglion cells are expressed RAGE under normal or diabetic conditions in vitro and in vivo [61, 62, 65, 66]. Yatamagishi and colleagues demonstrated pericytes apoptosis mediated via AGEs-RAGE interactions. It was proposed that AGEs-RAGE interactions induced generation of intracellular ROSs, which course overexpression of proapoptotic Bax protein in pericytes [67]. Schmidt studies demonstrated that AGEs after interaction with their cellular receptors are responsible for induction of oxidative stress, activation of nuclear factor kappa-light-chain-enhancer (NF- *k*B) both in vitro and in vivo [61, 62]. NF-*k*B is associated with transcriptional activation of genes associated with inflammatory responses [68]. Interestingly, persistent hyperglycemia leads to a gradual accumulation of AGEs in the BM and in pericytes in diabetic animal models, however, the retinal endothelial cells did not store AGEs. It was suggested that endothelium is capable to uptake AGEs directly from the blood stream through RAGE located on their luminal surface and further transfer the AGEs to subendothelial matrix and to pericytes. The preferential appearance of intracellular AGE deposits within pericytes and BM may affect their functions and lead to progression of DR [65]. Another study by Yamagishi demonstrated that in vitro exposure of retinal pericytes to AGEs retarded pericytes growth and induced apoptosis; moreover, these effects were cell-specific [66]. It was found that administration of an inhibitor of AGEs to diabetic animals prevented accumulation of AGEs in the retinal capillaries and significantly diminished pericyte loss, subsequent formation of microaneurysms, acellular capillaries, and capillary closure [69]. Furthermore, it was shown in vitro that AGEs induced VEGF overproduction by retinal pericytes, that is, additionally disturbed retinal microvascular homeostasis in concert with pericyte apoptosis [70]. Thereby, accumulation of AGEs significantly contributes to the development of diabetic retinopathy.

4.3 Activation of the protein kinase C (PKC) pathway

PKC activation has been shown to induce retinal vascular abnormalities in diabetes. Diacylglycerol (DAG) is the primary activator of PKC in physiology [4]. Increased total levels of DAG in DR were found [71]. Augmentation of DAG levels in diabetes can occur by several pathways. Hyperglycemia results in an increase of glucose flux through the glycolysis pathway, which in turn leads to enhanced de novo synthesis of DAG from glycolytic intermediates [72–74]. DAG can be gained as well from the hydrolysis of phosphatidylinositides, from the metabolism of phosphatidylcholine by phospholipase C [75]. Increased generation of DAG and the subsequent activation of PKC isoforms affect retinal functions in multiple different ways. Activation of DAG-PKC pathway is associated with cellular and vascular abnormalities in the retina such as increased endothelial permeability, basement membrane thickening, leucocyte adhesion, cytokine activation, abnormal angiogenesis, and excessive apoptosis [72]. Activation of PKC regulates gene expression via of phosphatidylinositol 3-kinase (PI3K) and mitogen-activated protein kinase (MAPK) pathways. Induced by phosphorylation, in response to extracellular signals, MAPK and PI3K regulate functions of a broad array of proteins involved in cell growth, proliferation, motility, adhesion, survival, apoptosis, and angiogenesis [76, 77]. Among the various PKC isoforms, the beta-isoform seems to be activated preferentially in the vasculatures of diabetic animals [78]. It was demonstrated that PKC beta-isoform plays a role in the VEGF-induced vascular permeability in the retina of diabetic animals and VEGF-induced proliferation of endothelial cells. Furthermore, PKC beta-isoform-selective inhibitors decreased VEGF-induced vascular permeability and endothelial cell growth [77, 78]. VEGF is a dimeric glycoprotein and has a crucial role in the development and progression of DR. In mammals, the VEGF family comprises seven members where VEGF-A typically, and below, referred to as VEGF. VEGF regulates cell functions via vascular endothelial growth factor receptor-1 (VEGFR-1) and VEGFR-2, which belongs to the receptor tyrosine kinase family and primarily implicated in angiogenesis [79]. Hypoxia is the major inducer of increased VEGF transcription in the retina via hypoxia inducible factor-1 (HIF-1) [44, 80]. In addition to hypoxia, a number of other factors can stimulate the overexpression of VEGF in DR, including oxidative stress and insulin-like growth factor [81]. The pathways by which these factors regulate upregulation of retinal VEGF transcription are not yet understood. However, it has been demonstrated that ROS can induce VEGF transcription by a mechanism involving the activity of signal transducer and activator of transcription factor 3 (STAT3) [82]. It was found that increased vessel permeability is correlated with increased ocular levels of VEGF [83]. It was suggested that VEGF-induced permeability results from triggering of a cascade of proteolytic activities on the endothelial cell surface. VEGF induces expression of urokinase plasminogen activator receptor (uPAR) that initiates cleavage of plasminogen by urokinase plasminogen activator (uPA). Subsequently, plasmin formation leads to activation of membrane-bound pro matrix metalloproteinase-9 pro (MMP-9) [84]. MMP-9 induces pericellular proteolysis affecting cell-cell and cell-BM attachment, producing leaky vessels and permitting to the endothelial cells to penetrate the underlying BM, migrate, and proliferate [85]. It was shown as well that VEGF increases microvascular permeability via increasing the intracellular calcium concentration in endothelial cells [86]. Growth of new blood vessels is induced by VEGF-VEGFRs mediated activation of MAPK cascades resulting in endothelium proliferation, migration, and tube formation [44]. Anti-vascular endothelial growth factor (anti-VEGF) drugs are viable treatment option for patients with diabetic macular edema and proliferative diabetic retinopathy [87, 88].

A role of PKC activation in the thickening of capillary basement membrane that is the prominent structural abnormality in the retinal microvessels in early DR was demonstrated. Treatment with PKC agonists stimulated type IV collagen expression and fibronectin accumulation that may increase the BM thickness [89, 90]. It was reported that inhibition of Na^+ -K^+ -ATPase by hyperglycemia was due to consecutive activation of PKC and cytosolic phospholipase A2 (cPLA2), inducing release of arachidonic acid and increased production of PGE2, which are known inhibitors of Na+,K(+)-ATPase [91]. Na^+-K^+-ATPase is a component of sodium pump, and it takes part in regulation of cellular contractility, MAPK transduction pathways, ROS formation, intracellular calcium levels. PKC takes part in sustaining of chronic inflammation in DR. A row of studies were demonstrated that activation of PKC in endothelial cells triggered upregulation of intercellular adhesion molecule 1 (ICAM-1) and vascular cell adhesion molecule (VCAM)-1 that increased adhesion of leukocytes to the vascular endothelium. PKC inhibitors prevented upregulation of ICAM -I and (VCAM)-1 and adherence of neutrophils to endothelial cells [92–96]. It was demonstrated that leukocytes trapped in retinal vasculature course capillary occlusion, vascular cell, and BM alterations in the animal diabetic model [97]. Being adhered to the vessel wall, leukocytes may release ROS, enzymes, and cytokines, which damage the endothelial cells and increase vascular permeability [98, 99]. Taking in account the significance of pathological events inducing by activation of PKC, inhibitors of PKC have been studied as potential therapeutic agents for the treatment of patients with microvascular complications associated with diabetes [100].

4.4 Increased flux through the hexosamine pathway

The hexosamine biosynthesis pathway (HBP) is a comparatively minor part of glycolysis. Hyperglycemic condition increases glucose flux through HBP. High availability of intracellular glucose leads to an excess amount of fructose-6-phosphate. The largest proportion of fructose-6-phosphate is utilized in the glycolytic pathway. Glutamine: fructose-6-phosphate aminotransferase (GFAT) regulates the entry of fructose-6-phosphate into the HBP. The major end product of the HBP is UDP-N-acetylglucosamine (UDP-GlcNAc) that catalyzes the addition of *O*-linked β-*N*-acetylglucosamine (*O*-GlcNAc) to serine and threonine residues of proteins [101]. O-GlcNAcylation is an important protein posttranslational modification (PTM) that involves the addition of *O*-GlcNAc moiety to the hydroxyl groups of serine and/or threonine residues of proteins. Such as phosphorylation, protein O-GlcNAc modification can directly modify protein functions and also lead to the changes of gene expression [102]. Under conditions of sustained hyperglycemia that occur in diabetes, GFAT is upregulated, fructose-6-phosphate flux increases through the HBP and results in increase of *O*-GlcNAc-modified proteins. There are studies showing an association between elevated flux through HBP and insulin resistance [103]. It was demonstrated that high levels of *O*-GlcNAcylation of proteins in the retinal endothelial cells and pericytes correlated with glucose concentration levels, but the physiological consequences of this mainly remain unknown [104]. O-GlcNAc protein modification dysregulation under hyperglycemia and/or ischemia may contribute to the pathogenesis of the DR and retinal neovascularization [104, 105]. Decreasing glucose flux through the HBP by preventing the biosynthesis of UDP-GlcNAc would appear to reduce glucose toxicity, but would also induce adverse effects. A lot of proteins including kinases, phosphatases, transcriptional factors, and metabolic enzymes can be O-GlcNAc modified, but the functional consequences of this modification remain unknown for most of these proteins and need to be clarified.

5. Retinal neural and glial cell impairment

The neural retina is transparent and largely undistinguished during clinical examination in contrast to retinal vessels. Nevertheless, the retina comprises a complex network of neurons and glia closely interconnecting with vasculature. The neurons: photoreceptors, bipolar cells, horizontal cells, amacrine cells, and retinal ganglion cells percept, integrate, and transmit visual signals into the brain. Glia comprises astrocytes, Müller cells (MCs), and microglial cells. MCs are the primary glial cells of the retina and play a pivotal role in retinal metabolism. It is now broadly acknowledged that in addition to the vascular alterations structural and functional detriment to nonvascular cells contributes to the pathogenesis of DR. Abnormalities of the neural retina have been found in experimental and human diabetes. There is evidence demonstrating an early neurodegeneration of photoreceptors in animal diabetic models [106]. Apoptosis of retinal ganglion cells has been observed as well in cases of short-term experimental diabetes and in humans with diabetes [107]. Decline of color sensitivity [108] and contrast sensitivity [109] are early signs of neural retinal malfunction that take place after only 2 years of diabetes. As glia maintenance functions of neurons and endothelium, apparently, glial reactive changes affect the function and survival both of vascular and of neuronal cells of the retina. It was detected that high glutamate levels in the retinas of diabetic animals as a consequence of MC reduced ability to convert glutamate into glutamine [110, 111]. Glutamate has been demonstrated to be toxic to neuronal cell [112, 113]. These findings suggested an early and probably persistent glutamate excitotoxicity in the retina during diabetes that courses neural degeneration. One of the early signs of retinal metabolic stress is the upregulation of glial fibrillary acidic protein (GFAP) in MCs and astocytes, which was detected in animals and in human patients with non-proliferative retinopathy [111, 114]. It was found that in activated MCs and astrocytes, VEGF expression was significantly increased [115, 116]. Glial cell proliferation is a well-recognized latest change in DR that induces epiretinal membrane formation, and fibrous tissue grows [43]. Microglia become activated early in diabetes in human and diabetic animal models [117]. It is supposed that diabetic conditions lead to an elevation of proinflammatory cytokine expression within the retina that induce microglia activation [118]. Being activated, microglia migrate to the source of inflammation and start to produce a wide range of proinflammatory cytokines, such as TNF- α, IL-6, IL-1, and IL-1, glutamate, ROS, NO, matrix metalloproteinases. All of these factors are implicated in the pathogenesis of DR, affect neuronal cell functions, and induce apoptosis [117–121]. It has been recognized that inflammation plays a pivotal role in pathophysiology of DR. Microglia, as highly sensitive to even low pathological changes in immune-effector cells in the retina, might be expected to have a significant role in the promotion and sustaining this inflammatory response.

6. Conclusions

Hyperglycemia induces a bewildering list of changes during DR in the retinal vasculature, neurons, and glia in animal models of diabetes and in diabetic patients. Apparently, increased flux of glucose and its metabolites affects a lot of cellular biochemical pathway driving a diverse nature of the changes. The main challenge for research studies is to identify those hyperglycemia-induced biochemical alterations that are significant in causing vascular and neural pathologies for the development of new effective ways for the treatment of DR.

Author details

Natalia Lobanovskaya
Department of Ophthalmology, East Viru Central Hospital, Kohtla-Järve, Estonia

*Address all correspondence to: natalia.lobanovskaya@ivkh.ee

References

[1] Atherton A, Hill DW, Keen H, Young S, Edwards EJ. The effect of acute hyperglycaemia on the retinal circulation of the normal cat. Diabetologia. 1980;**18**:233-237

[2] Kohner EM, Hamilton AMP, Saunders SJ, Sutcliffe BA, Bulpitt CJ. The retinal blood flow in diabetes. Diabetologia. 1975;**11**:27-33

[3] Pemp B, Polska E, Garhofer G, Bayerle-Eder M, Kautzky-Willer A, Schmetterer L. Retinal blood flow in type 1 diabetic patients with no or mild diabetic retinopathy during euglycemic clamp. Diabetes Care. 2010;**33**(9): 2038-2042

[4] Van den Enden MK, Nyengaard JR, Ostrow E, Burgan JH, Williamson JR. Elevated glucose levels increase retinal glycolysis and sorbitol pathway metabolism. Implications for diabetic retinopathy. Investigative Ophthalmology & Visual Science. 1995;**36**(8):1675-1685

[5] Williamson JR, Chang K, Frangos M, Hasan KS, Ido Y, Kawamura T, et al. Hyperglycemic pseudohypoxia and diabetic complications. Diabetes. 1993;**42**:801-813

[6] Kohner EM, Patel V, Rassam SMB. Role of blood flow and impaired autoregulation in the pathogenesis of diabetic retinopathy. Diabetes. 1995; **44**(6):603-607

[7] Kuchan MJ, Frangos JA. Shear stress regulates endothelin-I release via protein kinase C and cGMP in cultured endothelial cells. The American Journal of Physiology. 1993;**264**(1 Pt 2): H150-H156

[8] Gallis B, Corthals GL, Goodlett DR, et al. Identification of flow-dependent endothelial nitric-oxide synthase phosphorylation sites by mass spectrometry and regulation of phosphorylation and nitric oxide production by the phosphatidylinositol 3-kinase inhibitor LY294002. The Journal of Biological Chemistry. 1999;**274**:30101-30108

[9] Walshe TE, Ferguson G, Connell P, O'Brien C, Cahill PA. Pulsatile flow increases the expression of eNOS, ET-1, and prostacyclin in a novel in vitro coculture model of the retinal vasculature. Investigative Ophthalmology & Visual Science. 2005;**46**(1):375-382

[10] Chibber R, Molinatti PA, Wong JSK, Mirlees D, Kohner EM. The effect of aminoguanidine and tolrestat on glucose toxicity in bovine retinal capillary pericytes. Diabetes. 1994; **43**:758-763

[11] Klein R, Klein BE, Moss SE, Davis MD, DeMets DL. Is blood pressure a predictor of incidence and progression of diabetic retinopathy? Archives of Internal Medicine. 1989;**149**:2427-2432

[12] Klein R, Klein BEK, Moss SE, Davis MD, DeMets DL. The Wisconsin epidemiological study of diabetic retinopathy. I. Prevalence and risk of diabetic retinopathy when age at diagnosis is less than 30 years. Archives of Ophthalmology. 1984;**12**:520-526

[13] Knowler WC, Bennett PH, Ballintine EJ. Increased incidence of retinopathy in diabetics with elevated blood pressure. The New England Journal of Medicine. 1980;**302**:645-650

[14] Matthews DR, Stratton IM, Aldington SJ, Holman RR, Kohner EM. Risks of progression of retinopathy and vision loss related to tight blood pressure control in type 2 diabetes mellitus: UKPDS 69. Archives of Ophthalmology. 2004;**122**(11): 1631-1640

[15] Rasmussen KL, Laugesen CS, Datta N, Damm P, Mathiesen ER. Diabetic retinopathy during pregnancy. Ugeskrift for Laeger. 2008;**170**(50): 4117-4121

[16] Wang W, Lo ACY. Review. Diabetic retinopathy: Pathophysiology and treatments. International Journal of Molecular Sciences. 2018;**19**(6):1816

[17] Díaz-Flores L, Gutiérrez R, Madrid JF, Varela H, Valladares F, Acosta E, et al. Pericytes. Morphofunction, interactions and pathology in a quiescent and activated mesenchymal cell niche. Cellular and Molecular Biology. 2009;**24**(7):909-969

[18] Laties AM, Rapoport SI, McGlinn A. Hypertensive breakdown of cerebral but not of retinal blood vessels in rhesus monkey. Archives of Ophthalmology. 1979;**97**:1511-1514

[19] Beltramo E, Porta M. Pericyte loss in diabetic retinopathy: Mechanisms and consequences. Current Medicinal Chemistry. 2013;**20**(26):3218-3225

[20] Robison WG, Nagara M Jr, Tillis TN, Laver N, Kinoshira JH. Aldose reductase and pericyte-endothelial cell contacts in retina and optic nerve. Investigative Ophthalmology & Visual Science. 1989;**30**(11)

[21] Rucker HK, Wynder HJ, Thomas WE. Cellular mechanisms of CNS pericytes. Brain Research Bulletin. 2000;**51**:363-369

[22] Courtoy and Boyles. Fibronectin in the microvasculature: Localization in the pericyte-endothelial interstitium. Journal of Ultrastructure Research. 1983;**83**:258-273

[23] Fujimoto K. Pericyte-endothelial gap junctions in developing rat cerebral capillaries: A fine structural study. The Anatomical Record. 1995;**242**:562-565

[24] Larson DM, Carson MP, Haudenschild CC. Junctional transfer of small molecules in cultured bovine brain microvascular endothelial cells and pericytes. Microvascular Research. 1987;**34**:184-181

[25] Orlidge A, D'Amore PA. Inhibition of capillary endothelial cell growth by pericytes and smooth muscle cells. The Journal of Cell Biology. 1987; **105**:1455-1462

[26] Salomon D, Ayalon O, Patel-King R, et al. Extrajunctional distribution of N-cadherin in cultured human endothelial cells. Journal of Cell Science. 1992;**102**(Pt 1):7-17

[27] Armulik A, Genove G, Betsholtz C. Pericytes: Developmental, physiological, and pathological perspectives, problems, and promises developmental. Cell. 2011;**21**(2):0-215

[28] Frank RN, Turczyn TJ, Das A. Pericyte coverage of retinal and cerebral capillaries. Investigative Ophthalmology & Visual Science. 1990;**31**(6):999-1007

[29] Ueno M. Molecular anatomy of the brain endothelial barrier: An overview of the distributional features. Current Medicinal Chemistry. 2007; **14**:1199-1206

[30] Cunha-Vaz J, Bernardes R, Lobo C. Blood-retinal barrier. European Journal of Ophthalmology. 2011;**21**(Suppl. 6): S3-S9

[31] Antonetti DA, Barber AJ, Hollinger LA, Wolpert EB, Gardner TW. Vascular endothelial growth factor induces rapid phosphorylation of tight junction proteins occludin and zonula occluden 1. A potential mechanism for vascular permeability in diabetic retinopathy and tumors. The Journal of Biological Chemistry. 1999; **274**:23463-23467

[32] Naruse K, Nakamura J, Hamada Y, Nakayama M, Chaya S, Komori T, et al.

Aldose reductase inhibition prevents glucose-induced apoptosis in cultured bovine retinal microvascular pericytes. Experimental Eye Research. 2000; **71**:309-315

[33] Li W, Liu X, Yanoff M, Cohen S, Ye X. Cultured retinal capillary pericytes die by apoptosis after an abrupt fluctuation from high to low glucose levels: A comparative study with retinal capillary endothelial cells. Diabetologia. 1996;**39**:537-547

[34] Schalkwijk CG, Stehouwer CDA. Vascular complications in diabetes mellitus: The role of endothelial dysfunction. Clinical Science. 2005; **109**:143-159

[35] Cagliero C, Maiello M, Boeri D, Roy S, Lorenzi M. Increased expression of basement membrane components in human endothelial cells cultured in high glucose. The Journal of Clinical Investigation. 1988;**82**(2):735-738

[36] Roy S, Sala R, Cagliero E, Lorenzi M. Overexpression of fibronectin induced by diabetes or high glucose: Phenomenon with a memory. Proceedings of the National Academy of Sciences. 1990;**87**(1):404-408

[37] Dolgov W, Zaikina OE, Bondarenko MF, Repin VS. Aortic endothelium of alloxan diabetic rabbits: A quantitative study using scanning electron microscopy. Diabetologia. 1982;**22**:338-343

[38] Baumgartner-Parzer SM, Wagner L, Pettermann M, Grillari J, Gessl A, Waldhausl W. High-glucose–triggered apoptosis in cultured endothelial cells. Diabetes. 1995;**44**:1323-1327

[39] Kofler S, Nickel T, Weis M. The role of cytokines in cardiovascular diseases: Focus on endothelial response to inflammation. Clinical Science. 2005; **108**:205-213

[40] McLeod D, Marshall J, Kohner EM, Bird AC. The role of axoplasmic transport in the pathogenesis of retinal cotton-wool spots. The British Journal of Ophthalmology. 1977;**61**(3):177-191

[41] Arya M, Sorour O, Chaudhri J, Alibhai Y, Waheed NK, Duker JS, et al. Distinguishing intraretinal microvascular abnormalities from retinal neovascularization using optical coherence tomography angiography. Retina. 2020;**40**(9):1686-1695

[42] Kohner EM. Diabetic retinopathy. BMJ. 1993;**307**(6913):1195-1199

[43] Ohira A, de Juan E. Characterization of glial involvement in proliferative diabetic retinopathy. Ophthalmologica. 1990;**210**:187-195

[44] Penn JS, Madan A, Caldwell RB, Bartoli M, Caldwell RW, Hartnett ME. Vascular endothelial growth factor in eye disease. Progress in Retinal and Eye Research. 2008;**27**:331-371

[45] White NH, Cleary PA, Dahms W, et al. Beneficial effects of intensive therapy of diabetes during adolescence: Outcomes after the conclusion of the Diabetes Control and Complications Trial (DCCT). The Journal of Pediatrics. 2001;**139**(6):804-812

[46] Tarr JM, Kaul K, Chopra M, Kohner EM, Chibber R. Pathophysiology of diabetic retinopathy. International Scholarly Research Notices. 2013;**2013**:1-13

[47] Kinoshita JH. Mechanism initiating cataract formation proctor lecture. Investigative Ophthalmology & Visual Science. 1984;**13**:713-724

[48] Szwergold BS, Kappler F, Brown TR. Identification of fructose 3-phosphate in the lens of diabetic rats. Science. 1990;**247**(4941):451-454

[49] Chakrabarti AAFS, Nakajima T. Aldose reductase in the BB rat: Isolation,

immunological identifcation and localization in the retina and peripheral nerve. Diabetologia. 1987;**30**(4):244-251

[50] Drel VR, Pacher P, Ali TK, et al. Aldose reductase inhibitor fidarestat counteracts diabetes-associated cataract formation, retinal oxidative-nitrosative stress, glial activation, and apoptosis. International Journal of Molecular Medicine. 2008;**21**(6):667-676

[51] Akagi Y, Terubayashi H, Millen J, Kador PF, Kinoshita JH. Aldose reductase localization in dog retinal mural cells. Current Eye Research. 1986;**5**:883-886

[52] Sato S, Secchi EF, Lizak MJ, Fukase S, Ohta N, Murata M, et al. Polyol formation and NADPH-dependent reductases in dog retinal capillary pericytes and endothelial cells. Investigative Ophthalmology & Visual Science. 1999;**40**(3):697-704

[53] Akagi Y, Kador PF, Kuwabara T, et al. Aldose reductase localization in human retinal mural cells. Investigative Ophthalmology & Visual Science. 1983;**24**:1516-1519

[54] Akagi Y, Kador PF, Kwabara T, Kinoshita JH. Aldose reductase localisation in human retinal mural cells. Investigative Ophthalmology & Visual Science. 1983;**24**:1516-1519

[55] Kador F, Akagi Y, Terubayashi H, Wyman M, Kinoshita JH. Prevention of pericyte ghost formation in retinal capillaries of galactose-fed dogs by aldose reductase inhibitors. Archives of Ophthalmology. 1988;**106**(8):1099-1102

[56] Kador PF, Akagi Y, Takahashi Y, Ikebe H, Wyman M, Kinoshita JH. Prevention of retinal vessel changes associated with diabetic retinopathy in galactose-fed dogs by aldose reductase inhibitors. Archives of Ophthalmology. 1990;**108**(9):1301-1309

[57] Akita M, Mizuno K, Matsubara A, Nakano K, Kurono M. Effects of an aldose reductase inhibitor, SNK-860, on the histopathological changes of retinal tissues in a streptozotocin-induced diabetic rat model. Acta Medica Okayama. 1993;**47**(5):299-304

[58] Oates J, Mylari BL. Aldose reductase inhibitors: Therapeutic implications for diabetic complications. Expert Opinion on Investigational Drugs. 1999;**8**(12): 2095-2119

[59] Sorbinil Retinopathy Trial Research Group. A randomized trial of sorbinil, an aldose reductase inhibitor, in diabetic retinopathy. Archives of Ophthalmology. 1990;**108**:1234-1244

[60] Stitt AW, Frizzell N, Thorpe SR. Advanced glycation and advanced lipoxidation: Possible role in initiation and progression of diabetic retinopathy. Current Pharmaceutical Design. 2004; **10**(27):3349-3360

[61] Schmidt AM, Hasu M, Popov D, Zhang JH, Chen J, Yan SD, et al. Receptor for advanced glycation end products (AGEs) has a central role in vessel wall interactions and gene activation in response to circulating AGE proteins. Proceedings of the National Academy of Sciences. 1994;**91**(19):8807-8811

[62] Schmidt AM, Hori O, Brett J, Yan SD, Wautier JL, Stern D. Cellular receptors for advanced glycation end products. Implications for induction of oxidant stress and cellular dysfunction in the pathogenesis of vascular lesions. Arteriosclerosis and Thrombosis. 1994;**14**(10):1521-1528

[63] Mullarkey C, Edelstein D, Brownlee M. Free radical generation by early glycation products: A mechanism for accelerated atherogenesis in diabetes. Biochemical and Biophysical Research Communications. 1990; **173**:932-939

[64] Sakurai T, Tsuchiya S. Superoxide production from nonenzymatically glycated protein. FEBS Letters. 1988; **236**:406-410

[65] Stitt AW et al. Advanced glycation end products (AGEs) co-localize with AGE receptors in the retinal vasculature of diabetic and of AGE-infused rats. The American Journal of Pathology. 1997;**150**:523-528

[66] Yamagishi S, Hsu C-C, Taniguchi M, Harada S, Yamamoto Y, Ohsawa K, et al. Receptor mediated toxicity to pericytes of advanced glycosylation end products: A possible mechanism of pericyte loss in diabetic microangiopathy. Biochemical and Biophysical Research Communications. 1995;**213**:681-687

[67] Podestà F, Romeo G, Liu W, Krajewski S, Reed JC, Gerhardinger C, et al. Bax is increased in the retina of diabetic subjects and is associated with pericyte apoptosis in vivo and in vitro. American Journal of Pathology. 2000;**156**(3)

[68] Liu H, Lessieur EM, Saadane A, Lindstrom SI, Taylor PR, Kern TS. Neutrophil elastase contributes to the pathological vascular permeability characteristic of diabetic retinopathy. Diabetologia. 2019;**62**(12):2365-2374

[69] Hammes HP, Martin S, Federlin K, Geisen K, Brownlee M. Aminoguanidine treatment inhibits the development of experimental diabetic retinopathy. Proceedings of the National Academy of Sciences of the United States of America. 1991;**88**(24):11555-11558

[70] Yamagishi S, Amano S, Inagaki Y, Okamoto T, Koga K, Sasaki N, et al. Advanced glycation end products-induced apoptosis and overexpression of vascular endothelial growth factor in bovine retinal pericytes. Biochemical and Biophysical Research Communications. 2002;**290**(3):973-978

[71] Shiba T, Inoguchi T, Sportsman JR, Heath WF, Bursell S, King GL. Correlation of diacylglycerol level and protein kinase C activity in rat retina to retinal circulation. The American Journal of Physiology. 1993; **265**:E783-E793

[72] Das Evcimen N, King GL. The role of protein kinase C activation and the vascular complications of diabetes. Pharmacological Research. 2007; **55**:498-510

[73] Wolf BA, Easom RA, McDaniel ML, Turk J. Diacylglycerol synthesis de novo from glucose by pancreatic islets isolated from rats and human. The Journal of Clinical Investigation. 1990;**85**:482,190

[74] Xia P, Inoguchi T, Kern TS, Engerman RL, Oates PJ, King GL. Characterization of the mechanism for the chronic activation of diacylglycero–protein kinase C pathway in diabetes and hypergalactosemia. Diabetes. 1994;**43**:1122-1129

[75] Nishizuka Y. Intracellular signalling by hydrolysis of phospholipids and activation of protein kinase C. Science. 1992;**258**:607-614

[76] Clarke M, Dodson PM. PKC inhibition and diabetic microvascular complications. Best Practice & Research Clinical Endocrinology & Metabolism. 2007;**21**(4):573-586

[77] Xia P, Aiello LP, Ishii H, et al. Characterization of vascular endothelial factor's effect on the activation of protein kinase C, its isoforms, and endothelial cell growth. The Journal of Clinical Investigation. 1996;**98**(9): 2018-2026

[78] Aiello S, Bursell E, Clermont A, et al. Vascular endothelial growth factor-induced retinal permeability is mediated by protein kinase C in vivo and suppressed by an orally

effective-isoform-selective inhibitor. Diabetes. 1997;**46**(9):1473-1480

[79] Yancopoulos GD, Davis S, et al. Vascular-specific growth factors and blood vessel formation. Nature. 2000;**407**:242-248

[80] Wang GL, Semenza GL. Purification and characterization of hypoxia-inducible factor 1. The Journal of Biological Chemistry. 1995; **270**:1230-1237

[81] Ruberte J, Ayuso E, Navarro M, et al. Increased ocular levels of IGF-1 in transgenic mice lead to diabetes-like eye disease. Journal of Clinical Investigation. 2004;**113**(8):1149-1157

[82] Al-Shabrawey M, Bartoli M, et al. Mechanisms of Statin's protective actions in diabetic retinopathy: Role of NAD(P)H oxidase and STAT3. Investigative Ophthalmology & Visual Science. 2008;**49**(7):3231-3238

[83] Qaum T, Xu Q, et al. VEGF-initiated blood-retinal barrier breakdown in early diabetes. Investigative Ophthalmology & Visual Science. 2001;**42**:2408-2413

[84] Makowski GS, Ramsby ML. Binding of latent matrix metalloproteinase 9 to fibrin: Activation via a plasmin-dependent pathway. Inflammation. 1998;**22**:287-305

[85] Behzadian MA, Windsor LJ, et al. VEGF-induced paracellular permeability in cultured endothelial cells involves urokinase and its receptor. The FASEB Journal. 2003;**19**:19

[86] Bates DO, Curry FE. Vascular endothelial growth factor increases microvascular permeability via a Ca(2+)-dependent pathway. American Journal of Physiology—Heart and Circulatory Physiology. 1997;**273**(2): H687-H694

[87] Cai S, Bressler NM. Aflibercept, bevacizumab or ranibizumab for diabetic macular oedema: Recent clinically relevant findings from DRCR. net Protocol T. Current Opinion in Ophthalmology. 2017;**28**(6):636-643

[88] Gross JG, Glassman AR, Liu D, Sun JK, Antoszyk AN, Baker CW, et al. Diabetic retinopathy clinical research network. Five-year outcomes of panretinal photocoagulation vs intravitreous ranibizumab for proliferative diabetic retinopathy: A randomized clinical trial. JAMA Ophthalmology. 2018;**136**(10):1138-1148

[89] Fumo P, Kuncio GS, Ziyadeh FN. PKC and high glucose stimulate collagen alpha 1 (IV) transcriptional activity in areporter mesangial cell line. The American Journal of Physiology. 1994; **267**:F632-F638

[90] Studer RK, Craven PA, DeRubertis FR. Role for proteine kinase C in the mediation increased fibronectin accumulation by mesangial cells grown in high-glucose medium. Diabetes. 1993;**42**:118-126

[91] Xia P, Kramer RM, King GL. Identification of the mechanism for the inhibition of Na+ –K+ –ATPase by hyperglycemia involving activation of protein kinase C and cytosolic phospholipase A2. The Journal of Clinical Investigation. 1995;**96**:733-740

[92] Deisher TA, Haddix TL, Montgomery KF, Pohlman TH, Kaushansky K, Harlan JM. The role of protein kinase C in the induction of VCAM-1 expression on human umbilical vein endothelial cells. FEBS Letters. 1993;**331**:285-290

[93] Lane TA, Lamkin GE, Wancewicz E. Modulation of endothelial cell expression of intercellular adhesion molecule 1 by protein kinase C activation. Biochemical and Biophysical

Research Communications. 1989; **161**:945-952

[94] Miyamoto K, Hiroshiba N, Tsujikawa A, Ogura Y. In vivo demonstration of increased leukocyte entrapment in retinal microcirculation of diabetic rats. Investigative Ophthalmology & Visual Science. 1998;**39**:2190-2194

[95] Miyamoto K, Khosrof S, Bursell SE, et al. Prevention of leukostasis and vascular leakage in streptozotocin-induced diabetic retinopathy via intercellular adhesion molecule-1 inhibition. Proceedings of the National Academy of Sciences of the United States of America. 1999;**96**:10836-10841

[96] Nonaka A, Kiryu J, Tsujikawa A, et al. PKC-inhibitor (LY333531) attenuates leukocyte entrapment in retinal micro-circulation of diabetic rats. Investigative Ophthalmology and Visual Science. 2000;**41**(9):2702-2706

[97] Schroder S, Palinski W, Schmid-Schonbein GW. Activated monocytes and granulocytes, capillary nonperfusion, and neovascularization in diabetic retinopathy. The American Journal of Pathology. 1991;**139**:81-100

[98] Fantone JC, Ward PA. Role of oxygen derived free radicals and metabolites in leukocyte-dependent inflammatory reactions. The American Journal of Pathology. 1982;**107**(3): 397-418

[99] Janoff A, Schaefer S, Scherer J, Bean MA. Mediators of inflammation in leukocyte lysosomes: I. Mechanism of action of lysosomal cationic protein upon vascular permeability in the rat. The Journal of Experimental Medicine. 1965;**122**:841-851

[100] Shen GS. Selective protein kinase C inhibitors and their applications. Current Drug Targets. Cardiovascular & Haematological Disorders. 2003;**3**(4): 301-307

[101] Semba RD, Huang H, Lutty GA, Van Eyk JE, Hart GW. The role of O-GlcNAc signaling in the pathogenesis of diabetic retinopathy. Proteomics. Clinical Applications. 2014;**8**:218-231

[102] Love DC, Hanover JA. The hexosamine signaling pathway: Deciphering the "O-GlcNAc code". Science's STKE. 2005;**2005**:re13

[103] Buse MG. Hexosamines, insulin resistance and the complications of diabetes: Current status. American Journal of Physiology. Endocrinology and Metabolism. 2006;**290**(1):E1-E8

[104] Gurel Z, Sieg KM, Shallow KD, Sorenson CM, Sheibani N. Retinal O-linked N-acetylglucosamine protein modifications: Implications for postnatal retinal vascularization and the pathogenesis of diabetic retinopathy. Molecular Vision. 2013;**19**:1047-1059

[105] Luo B, Soesanto Y, McClain DA. Protein modification by O-linked GlcNAc reduces angiogenesis by inhibiting Akt activity in endothelial cells. Arteriosclerosis, Thrombosis, and Vascular Biology. 2008;**28**:651-657

[106] Park SH, Park JW, Park SJ, et al. Apoptotic death of photoreceptors in the streptozotocin-induced diabetic rat retina. Diabetologia. 2003;**46**(9): 1260-1268

[107] Barber AJ, Lieth E, Khin SA, et al. Neural apoptosis in the retina during experimental and human diabetes: Early onset and effect of insulin. The Journal of Clinical Investigation. 1998; **102**:783-791

[108] Daley M, Watzke R, Riddle M. Early loss of blue-sensitive color vision in patients with type I diabetes. Diabetes Care. 1987;**10**:777-781

[109] Sokol S, Moskowitz A, Skarf B. Contrast sensitivity in diabetes with and without background retinopathy. Archives of Ophthalmology. 1985; **103**:51-54

[110] Ishikawa A, Ishiguro S, Tamai M. Changes in GABA metabolism in streptozotocin-induced diabetic rat retinas. Current Eye Research. 1996; **15**:63-71

[111] Lieth E, Barber AJ, Xu B, et al. Glial reactivity and impaired glutamate metabolism in short-term experimental diabetic retinopathy. Diabetes. 1998; **47**:815-820

[112] Rothman SM, Olney JW. Glutamate and the pathophysiology of hypoxic-ischemic brain damage. Annals of Neurology. 1986;**L9**:105-111

[113] Vorwerk CK, Lipton SA, Zurakowski D, Hyman BT, Sabel BA, Dreyer EB. Chronic low-dose glutamate is toxic to retinal ganglion cells: Toxicity blocked by memantine. Investigative Ophthalmology & Visual Science. 1996;**37**:1618-1624

[114] Mizutani M, Gerhardinger C, Lorenzi M. Muller cell changes in human diabetic retinopathy. Diabetes. 1998;**47**:445-449

[115] Sueishi K, Hata Y, Murata T, Nakagawa K, Ishibashi T, Inomata H. Endothelial and glial cell interaction in diabetic retinopathy via the function of vascular endothelial growth factor (VEGF). Polish Journal of Pharmacology. 1996;**48**(3):307-316

[116] Llorián-Salvador M, Barabas P, Byrne EM, Lechner J, Augustine J, Curtis TM, et al. VEGF-B is an autocrine gliotrophic factor for Müller cells under pathologic conditions. Investigative Ophthalmology & Visual Science. 2020;**61**(11):35

[117] Zeng HY, Green WR, Tso MO. Microglial activation in human diabetic retinopathy. Archives of Ophthalmology. 2008;**126**:227-232

[118] Krady JK, Basu A, Allen CM, et al. Minocycline reduces proinflammatory cytokine expression, microglial activation, and caspase-3 activation in a rodent model of diabetic retinopathy. Diabetes. 2005;**54**(5):1559-1565

[119] Funatsu H, Yamashita H, Noma H, Mimura T, Yamashita T, Hori S. Increased levels of vascular endothelial growth factor and interleukin-6 in the aqueous humor of diabetics with macular edema. American Journal of Ophthalmology. 2002;**133**(1):70-77

[120] Langmann T. Microglia activation in retinal degeneration. Journal of Leukocyte Biology. 2007;**81**(6): 1345-1351

[121] Du XL, Edelstein D, Rossetti L, Fantus IG, Goldberg H, Ziyadeh F, et al. Hyperglycemia-induced mitochondrial superoxide overproduction activates the hexosamine pathway and induces plasminogen activator inhibitor-1 expression by increasing Sp1 glycosylation. Proceedings. National Academy of Sciences. United States of America. 2000;**97**:12222-12226

Chapter 2

High-Risk Diabetic Maculopathy: Features and Management

Maya G. Pandova

Abstract

A substantial group of patients with diabetic macular edema in our clinical practice is at high risk for profound and irreversible vision deterioration. Early identification of modifiable factors with long-term negative impact and their management, close monitoring and timely adjustments in the treatment can significantly reduce the probability of visual disability in the individual patient. This approach can also provide important guidelines for proactive decision making in order to avoid the risk of suboptimal response and unsatisfactory outcome.

Keywords: Retinal symptoms and signs, systemic risk factors, treatment options, management stages

1. Introduction

The introduction of intravitreal pharmacotherapy dramatically improved the visual prognosis of the patients with diabetic macular edema (DME). However, the pivotal randomized clinical trials demonstrated that a sizable proportion of the eyes remained with disabling visual acuity despite intensive treatment and vigorous monitoring for 2 years [1]. Moreover, after transition to standard clinical care for the next 3 years, the visual acuity worsened even in patients with significant vision gain [2]. Real-world studies on DME management from Europe, USA, Japan and Australia reveal significant differences in the registration, national policies and restrictions for the use of the medications. A common issue is a tremendous pressure on the ophthalmic care providers to reduce the cost of visits and treatment. This invariably has resulted in visual outcomes that were meaningfully inferior to those achieved in randomized controlled trials [3–8].

These data suggest that a substantial group of patients with diabetic macular edema in our clinical practice is at high risk for profound and irreversible vision deterioration. Early identification of modifiable factors with long-term negative impact and their management, close monitoring and timely adjustments in the treatment can significantly reduce the probability of visual disability in the individual patient. Such a systematic approach can also provide important guidelines for proactive decision making in avoiding the risk of suboptimal response and unsatisfactory outcome.

2. Low visual acuity at baseline

Post hoc analysis of the best-corrected visual acuity (BCVA) achieved in DRCR.net Protocol T randomized clinical trial after anti-VEGF treatment [1] demonstrated that 96–100% of eyes enrolled in the trial with BCVA 20/32 to 20/40 retained high vision after 6 months even in the presence of persistent edema. A small proportion - 8% of these eyes - deteriorated below 20/40 at the end of the first year and further 5–8% worsened after 2 years, and only if the edema was persistent. The outcome in eyes with baseline BCVA 20/50 to 20/320 was far less – through the 24th week 21–41% of them failed to improve over 20/50, and the results were worse if the edema was persistent – 31–51% of them had BCVA less than 20/40. By the end of the first year 11–30% of these eyes were still seeing below 20/40 and the outcome was worse if the edema was persistent – 33–46% remained in the low vision group. After 2 years of anti-VEGF treatment 17–25% of these eyes did not improve over 20/50 and their proportion reached 46% in eyes with persistent edema. Standard clinical care in the next three years resulted in vision deterioration by at least one Snellen line (4.8 letters) in the whole cohort and the proportion of eyes with BCVA less than 20/40 increased from 16% at the end of the second year to 27% [2]. The overall impression from the clinical trials and real-life practice is that significant vision gain is achievable even in eyes with low baseline vision at relatively low risk of severe vision loss, however it requires intensive treatment and the long-term outcome is often unstable. In contrast, eyes with higher visual acuity at baseline have much better chance to retain it in the next 2 and 5- year interval with appropriate management.

3. Imaging and biomarkers

Stereoscopic examination of the retina readily reveals signs predicting slow, limited visual response to treatment and tendency for recurrence:

Diffuse edema, ischaemic areas in the posterior pole, hard exudates close to the fovea and atrophic changes in the deep layers are often associated with **long-standing disease**. These changes persist if pharmacotherapy was provided occasionally and in long intervals.

Previous laser treatment close to the macula leaves chorioretinal scars that slowly progress towards the fovea, particularly if the photocoagulation spots were confluent and with high intensity.

PDR - active proliferative disease, signs of hypo- or nonperfusion and particularly the presence of retinal ischaemic areas in the equatorial zone and periphery indicate advanced microvascular damage and carry poor visual prognosis if left untreated. As noted in the secondary analysis of Protocol T patients, eyes with less than severe nonproliferative diabetic retinopathy (EDTRS severity levels 10 to 47) had 3.1 letters more visual acuity improvement after treatment for 2 years compared to patients with inactive advanced PDR and no prior panretinal photocoagulation [9].

Panretinal photocoagulation (PRP) for advanced PDR (EDTRS severity levels 61 to 75) at baseline in the same clinical trial was associated with approximately 3 letters less vision gain after 2 years [9]. This finding needs careful interpretation. Often, advanced PDR is associated with various stages of macular edema, and laser treatment that prevented the total blindness is such patients, was done years prior to the introduction of pharmacotherapy for the macular complication. On the other hand, confluent, high-intensity laser treatment applied over large areas in one or two sessions is associated with significant thermal trauma and can lead to inflammation, worsening of the macular edema, followed by atrophic changes and vision deterioration that may not respond to treatment.

Glistening, taut **epiretinal membranes** in the posterior pole with characteristic folds and retinal distortion require close monitoring - they may limit the vision gain in response to treatment, particularly in the presence of atrophic macular changes (**Figure 1**).

Anterior–posterior **vitreo-macular traction** can cause edema per se and will not respond to intravitreal treatment [10].

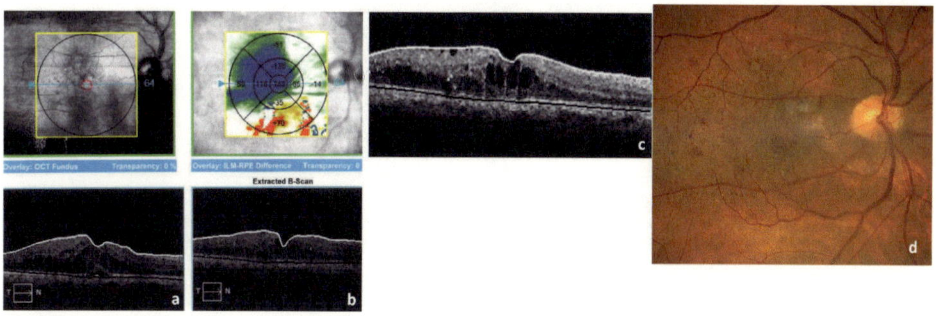

Figure 1.
63 years old male, DM for 23 years, DME, PDR. a –VA decreased from 20/40 to 20/80 in two month during decompensation of CAD and CABG -epiretinal membrane, lamellar macular hole, severe recurrence of intraretinal edema with macrocysts, subsensory fluid collection; b -after 5 anti-VEGF injection –persistent intraretinaledema, resolved subsensoryfluid, VA 20/40, c – 27 months and 9 anti-VEGF injections later – persistent intraretinal edema, hyperreflective foci, epiretinal membrane, lamellar macular hole, VA 20/40; d –persistent macrocysts, ischemic areas, hard exudates and microaneurisms.

4. Optical coherent tomography

Systematic analysis of OCT at the initial visit provides insight into the severity and duration of the disease and guides the appropriate choice of treatment and regimen.

The location, size and content of intra- and subretinal fluid collections: Cystic spaces exceeding 200 μm involving the outer nuclear layer (ONL) are seen in late stage of DME and have a worse impact on macular function than smaller cysts or cystoid formations occurring in inner retinal layers (**Figure 2b**). **Large cysts located in the perimacular area** tend to extend centrally with time (**Figure 3b** and **d**). Even though in the early phases the visual acuity is not severely deteriorated, in the presence of other risk factors treatment has to be initiated – these patients have excellent chances to retain good function without major fluctuations. Lack of retinal bridges between the cystic spaces in the inner and outer retina is a sign of long-standing severe disease and is associated with poor visual prognosis despite resolution of the fluid post treatment (**Figure 2d**). **Subfoveolar neurosensory detachment** is seen in cases with more severe edema and has been associated with more active inflammatory components of the disease (**Figure 1a**). These patients responded favorably in the pivotal clinical trials on anti VEGF and dexamethasone treatment with significant functional gains. This type of edema has a tendency to recur in chronic cases with interrupted intravitreal treatment, deterioration of the systemic disease or after cataract surgery (**Figure 4**).

Hyperreflective retinal foci appear as small lesions with size less than 30 μm with reflectivity similar to retinal nerve fiber layer and without back-shadowing over the underlying layers. They appear to represent subclinical lipoproteins that extravasate after breakdown of inner blood–retinal barrier, although there are suggestions that they might be activated microglial cell, and indicate chronicity and predominant inflammation in the eye. Increased number of the spots indicate tendency for recurrence of the edema and require close monitoring (**Figures 1c** and **7d**).

Hard exudates present in the OCT as hyperreflective intraretinal accumulations larger than 30 μm with back-shadowing. The deposits are thought to consist of lipoproteins and indicate advanced microvascular damage and chronicity. In severe cases they can form fibrotic lesions that are associated with visual decline, especially if located in or close to the macula (**Figure 5**) [11].

Disorganization of retinal inner (DRIL) and outer layers within the central 1 mm retinal zone may not be readily distinguishable if the edema is severe and

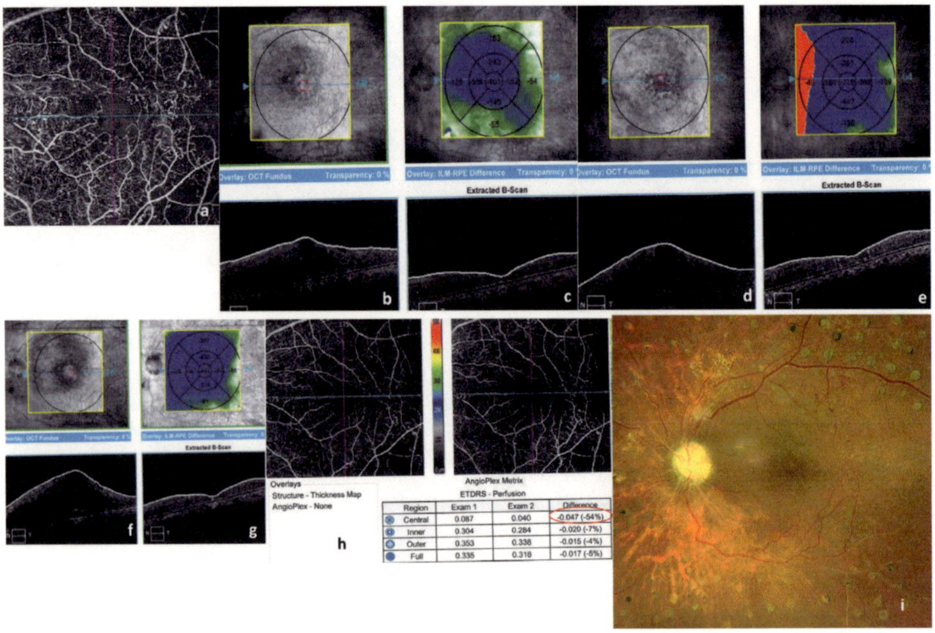

Figure 2.
58 years old male, nephropathy, diabetic foot, CAD, PDR, recurrent macular edema, neovascularglaucoma after glaucoma drainage implant (Ahmed valve). a –OCTA total retina –broad areas of hypoperfusion, microaneurisms, enlarged distorted foveolar avascular zone; b -severe recurrence during Leukemoid reaction, HbA1c 11%, VA 20/200; c -one week after anti-VEGF injection, VA 20/70; d – 3 months later -recurrence after treatment on Imatinib for 3 months, VA 20/100; e -one month after anti-VEGF injection, VA 20/50; f –recurrence during deteriorated foot ulcer, HbA1c 9% VA 20/150; g –one month after anti-VEGF intravitreal injection, VA 20/50; h –OCTA superficial plexus-decreased central perfusion by 54% in 6 months after 4 major recurrences; i –advanced OND pallor, macrocystsand atrophic areas in the macula, severe ischemia and NVE.

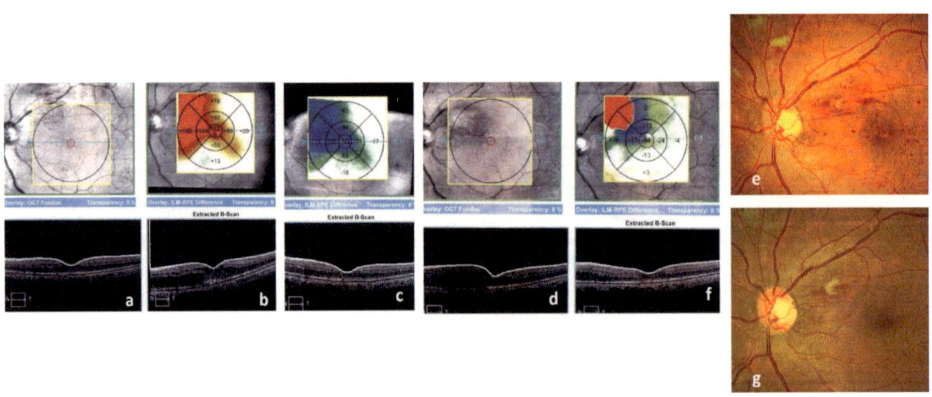

Figure 3.
60 years old female, 20 years of poorly controlled DM, arterial hypertension; multiple recurrences of perimacularedema, NPDR. a –One month after anti-VEGF injection, VA 20/20; b –treatment interrupted for 8 months, VA 20/30, 5 months after hysterectomy; c –one month later after anti-VEGF, VA 20/20; d, e–3 months later-new recurrent intraretinal edema progressing towards the macula, new ischemic areas, VA 20/30, f, g–one month after anti-VEGF injection and focal laser, persistent perimacular ischemia, VA 20/20.

associated epiretinal membranes and hyperreflective lesions, especially if there are media opacities (**Figure 2**). It is becoming evident in the course of the treatment after regression of the edema and explains the low visual acuity and minimal vision gain. DRIL has been attributed to macular capillary non-perfusion, the size and erosion

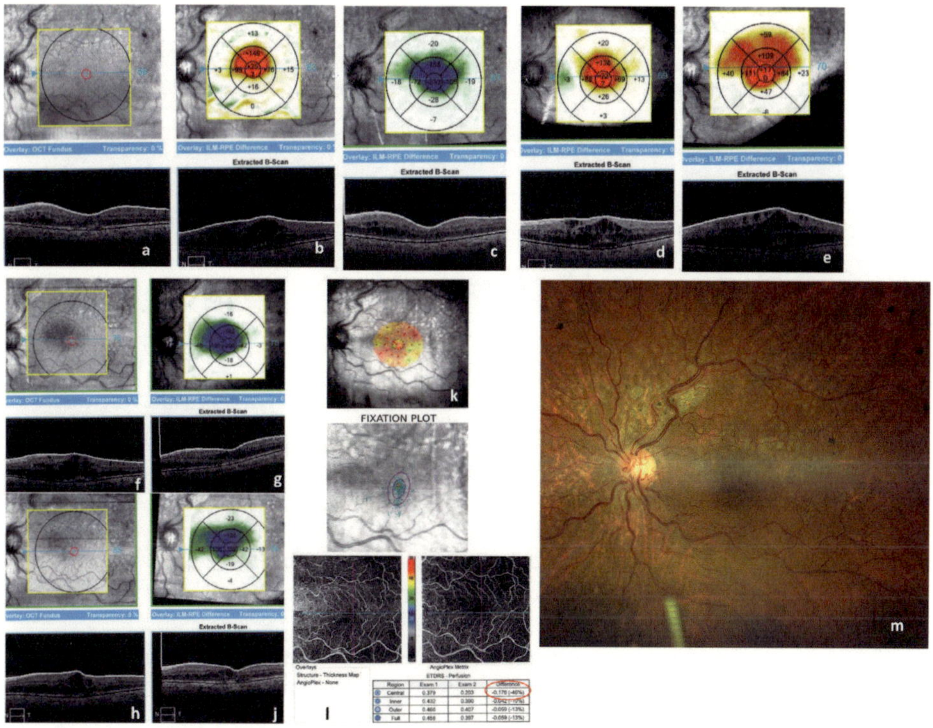

Figure 4.
57 years old female, DM for 25 years, sleeve gastrectomy, chronic cholecystitis, CAD, DME, PDR, secondary glaucoma. a –after 3 anti-VEGF injections and 1 OzurdexVA 20/60, cataract; b –deteriorated edema with subsensory fluid 14 days after phacemulsificationVA 20/60; c – 14 days after anti-VEGF injection, VA 20/30; d – recurrent edema during CABG, subsensory fluid, hyperreflective foci VA 20/40; e –severe edema after pyocele and sepsis, VA 20/40; f –recurrence after stroke, VA 20/30; g – 7 days after Ozurdex, VA 20/25; h –severe recurrence 3 months after the second Ozurdex, VA 20/40; j –rapid response to Iluvien, VA 20/25; k –microperimetry-decreased central retinal sensitivity, unstable central fixation; l -decreased central perfusion in the superficial plexus by 46% in 18 months; m –microcystic edema and hard exudates in the macula, stable PDR, visible Iluvien implant.

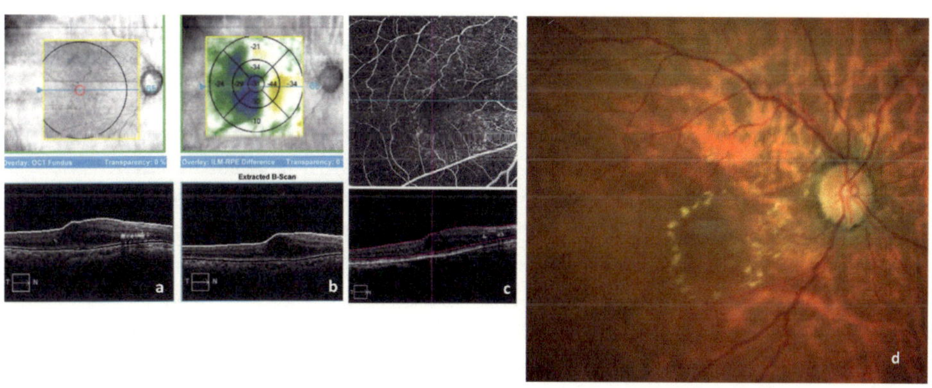

Figure 5.
70 years old female. Chronic macular edema, NPDR, chronic uveitis, secondary glaucoma for 12 years, poorly controlled diabetes, arterial hypertension, lost for follow up for 4 years. a –Three weeks after intensive topical steroids and antiglaucoma medications VA 20/250; b -after 4 anti-VEGF and focal laser –persistent macrocystic edema, regressing hard exudates, VA 20/50, c –OCTA –total retina-significant capillary dropout, enlarged irregular foveolar avascular zone; d –chronic edema, circinate hard exudates.

of the foveolar avascular zone and has been correlated with increasing severity of the retinopathy, especially in patients with proliferative disease (**Figure 6**). The presence of DRIL can be associated with disorganized outer retinal layer disruption,

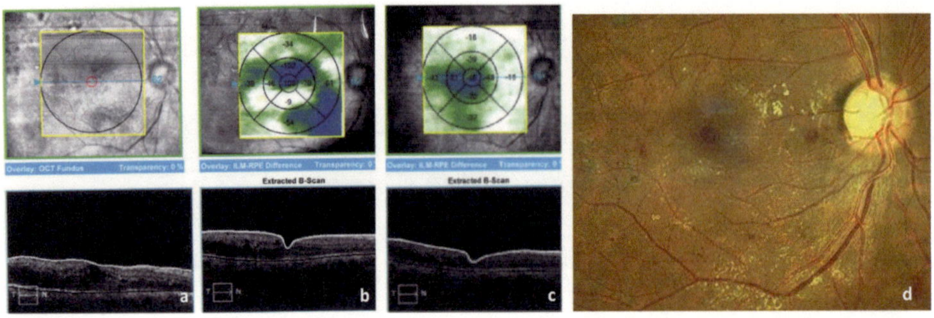

Figure 6.
60-years old female, 20 years of poorly controlled diabetes. Phacoemulsification and vitrectomy, choroidal effusions. a -Severe DME, epiretinal membrane, DRIL one month after surgery; b – 4 months later after 3 anti-VEGF injections –incomplete, unstable response; c – 6 months later after 2 Ozurdex implants –residual perimacular degenerative fluid spaces; d –persistent macular edema, mild DRIL, epiretinal membrane, hard exudates and microaneurisms.

specifically ellipsoid zone (EZ) and external limiting membrane (ELM). Moreover, Sun and colleagues have found that an increase in DRIL during 4 months predicted a decline of visual acuity by one line [12].

OCT assessment of the **vitreomacular adhesions and traction** is indispensable in the choice of treatment. The presence of anterior–posterior traction is considered an indication for pars-plana vitrectomy in eyes with DME, however other OCT findings - greater retinal thickness, presence of subretinal fluid, lack of external limiting membrane integrity and disruption of the ellipsoid zone - have been associated with a poorer final absolute BCVA [10]. Macular edema in eyes with lamellar holes associated with tangential traction needs careful consideration – it often responds favorably to intravitreal treatment and may remain stable, however should be monitored closely in the presence of active PDR and may eventually require surgical management (**Figure 1**).

5. Optical coherent tomography angiography

The contribution of OCTA in the assessment of high-risk DME is substantial. It will detect capillary dropout, microaneurisms and neovascularization in detailed 3-dimentional segments (**Figure 2a**) and provide quantitative estimates of the perfusion and vascular density by areas [13] (**Figure 4l**). A recent study demonstrated that although there was no significant difference in the superficial capillary plexus between anti-VEGF responders and poor responders, poor responders tended to show greater damage and more microaneurysms in the deep capillary plexus and a larger foveolar avascular zone (FAZ) area. The topographic location of the disrupted synaptic portion of the outer plexiform layer in SD OCT exactly corresponded to the nonflow area of the deep capillary plexus in OCTA [14]. The enlargement and irregularities of the FAZ have to be interpreted carefully in the presence of large central cysts as such findings could be associated with capillary displacement rather than ischemia, especially in eyes with retained inner and outer retinal morphology. OCTA assessment of patients with DME and neurosensory detachment demonstrated improvement in cysts area and perfusion density in the superficial and deep capillary plexus in response to treatment with Dexamethasone and ranibizumab [15]. Persistent microaneurisms and declining perfusion in the deep capillary plexus in another comparative work was associated with less vision gain and incomplete resolution of the edema after treatment with aflibercept [16].

6. Fundus autofluorescence

Short-wavelength FAF derives its signal mainly from lipofuscin in the RPE. Long wavelength autofluorescence or near-infrared FAF derives its signal from melanin, which is present in RPE and choroid. Intraretinal cysts in DME unmask the underlying RPE by displacing the luteal pigment in the fovea and this prevents the normal blockage of foveal FAF signal. Granular and patchy hyper- and hypo-autoflurescent lesions in the parafoveolar area have been described and correlated with foveolar cystoid spaces in DME patients. Larger area of hyper-autofluorescence in eyes with higher number of hyperreflective foci and presence of subfoveal neuroretinal detachment may indicate a prevalent inflammatory condition in DME with specific response to steroidal treatment [17, 18].

7. Microperimetry

Micoperimetry is able to quantify macular sensitivity and fixation pattern in an exact, fundus-related fashion, thus adding detailed information about the degree and pattern of macular function alteration (**Figure 4k**). It has been successfully used in the diagnosis and follow-up of different macular disorders, including age-related macular degeneration, myopic maculopathy, macular dystrophies, and diabetic macular edema. Vujosevic S et al. have demonstrated in a series of studies that macular sensitivity is significantly affected when diabetic macular edema develops and it deteriorates further in eyes at more severe stages of macular edema even in the absence of ischemia. The stability of the fixation is decreasing late in the disease and indicates advanced photoreceptor damage and chronicity [19].

8. Glaucoma in eyes with DME

In a recent meta-analysis of prospective cohort studies the pooled risk ratio of the association between primary open-angle glaucoma (POAG) and diabetes was 1.36 [20]. The prevalence of glaucoma in diabetics ranges from 4.96% to 14.6% with significant variations in geographic regions and racial groups. Moreover, there is a statistically significant association between the duration of diabetes and glaucoma [21]. Hou et al. compared rates of visual field (VF) loss and retinal nerve fiber layer thinning for patients with POAG and found no difference in progression between patients without and with type 2 diabetes and no detectable diabetic retinopathy. They also found that treated diabetes was linked to significantly slower loss of RNFL thickness [22].

The risk of ocular hypertension in a patient presenting with DME needs to be considered in the treatment choice. While anti-VEGF agents are generally safe, a key DRCR.net report on eyes with center-involved DME and no preexisting open-angle glaucoma treated on ranibizumab and monitored for 3 years demonstrated increase in the risk of sustained IOP elevation or the need for ocular hypotensive treatment after anti-VEGF treatment [23]. In patients with POAG and DME treated with ranibizimab and monitored for 24 months, Fursova et al. report a decrease in the functional and structural parameters of the retina and optic nerve, and a higher rate of progression of glaucomatous optic neuropathy compared to patients without DME. Long-term results have not revealed a significant deterioration in the structural parameters of the optic disc and retina as a consequence of anti-VEGF therapy [24].

Intravitreal steroids will induce hypertensive response in up to 50% of the eyes with DME. The MEAD Study reported that over 40% of eye required initiation of a topical ocular hypotensive agent and 0.3% of eyes required incisional glaucoma surgery after Ozurdex [25]. In the FAME Studies, 18.4% of eyes that were injected with the 0.2 μg Iluvien-FA per day implant developed an IOP higher than 30 mmHg and 4.8% underwent incisional glaucoma surgery [26]. After a follow-up of 5 years, 9% of eyes that had multiple injections of triamcinolone acetonide required a trabeculectomy [27]. An eye that does not develop substantial IOP elevation after a challenge course with a topical steroid may still respond with an IOP rise after Ozurdex or Iluvien, however in most cases it is well controlled on antiglaucoma medications [28].

Patients with refractive DME and well compensated glaucoma on one or two antiglaucoma drops responded favorably to both Ozurdex and Iluvien in our practice (**Figure 4**). An eye with advanced glaucoma on more than 2 medications is at a high risk of uncontrollable IOP and severe vision loss after intravitreal steroid, and glaucoma surgery has to be performed prior to the switch from anti-VEGF.

Neovascularization of the iris or neovascularization of the angle that ultimately lead to neovascular glaucoma is a consequence of long-standing ischemia in patients with PDR. The incidence of neovascular glaucoma is further increased in patients who have undergone vitrectomy and lensectomy. Breach of the posterior capsule from a complicated cataract extraction or even from Nd: YAG laser capsulotomy may allow angiogenic factors to gain access to the anterior segment more readily, accelerating formation of neovascularization. The management of DME in these eyes with intravitreal anti-VEGF provides temporary regression of the iris neovascularization, decrease in the PDR severity and facilitates the panretinal photocoagulation [29]. Early glaucoma surgery significantly improves the visual prognosis of DME in eyes with neovascular glaucoma, however they remain at high risk of IOP decompensation, reactivation of the PDR and recurrences of the macular edema and need prompt, often urgent treatment (**Figure 2**).

9. Uveitis

History of a previous uveitis episode or evidence of a chronic intraocular inflammation in a patient with DME heralds high rate of complications and difficult management (**Figure 5**). A large database from the UK was analyzed for the prevalence of acute uveitis over a six-year period among populations without (n = 889,856) and with diabetes (n = 48,584) and evaluated the impact of glycaemic control on disease risk. Poor glycaemic control increases the risk of acute uveitis, with patients that have an HbA1c over >11.3% almost 5 times more likely to have an event. Acute uveitis was also more common in those with proliferative retinopathy. The odds ratio (OR) for acute uveitis was significantly higher in patients with type 1 DM (OR 2.01), Black (OR 20.17) or Asian (OR 2.09) ethnicity, proliferative disease (OR 2.42) and escalated with increasing HbA1c, however the association with maculopathy was less - OR 1.15 [30]. In a cohort of middle-aged diabetic patients with uveitis, who were followed up for 4 years, 42% had final visual acuity worse than 6/18. In 53% of the eyes, the poor visual acuity was thought to be uveitis related, and a half of these eyes had clinically significant macular edema. Progression of diabetic retinopathy to proliferative stage occurred in 10% of the eyes. In patients with available HbA1c data, the levels were over 7.0% on almost all cases in the quiescent period and rose by 1.5–4% in the acute episodes. The authors conclude that uveitis occurring in patients with pre-existing diabetes can be associated with numerous ocular complications and recurrences. Macular involvement related to both the uveitis and the diabetes appears to be the main cause of reduced vision [31].

In clinical practice, diabetic patients with macular edema and uveitis have higher tendency to develop fibrinous exudates in the anterior chamber and posterior synechiae, particularly after intraocular surgery. They respond favorably to topical, periocular and intravitreal steroids and require close monitoring for intraocular pressure spikes. Interestingly, the IOP in many patients with uveitic glaucoma decreases in response to appropriate anti-inflammatory management; in the meantime the macular edema deteriorates, particularly if the patient is on systemic steroids or a biological agent and with significant fluctuations in the glucose levels. The recurrence of the edema may remain unnoticed in eyes with media opacities and active inflammation and is "discovered" once the uveitis subsides in the search for explanation of the poor vision - severe macrocysts in the macula are usually accompanied by exudative subsensory fluid collections. Early detection of the DME while the visual acuity is still reasonable and prompt intensive intravitreal treatment improve greatly the visual prognosis (**Figure 5**). These patients are very unstable - they present frequently with recurrent uveitis and macular edema in the course of each attack of their systemic inflammation or in periods of deteriorated metabolic control.

10. Cataract surgery and DME

Cataract surgery in diabetic patients has been associated with higher risk of complications, including postoperative macular edema (Irvine-Gass syndrome) and worsening of pre-existing DME (**Figure 4b**). The risk is high in patients with inconsistent previous treatment or chronic edema with incomplete response to intravitreal management. The prevalence is increased by intraoperative vitreous loss, vitreous traction at incision sites, vitrectomy for retained lens fragments, iris trauma, posterior capsule rupture, intraocular lens dislocation, early postoperative capsulotomy, iris-fixated intraocular lenses and placement of an anterior chamber intraocular lens and is further exaggerated by persistent postoperative inflammation [32, 33]. In clinical practice the edema is usually revealed late in the postoperative period and the differentiation between pseudophakic cystoid (Irvin-Gass) and macrocystic diabetic edema may not be very straightforward on OCT. The presence of hard exudates, atrophic changes and hypoperfusion in the posterior pole and some degree of retinopathy in an eye with low vision is more suggestive of a DME (**Figure 5**) while better vision and characteristic fluorescein angiography findings like retinal telangiectasis, capillary dilatation, and leakage from perifoveal capillaries in the early phase frames, and perifoveal hyperfluorescent spots classically described as a "petalloid" pattern in the late phase frames are suggestive of pseudophakic cystoid macular edema. While in most cases, acute pseudophakic CME spontaneously resolves with relatively good vision, the eyes with deteriorated DME after cataract surgery remain with low vision despite vigorous treatment on intravitreal anti-VEGF and steroids. There is a general consensus that DME and severe diabetic retinopathy should be stabilized before undergoing cataract extraction and proactive management is recommended in preparation for surgery. Recurrence or worsening of DME has been successfully prevented by preoperative or intraoperative ranibizumab [34] and triamcinolone acetonide (TA) [35], however the efficacy was short lasting and a sizable group of the eyes with TA develop elevated IOP. Dexamethasone implants have been used intraoperatively and postoperatively [36, 37], however if inserted 2 to 4 weeks prior to surgery they reach their peak activity at the time of the procedure and help control the postoperative inflammation. The initial improvement in visual acuity and decrease in the edema in the first 1–2 months start deteriorating in the next 2–3 months, yet these eyes respond favorably to repeated dexamethasone treatment [38].

11. Diabetic macular edema after vitrectomy

The development and use of smaller gauge instrumentation has been associated with a trend towards earlier surgical intervention for diabetic retinopathy. PPV indications include non-clearing vitreous hemorrhages, traction retinal detachment in PDR, and vitreoretinal interface abnormalities impeding macular edema resolution. The role of pars plana vitrectomy (PPV) for eyes with DME without traction elements is less clear. Debate still exists as to the necessity of ILM removal during vitrectomy for DME [39]. Several studies over the past 3 decades have established the structural improvements following vitrectomy in recalcitrant DME cases. Visual improvements however have not been as consistent and as significant as the reduction in retinal thickness following the procedure. Surgical intervention continues to be reserved for those cases that have had chronic and severe forms of DME when retinal damage is usually irreversible thereby compromising the results [40]. Vitrectomy itself is associated with morphological changes in the posterior pole. Detailed evaluation of the macular microstructure after vitrectomy has demonstrated deteriorated photoreceptor outer segment (PROS) length, ellipsoid zone (EZ) and external limiting membrane (ELM). The postoperative recovery was uneven – while PROS increased significantly after 12 months, ELM recovered but did not improve by 24 months when compared to baseline, and the EZ continued improving up to 24 months [41, 42]. Another factor contributing to lower postoperative visual results is post-vitrectomy cystoid macular edema that ranges between 5–47% and has been associated with combined cataract surgery, silicone oil tamponade and its removal, and removal of retained lens fragments in the diabetic eye. This inflammatory condition needs to be differentiated from a recurrence of pre-existing DME after PPV. The presence of dense hard exudates, disorganized retinal layers in the edematous macula, paramacular laser spots, capillary dropout on OCTA and persistent ischemic changes anywhere in the retina indicate the increased risk of poor postoperative vision, however, early intensive management on intravitreal steroids and anti-VEGF combined with careful laser treatment will significantly improve the prognosis (**Figure 6**). A recent meta-analysis estimated the overall pooled incidence of neovascular glaucoma (NVG) after PPV in PDR patients at 6%. The study showed a positive correlation for NVG after PPV in PDR patients with higher baseline IOP, preoperative iris neovascularization, lack of panretinal photocoagulation, preoperative or intraoperative combined cataract surgery, postoperative vitreous hemorrhage and a negative correlation with age [43]. Persistent macular edema in these eyes is a therapeutic challenge. Early glaucoma valve surgery with perioperative anti-VEGF, followed by appropriate intravitreal treatment can stabilize these eyes despite the grave prognosis, moreover that successful combined management of DME correlated closely with long-term recovery of photoreceptor integrity and visual outcome in patients with resolved DME in the presence of retained vascular density in the deep capillary plexus [44].

12. Age

The participants in Protocol T were enrolled at an average age of 61 years [45–58]. Secondary analysis of the baseline factors associated with visual outcome after 2 years of intensive anti-VEGF treatment revealed that even in such a relatively young cohort with every decade of age the scope of mean visual improvement decreased by 2.1 EDTRS letters. When the change in visual acuity over 2 years was estimated longitudinally as area under the curve (AUC), the improvement was reduced by 1.9 letters for each decade of life [9]. This association supports previous findings from DRCR.net Protocol I on treatment with a single anti-VEGF [59] and the RISE and RIDE trials where the odds of achieving at least a 15-letter gain at 2 years fell for every 5-year increase in the age of the patients.

13. Glycemic control

There is controversy on the correlation of HbA1c and visual response to anti-VEGF from large phase 3 trials. An analysis of ranibizumab-treated patients from the RISE and RIDE trials did not find an association between mean change in BCVA at weeks 52 and 100, with the baseline HbA1c [60]. This is in contrast to an analysis of aflibercept-treated patients from the VISTA and VIVID trials, which found that the mean improvement in VA at 2 years was dependent on HbA1c levels [61]. An exploratory analysis of DRCR.net Protocol T, in which participants were randomized to receive bevacizumab, ranibizumab, or aflibercept, found that the magnitude of vision improvement after anti-VEGF treatment decreased by 1 letter for each 1% increase in HbA1c levels at baseline [9]. More recently, lower HbA1c levels at baseline (7% or less) were significantly associated with greater reduction in central macular subfield thickness at one month after injection of bevacizumab or ranibizumab, however the change in BCVA after treatment did not have any correlation with the glycemic control [62]. Chen et al. reported that after one year of treatment on ranibizumab, only in the responder group the baseline level of HbA1c was significantly associated with the changes in BCVA and the final BCVA [63]. The common methodological issue with these trials and cohorts under observation is the estimate of glycemic control – HbA1c at baseline, only. There is a significant variability in the glucose plasma levels in diabetic patients. Its impact on microvascular complications in type 2 diabetes was investigated in a post-hoc analysis of 12 042 participants in both Action to Control Cardiovascular Risk in Diabetes (ACCORD) and the Veteran Affairs Diabetes Trial (VADT) that were observed for 84 to 87 months. Variability measures included coefficient of variation and average real variability for fasting glucose. Both indices were associated with development of future microvascular outcomes - higher risk of developing PDR that requires laser treatment - even after adjusting for other risk factors, including measures of average glycemic control (ie, cumulative average of HbA1c). Meta analyses of these 2 trials confirmed these findings and indicated fasting plasma glucose variation may be more harmful in those with less intensive glucose control [64]. A patient with DME and significant fluctuations in the plasma glucose, hypoglycaemic episodes and HbA1c over 7.5% needs close monitoring – even though the edema may respond structurally to intravitreal treatment, the visual outcome will be limited and very unstable. In addition to the ubiquitous dietary mistakes and sedentary lifestyle, often there are problems associated with ongoing infections, diabetic foot ulcers, non-ocular surgeries and systemic steroid treatment (**Figures 2** and **4**) Dynamic fasting and random plasma glucose and HbA1c re-assessment at the clinic and prior to intravitreal treatment are easy and useful in identifying these patients, particularly during worsening of the DME and diabetic retinopathy after periods of stabilization.

14. Cardiovascular disease

The association between cardiovascular disease and diabetic retinopathy was studied mainly in patients with mild retinal lesions. A recent meta-analysis was performed on 7604 individuals with type 2 diabetes from 8 prospective population-based surveys that were monitored for 5.9 years (3.2 to 10.1 years) where DME was identified in retinal photographs. DME was observed in 0.5% to 7.6% of the participants and was related to an increased risk of first-ever cardiovascular disease - incidence rate ratio 1.65 and fatal cardiovascular disease - incidence rate ratio 2.85. The incidence rate ratio for first-ever coronary heart disease was 1.57 and for fatal coronary heart disease - 3.55. These associations were consistent after multivariable adjustment for vascular risk factors, including smoking, systolic blood pressure, use of hypertension medication, total cholesterol level, and body mass index. When duration of diabetes, use of treatment for diabetes, and glycosylated hemoglobin level were included in the multivariable model, the relationship remained significant [65]. This analysis resonates with an early report on markers for subclinical cardiovascular disease in diabetic patients: CSME was associated with a high coronary artery calcium score (odds ratio, OR 2.86), low ankle-brachial index (OR 4.08) and high ankle-brachial index (OR 21.4) after adjusting for risk factors including hemoglobin A1c level and duration of diabetes, but there was significant association with carotid intima-media thickness or carotid stenosis, defined as >25% stenosis or presence of carotid plaque [66]. The diagnosis of CSME in these studies was based on fundus photographs; had OCT been used as a more sensitive imaging modality [13, 45, 67], the proportion of DME patients with increased cardiovascular risk could have been even higher. In clinical practice, confirmed or probable decompensated coronary artery disease is usually associated with more severe retinal ischemia, unstable response to treatment and higher risk of cardiovascular complications after intravitreal anti-VEGF if used in the course of an acute episode. The extent of macular edema and rate of its recurrence decrease notably after successful angioplasty or coronary bypass graft, however these patients remain at high risk as they are prone to new coronary heart attacks, severe infections and vision-threatening complications – neovascular glaucoma, ischemic diabetic optic neuropathy, vitreous hemorrhages and chronic macular edema (**Figures 1**, **3** and **4**).

15. Diabetic nephropathy and hemodialysis

Chronic kidney disease has been related with progression to PDR and DME in type 2 diabetic patients in advanced stages of their microvascular impairment. Systematic assessment of 2135 type 2 diabetic patients for 8 years revealed in 9.2% of new-onset DME identified in fundus photographs that had meaningful relationship with albumin/creatinine ratio below 31 mg/g at baseline, mean follow- serum creatinine levels and estimated glomerular filtration rate 30 and 45 mL/min/1.73 m2 [46]. This longitudinal study clearly emphasizes the importance of screening the DME patients for abnormal renal profile at baseline and throughout the whole follow up. A marked VEGF expression secondary to glomerular injury and elevated levels of serum VEGF in patients with advanced nephropathy could explain the incomplete and unstable response of their macular edema to intravitreal treatment. Introduction to hemodialysis of patients with end-stage renal disease and coexisting DME was associated with significant reduction in the central retinal thickness lasting over the next 12 months, to a level that eliminated the need for intravitreal treatment in 93.2% of the eyes. The fluid resolution was greater in eyes with subretinal detachment compared to spongelike swelling and macrocystic edema. A significant correlation between changes of BCVA and central retinal thickness at 12 months after hemodialysis initiation was found in the patients with good BCVA (over 20/50) but not in the patients with poor BCVA (less than 20/50) [47]. In clinical practice, a sizable group of patients with advanced renal decompensation

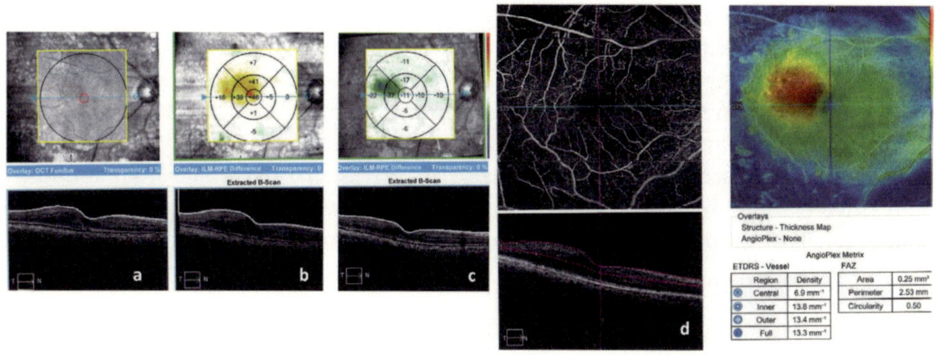

Figure 7.
59 years old male, DM for 25 years, renal failure, chronic hemodialysis, CAD, DME, PDR, recurrent anterior uveitis, recurrent iris neovascularization, secondary glaucoma. a, b -Perimacular edema progressing centrally during deterioration of CAD and CABG, VA 20/20, c – 6 months and 4 intravitreal injections later, VA 20/20, d - OCTA –superficial plexus, capillary dropout, microaneurisms, hyperreflectivefoci and distorted enlarged foveolar avascular zone.

had notable stabilization of their DME after induction of hemodialysis and needed less intensive management, however they remain at high risk for recurrences of the edema and severe retinal ischemia (**Figure 7**).

16. Treatment plan

Patients with DME at high risk for complications and vision loss require close monitoring at short intervals, intensive flexible treatment and arrangements for urgent visits and referrals. Very often, the patients present with multiple ophthalmic and systemic risk factors or develop them while they are under our care. Unrecognized and poorly treated complications and their exacerbations will readily explain the lack of results after "routine" management. Instead of labeling the patient as "non-responder" and giving up treatment altogether, or waiting for the inevitable vision deterioration in order to "start reacting", a "proactive" approach is more effective to achieve high and stable visual acuity, even in difficult patients.

17. Early start with high visual acuity

Initiation of treatment in high-risk eyes with BCVA better than 20/40 (Decimal 0.5, LogMAR 0.3) has resulted in better response and higher visual outcome in short- and long term. In our cohort of 152 eyes, 82.89% had BCVA 20/40 at their final visit after 3 to 8 years of management. Out of 126 eyes with BCVA 20/40 and better prior to treatment, 76.96% retained it through the follow up, however only 34.63% of the eyes with BCVA 20/50 and less could improve to 20/40 and better. Final BCVA 20/150 and less (the level of legal blindness in Kuwait) was seen in 4.82% of the eyes with high initial visual acuity and in 23.06% in the eyes with worse baseline vision.

18. Early start in eyes with perimacular edema

Recent or chronic edema close to the macula seldom affects the visual acuity, however it tends to progress centrally after major non-ocular surgeries, severe infections and exacerbations of cardiovascular and renal complications (**Figures 3**, **4** and 7). Early intravitreal treatment is usually effective and results in high visual acuity – in our cohort, 40% of the eyes with final BCVA 20/40 and better had significant perimacular edema at baseline. In eyes with more distant chronic lesions where persistent leakage and hypoperfusion are evident, intravitreal treatment can be followed by delicate focal laser once the edema has regressed. The classical perivascular technique of P. Hamilton performed with the 50 micrometer spot and minimal power settings applied in the temporal half of the posterior pole is suitable in severe chronic cases.

19. Severe NPDR and PDR in an eye with DME

Nowadays these patients seldom come without any previous treatment. Incomplete retinal laser and particularly interrupted intravitreal anti-VEGF injections for PDR have resulted in sight-threatening complications. PRP, primary vitrectomy or pharmacotherapy, alone or in combination, have been proposed with excellent outcome. The choice greatly depends on the ability of the patient to visit the clinic for regular follow up or emergency. Serious comorbidities and psychiatric diseases are associated with lengthy admissions and recuperation – and lack of eye treatment. Such patients will benefit from completion of the PRP and a longer-acting intravitreal medication while they are still ambulant. The main concern with PRP is the peripheral visual field (VF) loss associated with photocoagulation burns. A recent ad hoc review of DRCR.net Protocol S data reports decline of the pericentral and peripheral visual field 5 years after treatment with 20 ranibizumab injections to a level close to the pattern in eyes with PRP and 7 ranibizumab injections, suggesting that there are factors besides PRP associated with VF loss in eyes treated for PDR. In the longitudinal model describing total VF point score loss, the amount of loss depended on the type of laser treatment applied. On average, additional PRP sessions were associated with less VF loss than an initial PRP session, and endolaser application during vitrectomy was associated with more loss than an initial PRP session. The losses may be direct and immediate effects of heavier vs. lighter photocoagulation or reflections of delayed deleterious effects of the treatments, conditions associated with the persistence or return of neovascularization necessitating additional treatment, cataract progression, or, in the case of endolaser with vitrectomy, adverse effects of vitreous hemorrhage or the surgical procedure, such as cataract [48]. In practice, early, gradual and sparing laser technique with smaller spot size and less duration, particularly after intravitrel pharmacotherapy, is seldom associated with significant field loss – these defects appear after severe ischemia and correspond to non-perfusion areas.

20. Anti-VEGF medications as first choice

Abundant published data emphasize the safety of all off-label and approved drugs. Ranibizumab (Lucentis®, Novartis, Basel, Switzerland) and Aflibercept (EYLEA®; Bayer HealthCare, Berlin, Germany/Regeneron Pharmaceuticals Inc., Tarrytown, NY, USA) are preferable as initial treatment for eyes with DME and primary or secondary glaucoma, however the IOP needs close monitoring for spikes if larger volume has been injected intravitreally. This class of antibodies induces regression of the iris neovascularization and resolution of intraretinal edema and hemorrhages in eyes with PDR and this facilitates greatly the completion of PRP. An important consideration is the partial response and persistence of macular edema - data from Protocol T demonstrated chronic fluid in up to 65.9% of the eyes on bevacizumab, in 44.2% of the eyes on ranibizumab and

39.2% of the eyes on aflibercept after 2 years of treatment [1]. The number of intravitreal injections during the first year is decisive – in Protocol T, after the loading dose, the eyes that ended up with chronic edema had on average 3 injection from the 24th to 52nd week vs. 6 injections in eyes without chronic DME for the same period. Even though the eyes with chronic edema were given 4 to 6 injections during the second year, they remained with persistent fluid, unlike the eyes without fluid after the first year – they maintained relative stability on 2–3 injections during the second year [1]. The ability of a high-risk patient to complete such an intensive treatment, particularly if the edema is bilateral, needs to be discussed beforehand.

21. Intravitreal dexamethasone as first choice

The use of Dexamethasone intravitreal implant (0.7 mg) (Ozurdex, Allergan, Inc., Irvine, CA, USA) in eyes with DME, alone or in combination with anti- VEGF drugs, vitrectomy and retinal laser has been studied extensively since 2011. The implant provides rapid resolution of the macular fluid in all compartments that is sustained oved the next 2–4 months. It decreases the existing hard exudates and prevents the formation of new ones [49], and reportedly reduces the rate of progression of retinopathy [50]. Dexamethasone implant is selected as primary treatment in patients with recent and severe cardiovascular complications or pregnancy where the risk of systemic side effects from anti-VEGF injections needs to be avoided. Severe chronic maculopathy is often refractory to anti-VEGF management and a trial loading dose with these drugs may turn out to be an unnecessary delay. A dexamethasone implant as initial treatment might be a better choice for such patients, moreover that treatment–naïve eyes consistently fared better that eyes on long previous non-steroidal management. The main concerns are the formation of cataract in phakic eyes and elevation in the IOP. In the MEAD studies, the incidence of cataract-related side effects was 67.9% in the 0.7 mg dexamethasone implant and the rate of cataract surgery was 59.2%. In the same trial, an increase in IOP was observed in 27.7% of the eyes and 1.4% of them required a glaucoma procedure (trabeculoplasty, iridotomy, iridectomy, or trabeculectomy) [51]. A patient with advanced glaucoma, even well compensated on topical treatment or after glaucoma surgery, is at risk of developing further optic nerve disc damage and vision deterioration after a steroid- induced IOP spike. A short trial use of dexamethasone drops 4–5 times daily readily provokes a meaningful IOP elevation in a steroidal responder and foretells similar issues with the implant. In clinical practice, an increase in the IOP is observable a week after implantation and responds well to topical beta blockers and carbonic anhydrase inhibitors. The IOP needs monitoring for at least three months as in some cases it decreases after resolution of the implant, and in others it remains permanently high and requires consistent glaucoma care. The DME patients with glaucoma on intravitreal dexamethasone in our practice remained controlled on topical medications and none needed glaucoma surgery. The progression of cataract after several dexamethasone implants and the need for surgery as part of the vision rehabilitation has to be discussed with the high-risk patients beforehand - in most cases the possibility of good functional results outweigh the apprehension and fear (**Figures 4** and **6**). In vitrectomized eyes with aphakia, large iridectomies, zonulolysis, large peripheral defects in the posterior lens capsule and dislocated IOLs the implant tends to migrate in the anterior chamber and induce elevated IOP and corneal edema to a point that may require a corneal graft. A peribulbar depo-steroid might be a safer option in such complicated eyes.

22. Vitrectomy as first choice

The introduction of small gauge platforms and refined instrumentation have greatly improved the safety and reliability of PPV as primary treatment for eyes with DME and vitreomacular traction. The role of primary PPV for eyes with DME without traction elements is less clear. An earlier publication of Michalewska Z et al. [52] on 20-G vitrectomy and ILM removal, the multicenter trial of Iglicki M et al. [53] using 25-G PPV and ILM peeling and the report of Lin HC et al. [54] on 23-G vitrectomy with ILM peeling as a first line treatment for DME demonstrate substantial increase and stabilization of visual acuity, macular fluid resolution and rapid regression of hard exudates, without additional therapy up to 24 months post surgery. Prognostic factors associated with a greater visual gain include no history of prior macula laser treatment, lower hemoglobin A1c, recent onset of the edema and younger age, however delay of the procedure and damage of the IS/OS and ellipsoid zone at baseline had negative effect on the vision gain 12 and 24 months postoperatively. The complications after PPV can not be ignored – lamellar and full-thickness macular holes, non-resolving preretinal hemorrhages and rhegmatogenous retinal detachments have all been reported, and up to 50% of the phakic eyes develop significant cataract during the next 12 to 24 months that requires surgery compared to 7.14% of the eyes in the pharmacotherapy group [53]. These results suggest that earlier intervention with pars plana vitrectomy may be beneficial for treatment-naïve eyes, but they need to be replicated in larger prospective controlled trials.

23. Management of diabetes and its complications

Partnership and regular consultations with the diabetologist or treating physician are essential part of the management in high-risk DME patients. The adjustments or frank replacement of diabetic medications, provision of glycemic monitoring devices, lifelong screening for cardiovascular and renal complications, prompt referral to the necessary subspecialist create the foundation for better glycemic control, improved stability and less severe retinal complications. Regular measurements of HbA1c at the retinal clinic and RBS prior to intravitreal injections easily screen patients with unsatisfactory glycemic control and have become routine in our practice. Sudden worsening of the retinopathy and macular edema are often preceding serious systemic complications and a swift arrangement for medical assessment may prevent a major disability or even save the life of the patient (**Figure 1**). Discussing the medical background with a patient presenting with relapsing DME reveals sometimes bureaucratic and financial barriers to qualified medical care. Direct contacts with a dedicated medical team and suitable procedures for referral are particularly helpful in challenging situations that need consistent management. Holistic approach, continuous interest and candid conversations with the patients improve substantially the compliance and, in the long run, the outcome of DME treatment.

24. First outcome – review and adjustments of the treatment

Careful observation of high-risk eyes one week after the first anti-VEGF intravitreal injection reveals a degree of fluid resolution (**Figure 2c**) and its recurrence one month later. Rather than lack of response, this indicates ongoing retinal ischaemia and the need for tight metabolic control and management of systemic comorbidities. An early positive response on OCT may not be associated with immediate improvement of the visual acuity, however the monthly injections with the chosen drug need to be continued until the loading dose is completed. Meanwhile, if patient and physician have decided to perform further laser treatment for eyes with PDR and severe ischemia, it is split in suitable intervals. Intensive metabolic control - and the much needed changes in the diet – are usually followed by short episodes of hypoglycemia and deterioration of the retinopathy severity and recurrences of the edema. The patients need to be prepared for this difficult initial period in order to comply with the visits and procedures without anxiety and confusion. Monthly monitoring of eyes with advanced maculopathy is highly advisable – edema that is persistent after one or two anti-VEGF injections and is associated with large cysts, hyperreflective spots and particularly progressive disorganization in the outer retinal layers indicate severe disruption of the blood-retinal barrier and active inflammation. Extending the loading dose to 24 weeks will not provide better functional or anatomic outcomes and prompt transition to a dexamethasone implant at this point will be more beneficial (**Figure 4g**). At month 12, the probability of achieving a BCVA improvement of ≥10 letters was reported as 3.71 times greater after intravitreal dexamethasone vs. anti-VEGF treatment [55]. High-risk eyes with good response to anti-VEGF in terms of vision gain and fluid resolution by the end of the 3rd to 4th month, need sufficient number of injections and comprehensive medical care in the next years in order to maintain the outcome. Patients with high vision and completed intravitreal course in the first 2 years may present with recurrences - they are still at high risk – however they continue responding well to treatment and retain the acuity with minor variations.

An eye with a high-risk DME, good response to dexamethasone implant as initial treatment and well controlled IOP is already facing recurrence of the edema and deterioration of vision after 3 to 4 months (**Figure 4h**). Insertion of the implant at this point reduces the fluctuations in the edema and resulting detrimental changes in the outer retina. Improved metabolic control, successful cardio-vascular management and particularly, induction into hemodialysis are associated with more stable maculopathy – this allows increase the intervals between implants or even transition to anti-VEGF on "as needed" regimen.

25. Further management

The eyes with high-risk DME remain unstable even after they have responded well to intravitreal treatment. The patients often present with recurrences during and after severe systemic infections, major surgeries, trauma and stress. There are also fluctuations in the edema associated with variations in the metabolic control, ongoing ischemic events in patient with cardiac and renal complication and ocular surgeries. The visual acuity of a well treated diabetic eye is not severely affected by the new fluid in the first few months, however if left untreated, it causes gradual functional deterioration that may not be reversible. The management of these eyes is oriented towards early detection of the recurrences and timely treatment, in parallel with dynamic collaboration with the diabetologist in order to control the systemic complications.

Frequent assessment, sufficient number of intravitreal injections and adequate treatment of the retinopathy in the first 2 years are critical, and they need to continue for lifetime in order to maintain the visual outcome. The initial therapy needs modifications and combinations in response to the challenges of the disease.

A shift to a longer acting medication needs to be considered for eyes that can not remain stable for more than 45–60 days. There are some early results from the KITE and KASTREL studies on brolucizumab where 55.1% of the eyes in KESTREL and 50.3% of the eyes in KITE remained on a three-month dosing interval through year one, based on a treatment approach determined by disease activity assessment. If disease activity was detected, the patients were switched to two-month intervals through the end of the first year [56]. Faricimab, the first bispecific antibody to target both anti-Angiopoietin-2 and anti-vascular endothelial growth factor (VEGF) was investigated in YOSEMITE and RHINE trials as monotherapy for DME. More than 70% of patients achieved every-12-week or better dosing status at week 52--73.8% in the YOSEMITE study and 71.1% in the RHINE study with every 12-week and every-16-week dosing [57].

Temporary use of dexamethasone implants is convenient for systemically unstable patients or in preparation for major surgeries or ocular procedures - this will reduce the probability of severe inflammation and macular edema, provided the patient is able to use the antiglaucoma drops.

A patient with favorable response to dexamethasone is a good candidate for an intravitreal fluocinolone sustained-release Implant (**Figure 4g** and **m**). Two parallel, prospective, randomized, sham injection-controlled, double-masked, multicenter clinical trials (FAME trials) demonstrated significant reduction of the central macular thickness, mean BCVA improvement and a higher proportion of patients achieving a BCVA improvement of ≥15 letters in eyes with the implant vs. sham. The need of glaucoma surgery was 3.7% and 0.5% in the implant and sham groups, respectively [58]. A comparison of the effectiveness and safety of the fluocinolone acetonide intravitreal implant between the observational Iluvien Clinical Evidence study in the United Kingdom (ICE-UK) and the Fluocinolone Acetonide in Diabetic Macular Edema (FAME) randomized controlled trials (RCTs) in people with diabetic macular edema demonstrated statistically significant improvements in visual acuity 12 months after implantation in both the real-world study and in the RCTs. The improvement in vision and central retinal thickness in the RCTs was marginally greater than in the real-world study; however, recruits in the real-world study had more severe visual morbidity at baseline [68].

Flexible arrangements for walk-in visits or open appointments prevent delays in the evaluation of patients missing their regular review or presenting with a deterioration. Leaving a few empty slots for such unplanned patients in the daily schedule decreases the disorder in the medical retina clinic. A registry of the DME patients is useful in tracking any lapse in treatment of 3 months or longer that increases the probability of poorer outcome.

Author details

Maya G. Pandova
New Ahmadi KOC Hospital, Ahmadi, Kuwait

*Address all correspondence to: mayapandova@gmail.com

References

[1] Bressler NM, Beaulieu WT, Glassman AR, Blinder KJ, Bressler SB, Jampol LM, Melia M, Wells JA 3rd; Diabetic Retinopathy Clinical Research Network. Persistent Macular Thickening Following Intravitreous Aflibercept, Bevacizumab, or Ranibizumab for Central-Involved Diabetic Macular Edema With Vision Impairment: A Secondary Analysis of a Randomized Clinical Trial. JAMA Ophthalmol. 2018 Mar 1;136(3):257-269. doi: 10.1001/jamaophthalmol.2017.6565. Erratum in: JAMA Ophthalmol. 2018 May 1;136(5):601. PMID: 29392288; PMCID: PMC5885906.

[2] Glassman AR, Wells JA 3rd, Josic K, Maguire MG, Antoszyk AN, Baker C, Beaulieu WT, Elman MJ, Jampol LM, Sun JK. Five-Year Outcomes after Initial Aflibercept, Bevacizumab, or Ranibizumab Treatment for Diabetic Macular Edema (Protocol T Extension Study). Ophthalmology. 2020 Sep;127(9):1201-1210. doi: 10.1016/j.ophtha.2020.03.021. Epub 2020 Mar 29. PMID: 32402554; PMCID: PMC7483366.

[3] Ciulla TA, Bracha P, Pollack J, Williams DF. Real-world Outcomes of Anti-Vascular Endothelial Growth Factor Therapy in Diabetic Macular Edema in the United States. Ophthalmol Retina. 2018 Dec;2(12):1179-1187. doi: 10.1016/j.oret.2018.06.004. Epub 2018 Jul 29. PMID: 31047187.

[4] Shimura M, Kitano S, Muramatsu D, Fukushima H, Takamura Y, Matsumoto M, Kokado M, Kogo J, Sasaki M, Morizane Y, Kotake O, Koto T, Sonoda S, Hirano T, Ishikawa H, Mitamura Y, Okamoto F, Kinoshita T, Kimura K, Sugimoto M, Yamashiro K, Suzuki Y, Hikichi T, Washio N, Sato T, Ohkoshi K, Tsujinaka H, Kusuhara S, Kondo M, Takagi H, Murata T, Sakamoto T; Japan Clinical Retina Study (J-CREST) group. Real-world management of treatment-naïve diabetic macular oedema in Japan: two-year visual outcomes with and without anti-VEGF therapy in the STREAT-DME study. Br J Ophthalmol. 2020 Sep;104(9):1209-1215. doi: 10.1136/bjophthalmol-2019-315199. Epub 2019 Nov 29. PMID: 31784500; PMCID: PMC7577088.

[5] Van Aken E, Favreau M, Ramboer E, Denhaerynck K, MacDonald K, Abraham I, Brié H. Real-World Outcomes in Patients with Diabetic Macular Edema Treated Long Term with Ranibizumab (VISION Study). Clin Ophthalmol. 2020 Dec 2;14:4173-4185. doi: 10.2147/OPTH.S281501. PMID: 33299294; PMCID: PMC7720424.

[6] Holekamp NM, Campbell J, Almony A, Ingraham H, Marks S, Chandwani H, Cole AL, Kiss S. Vision Outcomes Following Anti-Vascular Endothelial Growth Factor Treatment of Diabetic Macular Edema in Clinical Practice. Am J Ophthalmol. 2018 Jul;191:83-91. doi: 10.1016/j.ajo.2018.04.010. Epub 2018 Apr 21. Erratum in: Am J Ophthalmol. 2018 Oct;194:192. PMID: 29684329.

[7] Stefanickova J, Cunha-Vaz J, Ulbig M, Pearce I, Fernández-Vega Sanz A, Theodossiadis P, Kodjikian L, Izmailov A, Muston D, Vassilev Z, Lamotte B, Tückmantel C, Friedl S, Altemark A, Schwarz HJ, Katz T; POLARIS study investigators. A noninterventional study to monitor patients with diabetic macular oedema starting treatment with ranibizumab (POLARIS). Acta Ophthalmol. 2018 Dec;96(8):e942-e949. doi: 10.1111/aos.13771. Epub 2018 Apr 25. PMID: 29696809; PMCID: PMC6585847.

[8] Ziemssen F, Wachtlin J, Kuehlewein L, Gamulescu MA, Bertelmann T, Feucht N, Voegeler J, Koch M, Liakopoulos S, Schmitz-Valckenberg S, Spital G;

OCEAN study group. Intravitreal Ranibizumab Therapy for Diabetic Macular Edema in Routine Practice: Two-Year Real-Life Data from a Non-interventional, Multicenter Study in Germany. Diabetes Ther. 2018 Dec;9(6):2271-2289. doi: 10.1007/s13300-018-0513-2. Epub 2018 Oct 4. PMID: 30288700; PMCID: PMC6250630.

[9] Bressler, S. B., Odia, I., Maguire, M. G., Dhoot, D. S., Glassman, A. R., Jampol, L. M., Marcus, D. M., Solomon, S. D., Sun, J. K., & Diabetic Retinopathy Clinical Research Network (2019). Factors Associated With Visual Acuity and Central Subfield Thickness Changes When Treating Diabetic Macular Edema With Anti-Vascular Endothelial Growth Factor Therapy: An Exploratory Analysis of the Protocol T Randomized Clinical Trial. JAMA ophthalmology, 137(4), 382-389. https://doi.org/10.1001/jamaophthalmol.2018.6786

[10] Schmidt-Erfurth U, Garcia-Arumi J, Bandello F, Berg K, Chakravarthy U, Gerendas BS, Jonas J, Larsen M, Tadayoni R, Loewenstein A. Guidelines for the Management of Diabetic Macular Edema by the European Society of Retina Specialists (EURETINA). Ophthalmologica. 2017;237(4):185-222. doi: 10.1159/000458539. Epub 2017 Apr 20. PMID: 28423385.

[11] Yoon CK, Sagong M, Shin JP, Lee SJ, Lee JE, Lee JE, Chung I, Jeong WJ, Pak KY, Kim HW. Title: efficacy of intravitreal dexamethasone implant on hard exudate in diabetic macular edema. BMC Ophthalmol. 2021 Jan 15;21(1):41. doi: 10.1186/s12886-020-01786-2. PMID: 33451297; PMCID: PMC7811249

[12] Sun JK, Radwan S, Soliman AZ, Lammer J, Lin MM, Prager SG, Silva PS, Aiello LB, Aiello LP: Neural retinal disorganization as a robust marker of visual acuity in current and resolved diabetic macular edema. Diabetes 2015;64:2560-2570

[13] Kwan, C.C., Fawzi, A.A. Imaging and Biomarkers in Diabetic Macular Edema and Diabetic Retinopathy. Curr Diab Rep 19, 95 (2019). https://doi.org/10.1007/s11892-019-1226-2

[14] Lee J, Moon BG, Cho AR, Yoon YH. Optical Coherence Tomography Angiography of DME and Its Association with Anti-VEGF Treatment Response. Ophthalmology. 2016 Nov;123(11):2368-2375. doi: 10.1016/j.ophtha.2016.07.010. Epub 2016 Sep 6. PMID: 27613201.

[15] Vujosevic S, Toma C, Villani E, Muraca A, Torti E, Florimbi G, Leporati F, Brambilla M, Nucci P, De Cilla' S. Diabetic macular edema with neuroretinal detachment: OCT and OCT-angiography biomarkers of treatment response to anti-VEGF and steroids. Acta Diabetol. 2020 Mar;57(3):287-296. doi: 10.1007/s00592-019-01424-4. Epub 2019 Sep 21. PMID: 31541333.

[16] Busch C, Wakabayashi T, Sato T, Fukushima Y, Hara C, Shiraki N, Winegarner A, Nishida K, Sakaguchi H, Nishida K. Retinal Microvasculature and Visual Acuity after Intravitreal Aflibercept in Diabetic Macular Edema: An Optical Coherence Tomography Angiography Study. Sci Rep. 2019 Feb 7;9(1):1561. doi: 10.1038/s41598-018-38248-1. PMID: 30733512; PMCID: PMC6367399.

[17] Yoshitake S, Murakami T, Uji A, Fujimoto M, Dodo Y, Suzuma K, Tsujikawa A. Granular lesions of short-wavelength and near-infrared autofluorescence in diabetic macular oedema. Eye (Lond). 2019 Apr;33(4):564-571. doi: 10.1038/s41433-018-0256-3. Epub 2018 Oct 31. PMID: 30382240; PMCID: PMC6462039.

[18] Vujosevic S, Torresin T, Bini S, Convento E, Pilotto E, Parrozzani R, Midena E. Imaging retinal inflammatory

biomarkers after intravitreal steroid and anti-VEGF treatment in diabetic macular oedema. Acta Ophthalmol. 2017 Aug;95(5):464-471. doi: 10.1111/aos.13294. Epub 2016 Oct 24. PMID: 27775223.

[19] Vujosevic S, Midena E, Pilotto E, Radin PP, Chiesa L, Cavarzeran F. Diabetic macular edema: correlation between microperimetry and optical coherence tomography findings. Invest Ophthalmol Vis Sci. 2006 Jul;47(7):3044-51. doi: 10.1167/iovs.05-1141. PMID: 16799051

[20] Zhao YX, Chen XW. Diabetes and risk of glaucoma: systematic review and a Meta-analysis of prospective cohort studies. Int J Ophthalmol. 2017 Sep 18;10(9):1430-1435. doi: 10.18240/ijo.2017.09.16. PMID: 28944204; PMCID: PMC5596230.

[21] Dharmadhikari S, Lohiya K, Chelkar V, Kalyani VK, Dole K, Deshpande M, Khandekar R, Kulkarni S. Magnitude and determinants of glaucoma in type II diabetics: A hospital based cross-sectional study in Maharashtra, India. Oman J Ophthalmol. 2015 Jan-Apr;8(1):19-23. doi: 10.4103/0974-620X.149858. PMID: 25709269; PMCID: PMC4333537.

[22] Hou H, Shoji T, Zangwill LM, Moghimi S, Saunders LJ, Hasenstab K, Ghahari E, Manalastas PIC, Akagi T, Christopher M, Penteado RC, Weinreb RN. Progression of Primary Open-Angle Glaucoma in Diabetic and Nondiabetic Patients. Am J Ophthalmol. 2018 May;189:1-9. doi: 10.1016/j.ajo.2018.02.002. Epub 2018 Feb 13. PMID: 29447914; PMCID: PMC5916320.

[23] Bressler SB, Almukhtar T, Bhorade A, Bressler NM, Glassman AR, Huang SS, Jampol LM, Kim JE, Melia M; Diabetic Retinopathy Clinical Research Network Investigators. Repeated intravitreous ranibizumab injections for diabetic macular edema and the risk of sustained elevation of intraocular pressure or the need for ocular hypotensive treatment. JAMA Ophthalmol. 2015 May;133(5):589-97. doi: 10.1001/jamaophthalmol.2015.186. PMID: 25719991; PMCID: PMC4496789.

[24] Fursova AZ, Gamza YA, Derbeneva AS, Vasilyeva MS. [Anti-angiogenesis therapy of diabetic macular edema in patients with primary open-angle glaucoma]. Vestn Oftalmol. 2020;136(6. Vyp. 2):185-194. Russian. doi: 10.17116/oftalma2020136062185. PMID: 33371648.

[25] Maturi RK, Pollack A, Uy HS, Varano M, Gomes AM, Li XY, Cui H, Lou J, Hashad Y, Whitcup SM; Ozurdex MEAD Study Group. INTRAOCULAR PRESSURE IN PATIENTS WITH DIABETIC MACULAR EDEMA TREATED WITH DEXAMETHASONE INTRAVITREAL IMPLANT IN THE 3-YEAR MEAD STUDY. Retina. 2016 Jun;36(6):1143-52. doi: 10.1097/IAE.0000000000001004. PMID: 26871523.

[26] Parrish RK 2nd, Campochiaro PA, Pearson PA, Green K, Traverso CE; FAME Study Group. Characterization of Intraocular Pressure Increases and Management Strategies Following Treatment With Fluocinolone Acetonide Intravitreal Implants in the FAME Trials. Ophthalmic Surg Lasers Imaging Retina. 2016 May 1;47(5):426-35. doi: 10.3928/23258160-20160419-05. PMID: 27183546.

[27] Gillies MC, Simpson JM, Gaston C, Hunt G, Ali H, Zhu M, Sutter F. Five-year results of a randomized trial with open-label extension of triamcinolone acetonide for refractory diabetic macular edema. Ophthalmology. 2009 Nov;116(11):2182-7. doi: 10.1016/j.ophtha.2009.04.049. Epub 2009 Oct 1. PMID: 19796823.

[28] Chawan-Saad J, Wu M, Wu A, Wu L. Corticosteroids for Diabetic

Macular Edema. Taiwan J Ophthalmol. 2019 Dec 13;9(4):233-242. doi: 10.4103/tjo.tjo_68_19. PMID: 31942428; PMCID: PMC6947754.

[29] Yan P, Qian C, Wang W, Dong Y, Wan G, Chen Y. Clinical effects and safety of treating diabetic macular edema with intravitreal injection of ranibizumab combined with retinal photocoagulation. Ther Clin Risk Manag. 2016 Apr 5;12:527-33. doi: 10.2147/TCRM.S99224. PMID: 27103811; PMCID: PMC4827417.

[30] Ansari AS, de Lusignan S, Hinton W, Munro N, Taylor S, McGovern A. Glycemic control is an important modifiable risk factor for uveitis in patients with diabetes: A retrospective cohort study establishing clinical risk and ophthalmic disease burden. J Diabetes Complications. 2018 Jun;32(6):602-608. doi: 10.1016/j.jdiacomp.2018.03.008. Epub 2018 Mar 23. PMID: 29656910.

[31] Oswal KS, Sivaraj RR, Murray PI, Stavrou P. Clinical course and visual outcome in patients with diabetes mellitus and uveitis. BMC Res Notes. 2013 Apr 29;6:167. doi: 10.1186/1756-0500-6-167. PMID: 23628425; PMCID: PMC3651352.

[32] Haddad NM, Sun JK, Abujaber S, Schlossman DK, Silva PS. Cataract surgery and its complications in diabetic patients. Semin Ophthalmol. 2014;29:329-337. doi: 10.3109/08820538.2014.959197.

[33] Chu CJ, et al. Risk Factors and Incidence of Macular Edema after Cataract Surgery: A Database Study of 81984 Eyes. Ophthalmology. 2016;123:316-323. doi: 10.1016/j.ophtha.2015.10.001

[34] Udaondo P, Garcia-Pous M, Garcia-Delpech S, Salom D, Diaz-Llopis M. Prophylaxis of macular edema with intravitreal ranibizumab in patients with diabetic retinopathy after cataract surgery: a pilot study. J Ophthalmol. 2011;2011:159436. doi: 10.1155/2011/159436. Epub 2011 Jun 16. PMID: 21772983; PMCID: PMC3136100.

[35] Tatsumi T, Oshitari T, Ando T, Takatsuna Y, Arai M, Baba T, Sato E, Yamamoto S. Comparison of the Efficacy of Sub-Tenon versus Intravitreal Triamcinolone Acetonide Injection during Cataract Surgery for Diabetic Macular Edema. Ophthalmologica. 2019;241(1):17-23. doi: 10.1159/000489716. Epub 2018 Jul 24. PMID: 30041252.

[36] Sze AM, Luk FO, Yip TP, Lee GK, Chan CK. Use of intravitreal dexamethasone implant in patients with cataract and macular edema undergoing phacoemulsification. Eur J Ophthalmol. 2015

[37] He Y, Ren XJ, Hu BJ, Lam WC, Li XR. A meta-analysis of the effect of a dexamethasone intravitreal implant versus intravitreal anti-vascular endothelial growth factor treatment for diabetic macular edema. BMC Ophthalmol. 2018;18:121. doi: 10.1186/s12886-018-0779-1.

[38] Kabanarou SA, Xirou T, Boutouri E, Gkizis I, Vasilias D, Bontzos G, Chatziralli I. Pre-operative intravitreal dexamethasone implant in patients with refractory diabetic macular edema undergoing cataract surgery. Sci Rep. 2020 Mar 26;10(1):5534. doi: 10.1038/s41598-020-62561-3. PMID: 32218471; PMCID: PMC7099086.

[39] Flikier S, Wu A, Wu L. Revisiting pars plana vitrectomy in the primary treatment of diabetic macular edema in the era of pharmacological treatment. Taiwan J Ophthalmol. 2019 Dec 13;9(4):224-232. doi: 10.4103/tjo.tjo_61_19. PMID: 31942427; PMCID: PMC6947753.

[40] Mansour SE, Browning DJ, Wong K, Flynn HW Jr, Bhavsar AR. The Evolving

Treatment of Diabetic Retinopathy. Clin Ophthalmol. 2020 Mar 4;14:653-678. doi: 10.2147/OPTH.S236637. PMID: 32184554; PMCID: PMC7061411.

[41] Miyamoto N, Ishida K, Kurimoto Y. Restoration of Photoreceptor Outer Segments up to 24 Months after Pars Plana Vitrectomy in Patients with Diabetic Macular Edema. Ophthalmol Retina. 2017 Sep-Oct;1(5):389-394. doi: 10.1016/j.oret.2017.01.017. Epub 2017 Apr 12. PMID: 31047566.

[42] Kogo J, Shiono A, Sasaki H, Yomoda R, Jujo T, Kitaoka Y, Takagi H. Foveal Microstructure Analysis in Eyes with Diabetic Macular Edema Treated with Vitrectomy. Adv Ther. 2017 Sep;34(9):2139-2149. doi: 10.1007/s12325-017-0598-4. Epub 2017 Aug 14. PMID: 28808926.

[43] Sun D, Lin Y, Zeng R, Yang Z, Deng X, Lan Y. The incidence and risk factors of neovascular glaucoma secondary to proliferative diabetic retinopathy after vitrectomy. Eur J Ophthalmol. 2020 Dec 18:1120672120980686. doi: 10.1177/1120672120980686. Epub ahead of print. PMID: 33334171.

[44] Moon BG, Um T, Lee J, Yoon YH. Correlation between Deep Capillary Plexus Perfusion and Long-Term Photoreceptor Recovery after Diabetic Macular Edema Treatment. Ophthalmol Retina. 2018 Mar;2(3):235-243. doi: 10.1016/j.oret.2017.07.003. Epub 2017 Sep 28. PMID: 31047592.

[45] Kang SW, Park CY, Ham D-I. The correlation between fluorescein angiographic and optical coherence tomographic features in clinically significant diabetic macular edema. Am J Ophthalmol. 2004;137(2):313-22.

[46] Hsieh Y, Tsai M, Tu S, Hsieh M. Association of Abnormal Renal Profiles and Proliferative Diabetic Retinopathy and Diabetic Macular Edema in an Asian Population With Type 2 Diabetes. JAMA Ophthalmol. 2018;136(1):68-74. doi:10.1001/jamaophthalmol.2017.5202

[47] Takamura Y, Matsumura T, Ohkoshi K, Takei T, Ishikawa K, Shimura M, Ueda T, Sugimoto M, Hirano T, Takayama K, Gozawa M, Yamada Y, Morioka M, Iwano M, Inatani M. Functional and anatomical changes in diabetic macular edema after hemodialysis initiation: One-year follow-up multicenter study. Sci Rep. 2020 May 8;10(1):7788. doi: 10.1038/s41598-020-64798-4. PMID: 32385333; PMCID: PMC7210956.

[48] Maguire MG, Liu D, Glassman AR, Jampol LM, Johnson CA, Baker CW, Bressler NM, Gardner TW, Pieramici D, Stockdale CR, Sun JK; DRCR Retina Network. Visual Field Changes Over 5 Years in Patients Treated With Panretinal Photocoagulation or Ranibizumab for Proliferative Diabetic Retinopathy. JAMA Ophthalmol. 2020 Mar 1;138(3):285-293. doi: 10.1001/jamaophthalmol.2019.5939. PMID: 31999300; PMCID: PMC7042909.

[49] Yoon CK, Sagong M, Shin JP, Lee SJ, Lee JE, Lee JE, Chung I, Jeong WJ, Pak KY, Kim HW. Title: efficacy of intravitreal dexamethasone implant on hard exudate in diabetic macular edema. BMC Ophthalmol. 2021 Jan 15;21(1):41. doi: 10.1186/s12886-020-01786-2. PMID: 33451297; PMCID: PMC7811249.

[50] Iglicki M, Zur D, Busch C, Okada M, Loewenstein A. Progression of diabetic retinopathy severity after treatment with dexamethasone implant: a 24-month cohort study the 'DR-Pro-DEX Study'. Acta Diabetol. 2018 Jun;55(6):541-547. doi: 10.1007/s00592-018-1117-z. Epub 2018 Mar 1. PMID: 29497837.

[51] Boyer DS, Yoon YH, Belfort R Jr, Bandello F, Maturi RK, Augustin AJ, Li XY, Cui H, Hashad Y, Whitcup SM; Ozurdex MEAD Study Group.

Three-year, randomized, sham-controlled trial of dexamethasone intravitreal implant in patients with diabetic macular edema. Ophthalmology. 2014 Oct;121(10):1904-14. doi: 10.1016/j.ophtha.2014.04.024. Epub 2014 Jun 4. PMID: 24907062.

[52] Michalewska Z, Stewart MW, Landers MB 3rd, Bednarski M, Adelman RA, Nawrocki J. Vitrectomy in the management of diabetic macular edema in treatment-naïve patients. Can J Ophthalmol. 2018 Aug;53(4):402-407. doi: 10.1016/j.jcjo.2017.10.011. Epub 2017 Dec 23. PMID: 30119796.

[53] Iglicki M, Lavaque A, Ozimek M, Negri HP, Okada M, Chhablani J, Busch C, Loewenstein A, Zur D. Biomarkers and predictors for functional and anatomic outcomes for small gauge pars plana vitrectomy and peeling of the internal limiting membrane in naïve diabetic macular edema: The VITAL Study. PLoS One. 2018 Jul 11;13(7):e0200365. doi: 10.1371/journal.pone.0200365. PMID: 29995929; PMCID: PMC6040739.

[54] Lin HC, Yang CM, Chen SN, Hsieh YT. Vitrectomy with internal limiting membrane peeling versus nonsurgical treatment for diabetic macular edema with massive hard exudates. PLoS One. 2020 Jul 31;15(7):e0236867. doi: 10.1371/journal.pone.0236867. PMID: 32735583; PMCID: PMC7394381.

[55] Busch C, Zur D, Fraser-Bell S, Laíns I, Santos AR, Lupidi M, Cagini C, Gabrielle PH, Couturier A, Mané-Tauty V, Giancipoli E, Ricci GD, Cebeci Z, Rodríguez-Valdés PJ, Chaikitmongkol V, Amphornphruet A, Hindi I, Agrawal K, Chhablani J, Loewenstein A, Iglicki M, Rehak M; International Retina Group. Shall we stay, or shall we switch? Continued anti-VEGF therapy versus early switch to dexamethasone implant in refractory diabetic macular edema. Acta Diabetol. 2018 Aug;55(8):789-796. doi: 10.1007/s00592-018-1151-x. Epub 2018 May 5. PMID: 29730822.

[56] Brown D, Wolf S, Garweg JG, et al. Brolucizumab for the treatment of visual impairment due to diabetic macular edema: 52-week results from the KESTREL & KITE studies. Presented at: The Association for Research in Vision and Ophthalmology (ARVO) 2021 Annual Meeting. May 2021.

[57] Wells JA "Efficacy, durability, and safety of faricimab in diabetic macular edema (DME): one-year results from the phase 3 YOSEMITE and RHINE trials," ARVO May 1, 2021.

[58] Campochiaro PA, Brown DM, Pearson A, Ciulla T, Boyer D, Holz FG, Tolentino M, Gupta A, Duarte L, Madreperla S, Gonder J, Kapik B, Billman K, Kane FE; FAME Study Group. Long-term benefit of sustained-delivery fluocinolone acetonide vitreous inserts for diabetic macular edema. Ophthalmology. 2011 Apr;118(4):626-635.e2. doi: 10.1016/j.ophtha.2010.12.028. PMID: 21459216.

[59] Bressler S, Qin H, Beck RW, Chalam KV, Kim JE, Melia M, Wells JA, for the Diabetic Retinopathy Clinical Research Network. Factors Associated with Changes in Visual Acuity and OCT Thickness at 1 Year after Treatment for Diabetic Macular Edema with Ranibizumab. Arch Ophthalmol. 2012 Sep;130(9):1153-1161

[60] Singh R. P., Habbu K., Ehlers J. P., Lansang M. C., Hill L., Stoilov I. The impact of systemic factors on clinical response to ranibizumab for diabetic macular edema. Ophthalmology. 2016;123(7):1581-1587. doi: 10.1016/j.ophtha.2016.03.038.

[61] Singh R. P., Wykoff C. C., Brown D. M., et al. Outcomes of diabetic macular edema patients by

baseline hemoglobin A1c: analyses from VISTA and VIVID. Ophthalmo logy Retina. 2017;1(5):382-388. doi: 10.1016/j.oret.2017.02.003.

[62] Wong WM, Chee C, Bhargava M, Chai C, Lin H, Zhao P, Ariadarma Mangunkusumo E, Naing T, Yuen YS, Wong TY, Su X, Lingam G. Systemic Factors Associated with Treatment Response in Diabetic Macular Edema. J Ophthalmol. 2020 Mar 19;2020:1875860. doi: 10.1155/2020/1875860. PMID: 32280516; PMCID: PMC7125481.

[63] Chen, YP., Wu, AL., Chuang, CC. et al. Factors influencing clinical outcomes in patients with diabetic macular edema treated with intravitreal ranibizumab: comparison between responder and non-responder cases. Sci Rep 9, 10952 (2019).

[64] Zhou JJ, Koska J, Bahn G, Reaven P. Fasting Glucose Variation Predicts Microvascular Risk in ACCORD and VADT. J Clin Endocrinol Metab. 2021 Mar 25;106(4):1150-1162. doi: 10.1210/clinem/dgaa941. PMID: 33367811; PMCID: PMC7993576.

[65] Xie J, Ikram MK, Cotch MF, Klein B, Varma R, Shaw JE, Klein R, Mitchell P, Lamoureux EL, Wong TY. Association of Diabetic Macular Edema and Proliferative Diabetic Retinopathy With Cardiovascular Disease: A Systematic Review and Meta-analysis. JAMA Ophthalmol. 2017 Jun 1;135(6):586-593. doi: 10.1001/jamaophthalmol.2017.0988. PMID: 28472362; PMCID: PMC5593137.

[66] Kawasaki R, Cheung N, Islam FM, Klein R, Klein BE, Cotch MF, Sharrett AR, O'Leary D, Wong TY; Multi-Ethnic Study of Atherosclerosis. Is diabetic retinopathy related to subclinical cardiovascular disease? Ophthalmology. 2011 May;118(5):860-5. doi: 10.1016/j.ophtha.2010.08.040. Epub 2010 Dec 18. PMID: 21168222; PMCID: PMC3087839.

[67] Lee J, Rosen R. Optical coherence tomography angiography in diabetes. Curr Diab Rep. 2016;16(12):123.

[68] Holden SE, Kapik B, Beiderbeck AB, Currie CJ. Comparison of data characterizing the clinical effectiveness of the fluocinolone intravitreal implant (ILUVIEN) in patients with diabetic macular edema from the real world, non-interventional ICE-UK study and the FAME randomized controlled trials. Curr Med Res Opin. 2019 Jul;35(7):1165-1176. doi: 10.1080/03007995.2018.1560779. Epub 2019 Jan 17. PMID: 30569759.

Chapter 3

Role of Inflammation in Diabetic Retinopathy

Anuj Sharma and Deepesh Arora

Abstract

As the global burden of diabetes is increasing there is a corresponding increase in the complications associated with the same. Diabetic retinopathy is a sight threatening complication of diabetes mellitus which was considered to be a microvasculopathy. Recent evidence however, has brought to light that inflammation may be a key player in the pathogenesis of this condition. Levels of inflammatory mediators like Hypoxia inducible factor, TNF-α, IL-6 and IL-1B amongst others have been noted to be elevated in the diabetic vitreous gel. The concept of the neurovascular unit better explains the changes that take place resulting in the breakdown of the blood retinal barriers and how these inflammatory mediators affect the morphology of the retina at a cellular level. Glial cells form a key instrument of this neurovascular structure and are also the cells from where the inflammatory response is initiated. Understanding of the pathogenesis of diabetic retinopathy will help us in finding targeted therapies which may provide long term benefits and possible cure. Few anti-inflammatory medications have shown promise albeit in a small clinical or experimental laboratory setting. However, future research may lead to better understanding of the disease and a better pharmacological intervention.

Keywords: pathogenesis of diabetic retinopathy, glial cells in diabetic retinopathy, retina inflammation, steroids, cytokines

1. Introduction

In the past few years, unhealthy lifestyle coupled with obesity has led to a rampant increase in the global burden of diabetes mellitus. As per WHO the global prevalence of the condition was 422 million in the year (2014) with 8.5% of adults aged more than 18 years suffering from this condition. Approximately 1.6 million deaths yearly are supposed to be caused by diabetes alone, this number excludes the mortality associated with cardiovascular events, renal disease and tuberculosis secondary to chronic hyperglycemia [1]. The global burden of diabetes is expected to swell to 642 million adults by the year 2040 with 75% of the affected individuals belonging to low and middle income countries. Diabetic retinopathy affects 1 in 3 adults with diabetes and is one of the major causes of blindness in the working-age population [2].

Diabetic retinopathy (DR) is a major microvascular complication of diabetes and it is categorised into a non-proliferative stage (NPDR) or proliferative stage (PDR) depending on the presence of retinal microvascular changes. The non-proliferative stage is characterised by the presence of microaneurysms, cotton wool spots, vascular tortuosity, retinal haemorrhage and lipid exudation while in the proliferative stage aberrant new blood vessels develop which are fragile and can extend into the posterior cortical vitreous [3]. Another important element in the vast conundrum of DR is diabetic macular edema (DME). It can occur across all levels of DR changes and compromises central vision. DME is the most common cause of diminished vision in an individual with DR [4].

2. The neurovascular unit in diabetic retinopathy

In recent years a concept of neurovascular unit in diabetic retinopathy has emerged. This is based on the findings that neurodegeneration is one of the earliest changes in a case of diabetic retinopathy. Indeed, a reduction in oscillatory potential in the electroretinogram is the first measurable change in retinal function, being recorded even in cases wherein there is no clinical change suggestive of DR. This indicates that neurodegeneration precedes microvascular abnormalities [5].

The retinal neurovascular unit includes the physical and biochemical interactions amongst the neurons, the vascular beds and the supporting cells of the retinal framework. The neural unit includes the ganglion cells and the glial cells while the vascular component of the unit is made up of the endothelial cells and the pericytes. The neurovascular unit reflects the inter-dependance of the vascular barrier and blood flow regulation on the glial cells, pericytes and neurons as well as their reciprocal dependance on vascular support. Together with the neurovascular unit the retinal pigment epithelium contributes to the formation of the blood retinal barrier [6]. The inner blood retinal barrier (iBRB) encompasses the endothelial cells of the retinal microvasculature which are covered by astrocytes, pericytes and muller cell end-feet. It regulates the transport across the retinal capillaries and maintain the micro-environment of the inner retina. The outer blood retinal barrier (oBRB) comprises the tight junctions of the neighbouring RPE cells and it serves as a filter for nutrients and solutes from the blood [7].

3. Histopathological changes in diabetic retinopathy

Diabetic retinopathy has been traditionally described as a microvasculopathy, however newer evidence has suggested that inflammation may provide a substantial role in the histopathological changes that are noted in the disease.

3.1 Microvascular changes

Retinal ischemia is the initiator that propels the plethora of changes that occur in DR. In the initial stages, prior to even the development of visually significant vascular alterations, there is a disruption of vascular auto-regulation which leads to oxygen and nutrient deprivation in the inner retinal layers [8].

Retinal vascular basement membrane thickening is present in the early stages of the disease and is mediated by hyperglycemia. Impaired sugar levels lead to an up-regulation of extracellular matrix proteins, collagen and fibronectin [9]. This thickening of the basement membrane may lead to an impairment in cell to cell communication between the endothelium, pericytes, glial cells and the retinal immune cells, ultimately leading to a loss of function [10]. Loss of pericytes leads to a weakening of the capillary wall; this ultimately results in the development of areas of out-pouching labelled as microaneurysms (MA), which are amongst the first clinically detectable signs of DR [11].

A progressive occlusion of the retinal capillaries is noted on histopathological evaluation of post-mortem specimens. Stitt et al. [10] evaluated trypsin digest preparations of these capillaries and noted them to be acellular tubes of naked basement membrane without endothelial cells. The loss of endothelial cells can be attributed to pericyte death which ultimately culminates into breakdown of the inner blood retinal barrier.

The breakdown of the inner blood retinal barrier would lead accumulation of fluid and exudates in the retinal layers contributing to diabetic macular edema (DME). Fluid exuding out from the superficial capillary plexus leads to accumulation of fluid in the inner nuclear layer while that exuding out from the deep capillary plexus is believed to collect in the outer plexiform layer. Cystoid spaces noted in the macula appear due to liquefaction and necrosis of the muller cells and the production of prostaglandins and inflammatory cytokines [12].

3.2 Neuroglial changes

The muller cells, astrocytes and microglial cells are present in close vicinity of the retinal blood vessels and help to maintain retina homeostasis. Muller cells play a central role in the retinal metabolism and hence are susceptible to the metabolic alterations of diabetes. An increased production of glial fibrillary acidic protein (GFAP) by the muller cells is noted in the early part of the disease, which plays a key role in gliosis. This is indicative of a state of glial hypertrophy [13].

Microglial cells are the resident inflammatory cells of the retina which get activated in DR. In the early stages of mild DR a hypertrophy of the microglia is noted and the cells are settled along the retinal plexiform layers. When the DR progresses into a proliferative stage the microglial cells are found to be extensively distributed in areas of retinal ischemia and neovascularisation [14]. A strong tendency of the microglial cells to invade the outer retinal layers is also noted in prolonged DR [15].

3.3 Neuronal changes

Overt degeneration of retinal neurons during diabetes is a concept that was first described in the 1960s in post-mortem patient samples. By the late 1990s experimental evidence reinforced this finding by demonstrating that depletion of some neuronal populations occurred in diabetic rodent models, possibly even prior to appearance of obvious microvascular lesions. Apoptosis of the retinal ganglion cells (RGCs) is histologically noted in diabetic retinas. This also accounts for the diminished thickness of the retinal nerve fibre layer on optical coherence tomography (OCT). It is believed that hyperglycemia induces a down-regulation of neuronal growth factors thereby contributing to programmed cell death [16].

3.4 Immune cell activation

Histological evaluation of blood vessels, early in the course of DR, have shown increased interaction between leukocytes and endothelial cells. This phenomenon called leukostasis is characterised by an adherence of monocytes and neutrophils to the endothelial lining of the blood vessels. This leads to blockage of the thin retinal capillaries and areas of retinal non-perfusion [17].

3.5 Retinal pigment epithelium and choroid

The changes are not only localised to the inner retinal layers but also extend to the RPE and the choroid compromising the outer blood retinal barrier. RPE dysfunction and leakage from the choriocapillaris is noted leading to outer retinal edema and impaired clearance of fluid [18].

Choroidal atrophy has been noted in cases of long standing DR, with a diminished choroidal thickness noted on OCT evaluation. This thinning of the choroid have been linked to HbA1c levels and may lead to choroidal neovascular membranes or intra-choroidal microvascular abnormalities [19].

4. Inflammation in DR

4.1 What is inflammation?

Inflammation is non-specific response of the the body to injury or stress which includes a variety of molecular and cellular mediators. Tissue stress may lead to de-inhibition of the transcription factor nuclear factor kappa beta (NF-κB) which stimulates the production of acute phase proteins, pro-inflammatory cytokines and chemokines such as TNF-α, IL-6 and IL-1B amongst others. These pro-inflammatory mediators play a major role in the unfolding of the inflammatory processes with recruitment and activation of monocytes and leukocytes. Inflammation usually resolves spontaneously in a coordinated manner, however when this fails to happen the beneficial effect of inflammation is lost and consequences ensue.

4.2 Inflammation in pathogenesis of diabetic retinopathy

If we consider diabetic retinopathy to be a disease mediated via the inflammatory pathway then anti-inflammatory medications should provide some degree of safety. This was noted in 1964 by Powell and Field who reported that patients with rheumatoid arthritis on high dose aspirin therapy tended to have a less severe form of DR [20]. Histological features of DR were less commonly noted in dogs wherein aspirin was initiated in a dose of 20-25 mg/kg/day shortly after the diagnosis of diabetes mellitus and continued for a period of 5 years [21].

Increased concentrations of inflammatory cytokines such as IL-1, IL-6, IL-8, TNF-α and MCP-1—have been reported in ocular tissues from non-proliferative DR (NPDR) patients. The accumulation of these cytokines is believed to lead to early neuronal cell death. Cytokines such as MIP-1, IL-3 and IL-1 are believed to have a role in the angiogenesis. Thus inflammation may contribute towards and precede the development of neovascularisation [22]. Cylco-oxygenase-2 (COX-2) is expressed in the retinal astrocytes in human diabetic retinas. Prostanoids generated from COX-2 lead to an increased expression of VEGF and other pro-angiogenic factors, thereby contributing to development of proliferative diabetic retinopathy [23].

In case of diabetic macular edema (DME) levels of pro-inflammatory molecules Vascular Endothelial Growth Factor (VEGF) and IL-6 are noted to be elevated as per different studies. In particular DME associated with sub-retinal fluid on OCT shows elevated levels of these cytokines [24].

4.3 Diabetes and inflammation

The signal for the initiation of inflammation in a diabetic retina is believed to be metabolic in origin. Cell death was proposed as one of the causes, however, retinal cell death in DR is primarily via apoptosis and hence may not be associated with an inflammatory response. Certain factors that contribute directly or indirectly to increased inflammation are summarised below:

4.3.1 Hyperglycemia

Presence of hyperglycemia is linked with a pro-inflammatory environment. Retinal cells when incubated in high glucose environment led to increased production of iNOS, COX-2 and leukotrienes [25]. Furthermore, Joussen et al. in 2004 demonstrated diabetic retinopathy like disease following a sugar rich diet in laboratory mice. This was associated with leukostasis and increased vascular permeability [26].

4.3.2 Oxidative stress

Diabetes is known to produce oxidative stress at a molecular level. Two months of diabetes in rats led to a significant increase in levels of IL-1 and NF-κB. This increase is inhibited by antioxidants. It is believed that oxidative stress induced increase in retinal permeability and inflammation is mediated via the WNT signalling pathway [27].

4.3.3 Lipids

Diabetes results in a decrease in the levels of poly-unsaturated fatty acids especially docosohexanoic acid (DHA) and these changes are associated with chronic inflammation. Long term administration of omega 3 fatty acids has been linked to retinal capillary degeneration. DHA, resolvins and autocoids have shown to have critical anti-inflammatory properties. Li et al. noted that administration of statins (HMG-CoA inhibitor) inhibited diabetes induced changes in the blood retinal barrier [28].

4.3.4 Age

Interaction between the advanced glycation end-products (AGE) with its receptor (RAGE) is known to have pro-inflammatory consequences. Pharmacological inhibition of RAGE signalling led to a significant decrease in retinal capillary degeneration and other early lesion of DR in animal models [29].

4.3.5 Hypertension

Hypertension is a main secondary risk factor associated with DR. Silva et al. [30] in 2007 found an increased expression of VEGF and ICAM-1 in an experimental model in rats who were in a prehypertensive or hypertensive group. They concluded that hypertension led to an increased inflammatory response in the diabetic retina and consequently worsened retinopathy.

4.4 Inflammatory mediators involved

A variety of factors are involved in the cascade of the inflammatory process in a diabetic retina. It has been seen that intravitreal levels of cytokines, chemokines and growth factors change under inflammation leading to increased secretion from endothelial cell and development of neovascularization. The major factors are highlighted below:

4.4.1 Growth factors

4.4.1.1 Vascular endothelial growth factor (VEGF)

It is known that VEGF is the principal target of pharmacologic intervention for proliferative diabetic retinopathy and studies have confirmed elevated levels of VEGF in vitreous samples in DR causing increased vascular permeability [31, 32], stimulates angiogenesis because of its mitogenic effect on endothelial cells, and enhances endothelial cell migration and survival [33, 34] and their production increases markedly under conditions of hypoxia [35]. Intercellular adhesion molecule-1 (ICAM-1) is involved in inflammation and acts as a local intensifying signal in the pathological processes associated with chronic eye inflammation. It has been seen that VEGF increases ICAM-1 and leukocyte adhesion to vessel wall and elevated ICAM-1 and cell adhesion molecule-1 synthesis in retina. It further increases ICAM-1 in endothelial cells and this in turn leads to activation and increased production of cytokines and leukocyte activation [36], these cytokines initiate and mediate the inflammatory response and stimulate further release of VEGF [37]. Various studies have strongly indicated that the increased level of ICAM-1 generally exists in the patients with DR and it may associated with the severity of DR [38]. Placental growth factor (PGF), member of VEGF family, binds to VEGF- and neuropilin-receptor sub-types. PGF induces a range of neural, glial and vascular cell responses that are distinct from VEGF-A. As its expression is associated with pathological angiogenesis and inflammation, its blockade does not affect the healthy vasculature [39]. High levels of PGF have been found in aqueous humour, vitreous and in retina of patients especially those with diabetic retinopathy (DR). Results suggest that anti-PGF therapy might have advantages over anti-VEGF treatment, and that it may have clinical applications as a standalone treatment or in combination with anti-VEGF [39]. Low concentrations of VEGF have been seen to rise with PGF stimulating endothelial cell proliferation, migration, and angiogenesis [40]. Higher levels of PGF in vitreous are seen in DR and these levels are correlated well with VEGF levels [41].

4.4.1.2 Tenascin-C (TNC)

Tenascin-C is an extracellular matrix protein and plays an important role in cell growth and adhesion, playing an equally involved in angiogenesis, oncogenesis, wound repair and inlflammation [42, 43]. Studies have shown that TNC is involved in the pathogenesis of ischemic proliferative retinopathy. Elevated levels have been detected in PDR vitreous humour. mRNA and protein expression of TNC has been found in pre-retinal fibrovascular membranes excised from PDR patients [44]. Extracellular matrix (ECM) synthesis plays an important part in the pathogenesis of the intravitreal membranes and is thus characteristic of both proliferative vitreoretinopathy (PVR) and early stages of proliferative diabetic retinopathy (PDR). Hence it is clear that TNC plays a role in the development of epiretinal PVR and PDR membranes by controlling cell adhesion and regulating extracellular matrix formation formation [45].

4.4.1.3 Insulin like growth factor

It is known that IGF-1 is has a significant role in pathogenesis of DR as it is involved in regulation along with influencing growth, maturation and functioning of blood vessels. It also activates VEGF in human RPE cell and receptors which are actively involved in development of vitreo-retinal disorders [46, 47]. Insulin-like growth factor-I (IGF-I) is known to enhances insulin action in normal subjects and in both type 1 and 2 diabetes. It is associated with significant side effects in a high percentage of patients. Simultaneous administration of IGF binding protein-3 with IGF-I limits IGF-I inducible side effects, but it does not downgrade the ability of IGF-I to enhance protein synthesis and bone accretion [48]. Severity of DR in patients with type 1 diabetes is inversely related to serum IGF-1 levels. Low IGF levels are an indicator for closer follow-up and strict management of diabetes and retinopathy [49].

4.4.1.4 Basic fibroblast growth factor

Amongst the factors which play a role in mitogen and antigenic activity involving survival and maturation of glial cells and neuron, basic fibroblast growth factor (bFGF) play an important role [50]. Neurotrophic factors synthesised from glial cell line stimulates Muller cells which produce bFGF, which initiates endothelial cell proliferation and VEGF production [51, 52]. Studies have detected presence of two growth factors in same cells of ocular neovascular membrane suggesting more than one growth factor may contribute to defective angiogenesis. Growth factors are not exclusively seen in neovascular tissues and are not localised mainly in the vascular endothelium as shown by this study which detected their presence in choroidal neovascular membranes also [53]. Another study documented increased levels of basic fibroblast growth factor in vitreous specimens from patients with proliferative diabetic retinopathy, particularly those with active proliferative retinopathy [54]. Various studies have shown that bFGF, nerve growth factor, and glial cell line-derived neurotrophic factor are also part of process involved in the formation of epiretinal membranes in PDR [55]. This confirms that both vegf and basic fibroblast growth factor are present in diabetic eyes and part of process causing PDR.

4.4.1.5 Aminopeptidase

Adipocytes are involved in production of a polypeptide hormone named aminopeptidase, which circulates at very high levels in the bloodstream, exerts anti-inflammatory effect. It also expresses an anti-atherosclerotic effect and inhibits intimal thickening and vascular smooth muscle cell proliferation in injured arteries [56]. Angiogenesis, a neo-vessel formation from pre-existing micro-vessels requires sequential steps involving detachment of pre-existing pericytes for vascular destabilisation, extracellular matrix turnover, migration, proliferation, tube formation by endothelial cells, and reattachment of pericytes for vascular stabilisation. Aminopeptidases has been found to regulate the N-terminal modification of proteins and peptides for maturation, activation or degradation, and thereby relate to a variety of biological processes. Three types of aminopeptidases which have been reported are involved in angiogenesis. They include type 2 methionine aminopeptidase, aminopeptidase N, and adipocyte-derived leucine aminopeptidase/puromycin insensitive leucyl-specific aminopeptidase [57]. It has been documented and shown by Costagliola et al. [58] that APN levels in aqueous humour of patients with type 2 diabetes, PDR, and macular edema are higher than in aqueous of control subjects.

4.4.1.6 Connective tissue growth factor

Connective tissue growth factor, also known as CCN2, is a cysteine-rich matricellular protein forms part of control on biological processes, such as cell proliferation, differentiation, adhesion and angiogenesis, as well as multiple pathologies, such as tumour development and tissue fibrosis [59]. Possible role of CTGF, CD105, and gelatinase B in the pathogenesis of proliferative vitreo-retinal disorders has been suggested by various studies [60]. It has been see that both CTGF and VEGF levels are elevated in PDR patients and CTGF could help in development of proliferative membranes in PDR though plays no role in retinal neovascularization [61].

4.4.1.7 Hepatocyte growth factor

Its has been seen that HCG and its receptor unit control motility, growth and morphogenesis of various cell types and possess angiogenic activity [62]. Data indicates that HGF is a pro-permeability, pro-inflammatory, and pro-angiogenic factor and along with its activator is found increased in ischemic retina providing support for a potential role of HGF in macular edema and in ischemic retinopathies such as diabetic retinopathy [63]. Elevated levels of HCG in aqueous have been found to be directly related to degree of PDR [64].

4.4.1.8 Stem cell factor

EPO is a glycoprotein which is multifunctional, produced in foetal liver and adult kidney when exposed to hypoxic conditions [65]. It possess anti-inflammatory, antioxidant, pro-angiogenic properties [66–68]. Some studies have also documented neuro-protective and anti-apoptotic properties [69, 70]. The mechanisms controlling the expression of the gene encoding for the hormone erythropoietin (EPO) are exemplary for oxygen-regulated gene expression. In humans and other mammals, hypoxia modulates EPO levels by increasing expression of the EPO gene [71]. Expression of EPO is mediated by HIF-1α which simultaneously stimulates VEGF secretion [72]. The hormone erythropoietin (EPO) maintains red blood cell mass by promoting the survival, proliferation and differentiation of erythrocytic progenitors. Circulating EPO originates mainly from fibroblasts in the renal cortex. EPO production is controlled at the transcriptional level. Hypoxia attenuates the inhibition of the EPO promoter by GATA-2 [73]. In patients with PDR, both EPO and VEGF are up-regulated into the vitreous each acting independently [74]. It has been seen that inhibition of EPO or VEGF leads to suppression of retinal neovascularization, results are best when both are suppressed together and in vitro inhibition of EPO leads to attenuation of endothelial cell proliferation in PDR [75].

4.4.2 Transcription factors

4.4.2.1 Nuclear factor kappa beta (NF-κB)

NF-κB is a pro inflammatory transcription factor and a regulator of inflammation related to immune responses, cellular proliferation and cell apoptosis [76]. It is located in endothelial and retinal pericytes and released on exposure to hypoxia and hyperglycemia and thereafter releases cytokines, chemokines, and other pro-inflammatory molecules [59]. Once NF-κB is activated it leads to production of cytokines, chemokines and other pro-inflammatory molecules [77]. Studies have shown a relation between NF-κB activation and downstream up-regulation of vascular endothelial growth factor (VEGF) in DR. VEGF SNPs i.e., RS2010963 C allele and RS3025039 T allele might be strongly associated with PDR occurrence and in turn regulating VEGF expression in PDR subjects [78]. NF-κB is also involved in the formation of both glial and vascular endothelial cellular components, and that these two cell types might have functional interactions that lead to the enlargement of intraocular proliferative membranes namely ERM [79]. Receptor activator of NF-κB ligand (RANKL) is a member of the tumour necrosis factor (TNF) superfamily. RANKL increases endothelial permeability and induces angiogenesis, suggesting its critical roles in the vasculature. Hence the use of an RANKL blockade as a potential therapeutic approach against ischemic retinopathies is confirmed [80]. It is important to remember that the signal related to RANKL plays a role in the pathogenesis of insulin resistance and suggests a link between inflammation and the pathogenesis of type 2 diabetes mellitus [81].

4.4.2.2 Hypoxia inducible factor

Adapting to hypoxic conditions leads to cellular and tissue transcriptional induction involving genes that participate in angiogenesis, glucose metabolism, and cell proliferation and survival. The principal factor mediating this response is the hypoxia-inducible factor-1 (HIF-1), an oxygen-sensitive transcriptional activator. It consists of a constitutively expressed subunit HIF-1β and an oxygen-regulated subunit HIF-1α [82]. It has been shown that diabetic factors result in HIF-1 production and angiogenesis and Treins et al. [83] showed that insulin-like growth factor-1 (IGF-1) stimulates accumulation of HIF-1 in human retinal pigment epithelial cells. As HIF-1 becomes active it activates several genes, including the genes for IL-6, IL-8, and pro-angiogenic growth factors. It has also been shown that acute intensive insulin therapy exacerbates the diabetic induced BRB breakdown through HIF-1 and VEGF [84] and presence of HIF-1α has been demonstrated in diabetic epiretinal membrane [85]. NF-κB controls the expression and synthesis of HIF-1 in response to inflammatory stimuli. Hypoxia activates NF-κB that binds promoter of HIF-1, stimulates the production of IL-6 and IL-8 in the vitreous of patients with PDR. HIF-1α, Ang-2 and VEGF seem to play an important role in the pathogenesis of PDR and simultaneously provide adverse angiogenic milieu in PDR epiretinal membranes favouring aberrant neovascularisation and endothelial abnormalities [84].

4.4.3 Cytokines

4.4.3.1 Interleukin-6 (IL-6)

IL-6 is a cytokine regulates the expression of matrix metalloproteinases (MMPs) which is a primary constituent of the vitreous [86, 87] and it also regulates immune response, increases permeability of vessels and initiates angiogenesis [88, 89]. Studies, have indicated that IL-8, VEGF-A, and PlGF demonstrated a strong correlation in vitreous and aqueous of patients with PDR. The aqueous may serve as a proxy for vitreous for some cytokines involved in PDR. More recently anti-VEGF injections have been able to decrease VEGF-A levels in aqueous, however they did not significantly affect other cytokines, indicating a need for other targeted therapies in PDR management [90]. Role of IL-6 in neovascularization, a key clinical feature of DR, is shown in studies that show IL-6 can not only promote angiogenesis directly but support angiogenesis by inducing expression of VEGF, an angiogenic factor [91]. Hence, the role of IL-6 and IL-8 as angiogenic and factor for causing neovascularization is supported.

4.4.3.2 IL-1β

Macrophages produce IL-1β which is an inflammatory cytokine mainly which can further activate the transcriptional factor NF-κB, which plays an important role in transcription of inflammatory cytokines [92]. Furthermore TNF-α and recombinant IL-1β seem to stimulate human retinal pigment epithelium cells leading to secretion of IL-6 and IL-8 [93]. It has been seen in studies that TNF-α and IL-1β promote angiogenic activity leading to stimulation and synthesis of collagen glial cells, and fibroblasts leading to proliferation and contraction promoting angiogenesis and ocular neovascularization [94]. It has been observed that invading microorganisms activate the inflammatory response by secreting pro-inflammatory cytokines particularly IL-1β. IL-1-responsive genes initiate and coordinate local inflammation and also attract and activate cells of the adaptive immune system at sites of infection eventually leading these signals to activate NALP3-inflammasome pathway, which plays a central role in acute and chronic sterile inflammation [95]. Studies assessing inflammatory mechanisms involving NLRP3 inflammasome were carried out using akimbo mouse, revealing an increased vascular leakage, reduced retinal thickness, and function in Akimba retina. High levels of IL-1β along with increased NLRP3, ASC, and Caspase-1 at mRNA and protein levels were seen suggesting a critical role for NLRP3 inflammasome in akimbo retina depicting advanced stages of DR pathogenesis [96]. Other studies have shown elevated levels in aqueous of IL-6 and macular thickness indicating IL-6 may play a central role in the development of diabetic macular edema [97].

4.4.3.3 TNF-alpha

TNF-α, a cytokine with tumour necrosis activity is produced by various types of cells which includes macrophages, is recognised as an important host defence factor that affects malignant and normal cells. It is synthesised by T cells and macrophages and its expression is regulated by NF-κB [98]. It also plays the role of inflammatory mediator of neuronal cell after cerebral ischemic trauma and also a similar role in retinal tissue [99]. Besides increasing endothelial cell permeability [100]. TNF-α is also involved in stimulating leukocyte adhesion and inducing oxidation and simultaneous production of reactive oxygen due to the death of retinal ganglion cells and degeneration of the optic nerve [101]. High pharmacological doses of TNF-α combined with chemotherapy has been seen to regress intractable tumours. Evidence demonstrates that pathophysiological concentrations of endogenous TNF-α could act to promote tumour genesis and growth [102]. In diabetic retinopathy pro-inflammatory mediators regulated by cytokines, such as TNF-α, IL-1β and growth factors leads to further progression of these processes, leading to vaso-permeability (diabetes macular edema) and/or pathological angiogenesis (proliferative diabetic retinopathy) [103]. Diabetic patients have shown higher TNF-α levels in vitreous/serum ratio compared to non-diabetics [104]. Strong correlation between plasma TNF-α levels and severity of DR has been documented [105]. It has been documented that TNF-α is expressed in the endothelial cells and stromal cells of the fibrovascular membranes of diabetic patients with PDR [106]. Studies have confirmed the presence of vascular endothelial growth factor (VEGF) and TNF-α in epiretinal membranes in proliferative eye disease [107]. Recent studies assessing the impact of anti-TNF agents on intermediary metabolism suggest that TNF-α blockade could improve insulin resistance and lipid profiles in patients with chronic inflammatory disease [108].

4.4.3.4 HMGB1

HMGB1 though secreted from numerous sites in the retina, including the ganglion cell layer, inner nuclear layer, outer nuclear layer, inner and outer segment of the photoreceptors, and retinal pigment epithelial cells [109, 110]. It is a protein that stabilises the formation of nucleosomes and gene transcription [111]. Studies indicate that HMGB1 is released from activated innate immune cells or necrotic cells and functions as an important mediator of endotoxaemia, sepsis, arthritis, and local inflammation hence agents that inhibit HMGB1 release or action, confer significant protection against endotoxaemia, sepsis, and arthritis in animal models and thus hold potential for the clinical management of various inflammatory diseases [112]. HMGB1 functions as a cytokine that amplifies the effect of the receptor for AGE

(RAGE) axis and mediates the secretion of survival factors such as VEGF-A, to counteract the effects of oxidative stress. HMGB1 is thought to contribute to the accelerated micro and macro-vasculopathy seen in diabetes [113]. Its level has been detected on higher side in vitreous in patients with PDR and has been detected in endothelial and stromal cells of ERM in PDR patients [114].

4.4.4 Chemokines

Chemokines constitute a family of chemoattractant cytokines and are subdivided into four families on the basis of the number and spacing of the conserved cysteine residues in the N-terminus of the protein. They seem to play a role in selectively recruiting monocytes, neutrophils, and lymphocytes, along with inducing chemotaxis through the activation of G-protein-coupled receptors.

4.4.4.1 Monocyte chemoattractant protein-1 (MCP-1/CCL2)

Monocyte chemoattractant protein-1 (MCP-1/CCL2) is considered one of the key chemokines that regulate migration and infiltration of monocytes/macrophages [115]. The expression of MCP-1 is regulated by NF-κB and MCP-1 can induce VEGF production [116]. Both CCL2 and its receptor CCR2 have been demonstrated to be induced and involved in various diseases [115]. Diabetic patients have shown elevated levels of MCP-1 in vitreous and its levels are higher in the vitreous than in the serum indicating local production of MCP-1 [117]. Studies have shown that there is a significant association between the vitreous MCP-1 levels and DR severity [118]. The MCP-1 is also a potent chemotactic factor for monocytes and macrophages that can stimulate them to produce superoxide and other mediators. Following hyperglycemia, retinal pigment epithelial (RPE) cells, endothelial cells, and Müller's glial cells are of utmost importance for MCP-1 production, and vitreous MCP-1 levels rise in patients with DR. Increased expression of the MCP-1 in the eyes can also play a significant role in the pathogenesis of DR [119]. Interferon-gamma inducible protein 10 (IP-10) is a CXC chemokine that is expressed at higher levels in the vitreous of diabetic patients [120], and its vitreous levels are higher than its serum levels [121]. Anti-inflammatory cytokines such as IL-10 and IL-13 may be involved more in the pathogenesis of DR and CRVO than in other diseases and both cytokines and chemokines may be correlated to VEGF in the vitreous fluid and the inflammatory reaction may be more active in CRVO than in DR [122].

4.4.4.2 Monokine

Monokine which is induced by interferon-gamma (MIG) is a chemoattractant for activated T cells and also has angiostatic activity [123]. In their study Wakabayashi et al. reported that MIG could play an role in the pathogenesis of DR and works in cooperation of VEGF in the progression of pathological angiogenesis in DR. The authors have detected higher levels of MIG in vitreous of DR patients [123]. Elevated MIG levels are could be in response to the up-regulation of angiogenic factors such as VEGF. The alternative mechanism could be in play in DR which results in chemotaxis of leukocytes rather than in carrying out its angiostatic functions [26].

4.4.4.3 Stromal cell-derived factor-1

Stromal cell-derived factor-1 (SDF-1) is a chemokine that is up-regulated in response to tissue damage and is involved in stimulation and mobilisation of cells involved in tissue repair and cellular migration, differentiation, and proliferation of endothelial progenitor cells [124]. SDF-1 repairs after ischemic injury by binding to its receptor, CXCR4 and recruits the progenitors of endothelial cells from the bone marrow. The levels off SDF-1 in vitreous have been found to be on higher side in DME and PDR patients [125]. Studies have demonstrated that inhibiting the N-(carboxymethyl)lysine-induced TPL2/ATF4/SDF1 axis can effectively prevent diabetes mellitus-mediated retinal microvascular dysfunction and this signalling axis could include the therapeutic potential for other diseases involving pathological neovascularization and or macular edema [126].

4.4.4.4 Fractalkine

Fractalkine (CX3CL1) is an intriguing chemokine that plays a central role in the nervous system. Expression of CX3CL1 on neurons and its receptor CX3CR1 on microglia facilitates a privileged interaction, playing important roles in regulating the function and maturation of these cells. CX3CL1 is reported to have neuroprotective and anti-inflammatory activities [127]. Studies suggest that dysregulated microglial activation via loss of FKN/CX3CR1 signalling disrupts the vascular integrity in retina during systemic inflammation [128].

4.4.4.5 Macrophage migration inhibitory factor

Macrophage migration inhibitory factor (MIF) is a chemokine that stimulates macrophages causing their recruitment at sites of inflammation, increasing their adherence, motility, and phagocytosis. It also prevents random migration of macrophages [129]. Studies indicate increased levels of MIF in the vitreous of patients with PDR and a significant association between MIF levels and grades of fibrous proliferation, suggesting the possibility that MIF may play a part in the development of the proliferative phase of PDR [130].

4.4.5 Intercellular adhesion molecule-1 (ICAM1)

ICAM-1 is a cell surface glycoprotein, which serves as an adhesion receptor that is known for regulating leukocyte recruitment from circulation to sites of inflammation. In addition to vascular endothelial cells, ICAM-1 expression is also induced on epithelial and immune cells in response to inflammatory stimulation. ICAM-1 also serves as a biosensor to transduce outside-in-signalling via association of its cytoplasmic domain with the actin cytoskeleton following ligand engagement of the extracellular domain. Thus, ICAM-1 has emerged as a master regulator of many essential cellular functions both at the onset and at the resolution of pathologic conditions [131]. Increased expression of adhesion molecule leads to activation of RAGE, oxidative stress, vascular leakage in the diabetic retina, capillary non perfusion, and damage of endothelial cells and the adhesion of leukocytes to the endothelium and expression of retinal vascular adhesion molecules such as VEGF [132]. ICAM-1 is the primary adhesion molecule involved in DR and its levels in vitreous are elevated in patients with active PDR [114].

5. Therapy aimed at inflammatory targets

Maintenance of a good glycemic control is considered to be the most important modifiable factor influencing the stage and progression of diabetic retinopathy. However, inhibition of retinal inflammation may also reduce the degree of retinopathy despite the presence of a hyperglycaemic state. High-dose aspirin, COX-2 inhibitors and corticosteroids have been used, either experimentally in animal models or therapeutically in humans, and found to have a beneficial effect in reducing DR changes. However, these drugs are associated with unfavourable side effects especially when used over a long-term course. Hence other alternatives should be looked at. These alternatives can include RAGE inhibitors, minocycline, derivatives of salicylates and inhibitors of TNF-α and 5-lipoxygenase. Salicylates inhibit the nuclear migration and possibly activation of NF-κB in retinal neurons [133]. Evidence is accumulating showing that lipid supplementation with omega 3 polyunsaturated fatty acids (especially DHA) has a beneficial effect in DR [134].

Retinal inflammatory changes in diabetics have been found to be inhibited by therapies wherein the primary target is at a different site. The antihypertensive telmisartan, angiotensin receptor blocker (Type I receptor) was found to suppress retinal leukostasis and expression of VEGF and ICAM-1 [135]. Similarly, in diabetic animal models, Candesartan reduces the presence of acellular retinal capillaries, iNOS and nitric oxide [136]. The beneficial effect of statins on DR has also been reported by Kang et al. in 2019 [137]. The authors evaluated patients with diabetes and dyslipidemia and found that statin use was associated with a decreased prevalence of DR and a lower need for invasive therapy for vision threatening diabetic retinopathy complications. This therapeutic benefit can be attributed to the pleiotropic property of statins, which also function as anti-inflammatory agents. Tuuminen et al. [138] found a decreased intravitreal levels of pro-angiogenic factors, transforming growth factor B1 and matrix metalloproteinase 9 in individuals treated with simvastatin.

The role of salicylates in DR has been studied extensively, following the initial reports by Powell and Field in 1964 [20]. Administration of aspirin in animal models has found to reduce retinal capillary degeneration but conflicting results were reported in human trials. The Early Treatment Diabetic Retinopathy Study (ETDRS) is particularly of note in this case. The ETDRS report number 8 results indicated that aspirin has no clinically beneficial effect on the progression of retinopathy in individuals taking 650 mg of aspirin per day [139]. However, we have to take into account that the anti-inflammatory dose of aspirin is much higher than what was being administered in the study. Salicylates have shown to reduce insulin resistance in the retina in a Type II diabetic rat model as per Jiang Y and co-workers [140].

TNF-α is a key molecule in the inflammatory puzzle thus it serves as an attractive pharmacological target. Subcutaneous injection of TNF-α trap (Eternacept) was found to significantly reduce retinal inflammation, retinal cell injury and vascular permeability in diabetic rats [141]. However, no clinical trials have reported this effect till date. A small pilot study of 4 patients who were administered Infliximab (TNF-α antibody) showed a decrease in central macular thickness and a corresponding improvement in visual acuity [142].

Inhibition of leukostasis is another mechanism that can be targeted in anti-inflammatory therapy for DR. Leukocyte function associated antigen-1 (LFA-1) is an integrin molecule and is extremely important for leukocyte-endothelial cell interactions. SAR-1118 is a topical antagonist of LFA-1 and has shown a dose dependant reduction of leukostasis and vascular leakage in a diabetic rat model [143]. Anti CD49a neutralising antibody blocks the interaction between very late antigen-4 (VLA-4) and VCAM-1 and has also shows efficacy in reducing leukostasis [144].

Apart from their antibiotic activity both Minocycline and Doxycycline are known to possess neuro-protective and immunomodulatory properties, such as inhibiting production of NO, prostaglandins, TNF-α and caspases [145]. A small study of minocycline in 5 patients with DME showed improvement in visual acuity with reduction in macular edema [146]. Another study involving doxycycline demonstrated an improvement in perimetric parameters in individuals with severe NPDR or PDR [147].

Photobiomodulation is another prospective therapy which has shown promise in a small clinical study of patient with non-centre involving diabetic macular edema [148]. It consists of series of brief illumination with specific wavelengths of light emitted from a laser. It has shown to affect the signalling pathways within the cells and inhibits diabetes induced leukostasis, ICAM-1 expression and production of reactive oxygen species [149].

6. Conclusion

Studies carried out both in diabetic patients and experimental animal models of diabetic retina have shown that the diabetic milieu promotes an increased local expression of inflammation. Unlike, uveitis however this inflammation is not clinically apparent and is noted at a molecular level. Critically located between the vasculature and neurons of the retina, Glial cells have a key role in closely regulating the retinal microenvironment. Recent findings implicate that these cells also responsible in the initiation of the inflammatory cascade.

It is possible that inflammation does not perfectly describe all the changes that ultimately occur in diabetic retinopathy, but it does seems to describe the pathogenesis of the retinopathy better than the previous concept of microvasculopathy. It is likely that this concept will become better focused with future research.

Author details

Anuj Sharma* and Deepesh Arora
Retina Services, Amritsar Eye Clinic, Dehradun, India

*Address all correspondence to: dr.anuj18@gmail.com

References

[1] WHO. Diabetes. Available from: https://www.who.int/news-room/fact-sheets/detail/diabetes [Accessed 10 August, 2021].

[2] Wong T, Y, Sabanayagam C: Strategies to tackle the global burden of diabetic retinopathy: From epidemiology to artificial intelligence. Ophthalmologica 2020;243:9-20. DOI:10.1159/000502387

[3] Wilkinson CP, Ferris FL, Klein RE, Lee PP, Agardh CD, Davis M, Dills D, Kampik A, Pararajasegaram R, Verdaguer JT. Proposed international clinical diabetic retinopathy and diabetic macular edema disease severity scales. Ophthalmology. 2003;110: 1677-1682.

[4] Mitchell P, Annemans L, Gallagher M, et al. Cost-effectiveness of ranibizumab in treatment of diabetic macular oedema (DME) causing visual impairment: evidence from the RESTORE trial.

[5] E Lieth, AJ Gardner Tw Fau-Barber, DA Barber Aj Fau-Antonetti, DA Antonetti. Retinal neurodegeneration: early pathology in diabetes. Graefes Arch. Clin. Exp. Ophthalmol., 28 (1) (2000), pp. 3-8

[6] T.W. Gardner, J.R. Davila. The neurovascular unit and the pathophysiologic basis of diabetic retinopathy. Graefes Arch Clin Exp Ophthalmol, 255(1);2017:1-6.

[7] A. Das, P.G. McGuire, S. Rangasamy. Diabetic macular edema: Pathophysiology and novel therapeutic targets. Ophthalmology, 122 (7) (2015), pp.1375-1394

[8] VA Alder, EN Su, DY Yu, SJ Cringle, PK Yu. Diabetic retinopathy: Early functional changes. Clinical and Experimental Pharmacology and Physiology, 24 (9-10) (1997), pp. 785-788

[9] S. Roy, J. Ha, K. Trudeau, E. Beglova. Vascular basement membrane thickening in diabetic retinopathy. Current Eye Research, 35 (12) (2010), pp. 1045-1056.

[10] AW Stitt, TM Curtis, M Chen, RJ Medina, G.J. McKay, A. Jenkins, N. Lois. The progress in understanding and treatment of diabetic retinopathy. Progress in Retinal and Eye Research, 51 (2016), pp. 156-186.

[11] T.M. Curtis, T.A. Gardiner, A.W. Stitt. Microvascular lesions of diabetic retinopathy: Clues towards understanding pathogenesis? Eye (London), 23 (7) (2009), pp. 1496-1508.

[12] R. F. Spaide, Retinal vascular cystoid macular edema:Review and new theory. Retina, vol. 36, no. 10, pp. 1823-1842, 2016.

[13] Mizutani M, Gerhardinger C, Lorenzi M. Müller cell changes in human diabetic retinopathy. Diabetes. 1998;47:445-449.

[14] M Karlstetter, R Scholz, M Rutar, WT Wong, JM Provis, T. Langmann Retinal microglia:just bystander or target for therapy? Prog. Retin. Eye Res., 45 (2015), pp. 30-57

[15] Elisabeth Rungger-Brändle, André A. Dosso, Peter M. Leuenberger; Glial Reactivity, an Early Feature of Diabetic Retinopathy. Invest. Ophthalmol. Vis. Sci. 2000;41(7): 1971-1980.

[16] R. Simo, C. Hernandez. Novel approaches for treating diabetic retinopathy based on recent pathogenic evidence. Progress in Retinal and Eye Research, 48 (2015), pp. 160-180.

[17] R. Chibber, B.M. Ben-Mahmud, S. Chibber, E.M. Kohner. Leukocytes in diabetic retinopathy. Current Diabetes Review, 3 (1) (2007).

[18] E.A. Runkle, D.A. Antonetti. The blood-retinal barrier: Structure and functional significance Methods in Molecular Biology, 686 (2011), pp. 133-

[19] J. Cao, S. McLeod, C.A. Merges, G.A. Lutty. Choriocapillaris Degeneration and Related Pathologic Changes in Human Diabetic Eyes Archives of Ophthalmology, 116 (5) (1998).

[20] Powell EDU, Field RA. Diabetic retinopathy in rheumatoid arthritis. Lancet 1964; 2:17-18.

[21] Kern TS, Engerman RL. Pharmacological inhibition of diabetic retinopathy: Aminoguanidine and aspirin. Diabetes 2001;50:1636-1642.

[22] Demircan, N.; Safran, B.G.; Soylu, M.; Ozcan, A.A.; Sizmaz, S. Determination of vitreous interleukin-1 (IL-1) and tumour necrosis factor (TNF) levels in proliferative diabetic retinopathy. Eye (London) 2006, 20,1366-1369.

[23] Cheng T, Cao W, Wen R, Steinberg RH, LaVail MM. Prostaglandin E2 induces vascular endothelial growth factor and basic fibroblast growth factor mRNA expression in cultured rat Muller cells. Invest Ophthalmol Vis Sci. 1998; 39:581-591.

[24] Sonoda S, Sakamoto T, Yamashita T, Shirasawa M, Otsuka H, and Sonoda Y. Retinal morphologic changes and concentrations of cytokines in eyes with diabetic macular edema. Retina, vol. 34, no. 4, pp. 741-748, 2014.

[25] Talahalli R, Zarini S, Sheibani N, Murphy RC, Gubitosi-Klug RA. Increased synthesis of leukotrienes in the mouse model of diabetic retinopathy. Invest Ophthalmol Vis Sci. 2010; 51:1699-1708.

[26] Joussen AM, Poulaki V, Le ML, Koizumi K, Esser C, Janicki H, Schraermeyer U, Kociok N, Fauser S, Kirchhof B, Kern TS, Adamis AP. A central role for inflammation in the pathogenesis of diabetic retinopathy. Faseb J. 2004; 18:1450-1452.

[27] Chen Y, Hu Y, Zhou T, Zhou KK, Mott R, Wu M, Boulton M, Lyons TJ, Gao G, Ma JX. Activation of the Wnt pathway plays a pathogenic role in diabetic retinopathy in humans and animal models. Am J Pathol. 2009; 175:2676-2685.

[28] Li J, Wang JJ, Chen D, Mott R, Yu Q, Ma JX, Zhang SX. Systemic administration of HMG-CoA reductase inhibitor protects the blood-retinal barrier and ameliorates retinal inflammation in type 2 diabetes. Exp Eye Res. 2009a; 89:71-78

[29] Li G, Tang J, Du Y, Lee CA, Kern TS. Beneficial effects of a novel RAGE inhibitor on early diabetic retinopathy and tactile allodynia. Mol Vis. 2011;17:3156-3165.

[30] Silva KC, Pinto CC, Biswas SK, de Faria JB, de Faria JM. Hypertension increases retinal inflammation in experimental diabetes: A possible mechanism for aggravation of diabetic retinopathy by hypertension. Curr Eye Res. 2007 Jun;32(6):533-541.

[31] Schwartzman M.L., Iserovich P., Gotlinger K., Bellner L., Dunn M.W., Sartore M., Grazia P.M., Leonardi A., Sathe S., Beaton A., et al. Profile of lipid and protein autacoids in diabetic vitreous correlates with the progression of diabetic retinopathy. Diabetes. 2010;59:1780-1788.

[32] Othman A., Ahmad S., Megyerdi S., Mussell R., Choksi K.,

Maddipati K.R., Elmarakby A., Rizk N., Al-Shabrawey M. 12/15-Lipoxygenase-derived lipid metabolites induce retinal endothelial cell barrier dysfunction: Contribution of NADPH oxidase. PLoS ONE. 2013;8:e57254.

[33] Carmeliet P., Moons L., Luttun A., et al. Synergism between vascular endothelial growth factor and placental growth factor contributes to angiogenesis and plasma extravasation in pathological conditions. Nature Medicine. 2001;7(5):575-583.

[34] Dull R. O., Yuan J., Chang Y. S., Tarbell J., Jain R. K., Munn L. L. Kinetics of placenta growth factor/vascular endothelial growth factor synergy in endothelial hydraulic conductivity and proliferation. Microvascular Research. 2001;61(2):203-210.

[35] Levy A. P., Levy N. S., Wegner S., Goldberg M. A. Transcriptional regulation of the rat vascular endothelial growth factor gene by hypoxia. The Journal of Biological Chemistry. 1995;270(22):13333-13340.

[36] Melder R. J., Koenig G. C., Witwer B. P., Safabakhsh N., Munn L. L., Jain R. K. During angiogenesis, vascular endothelial growth factor and basic fibroblast growth factor regulate natural killer cell adhesion to tumor endothelium. Nature Medicine. 1996;2(9):992-997.

[37] Wang J., Xu E., Elliott M. H., Zhu M., Le Y.-Z. Müller cell-derived VEGF is essential for diabetes-induced retinal inflammation and vascular leakage. Diabetes. 2010;59(9):2297-2305.

[38] Yao Y, Du J, Li R, Zhao L, Luo N, Zhai JY, Long L. Association between ICAM-1 level and diabetic retinopathy: A review and meta-analysis. Postgrad Med J. 2019 Mar;95(1121):162-168.

[39] Van Bergen T, Etienne I, Cunningham F, Moons L, Schlingemann RO, Feyen JHM, Stitt AW. The role of placental growth factor (PlGF) and its receptor system in retinal vascular diseases. Prog Retin Eye Res. 2019 Mar;69:116-136.

[40] Ziche M., Maglione D., Ribatti D., et al. Placenta growth factor-1 is chemotactic, mitogenic, and angiogenic. Laboratory Investigation. 1997;76(4): 517-531.

[41] Spirin K. S., Saghizadeh M., Lewin S. L., Zardi L., Kenney M. C., Ljubimov A. V. Basement membrane and growth factor gene expression in normal and diabetic human retinas. Current Eye Research. 1999;18(6): 490-499.

[42] Chiquet-Ehrismann R., Mackie E. J., Pearson C. A., Sakakura T. Tenascin: An extracellular matrix protein involved in tissue interactions during fetal development and oncogenesis. Cell. 1986;47(1):131-139.

[43] Canfield A. E., Schor A. M. Evidence that tenascin and thrombospondin-1 modulate sprouting of endothelial cells. Journal of Cell Science. 1995;108(2):797-809.

[44] Kubo Y, Ishikawa K, Mori K, Kobayashi Y, Nakama T, Arima M, Nakao S, Hisatomi T, Haruta M, Sonoda KH, Yoshida S. Periostin and tenascin-C interaction promotes angiogenesis in ischemic proliferative retinopathy. Sci Rep. 2020 Jun 9;10(1):9299.

[45] Hagedorn M, Esser P, Wiedemann P, Heimann K. Tenascin and decorin in epiretinal membranes of proliferative vitreoretinopathy and proliferative diabetic retinopathy. Ger J Ophthalmol. 1993 Feb;2(1):28-31.

[46] Whitehead M, Wickremasinghe S, Osborne A, Van Wijngaarden P, Martin KR. Diabetic retinopathy: A complex pathophysiology requiring

novel therapeutic strategies. Expert Opin Biol Ther. 2018;18:1257-1270.

[47] Wang W, Lo ACY. Diabetic retinopathy: Pathophysiology and treatments. Int J Mol Sci. 2018; 19:1816.

[48] Clemmons DR, Moses AC, McKay MJ, Sommer A, Rosen DM, Ruckle J. The combination of insulin-like growth factor I and insulin-like growth factor-binding protein-3 reduces insulin requirements in insulin-dependent type 1 diabetes: Evidence for in vivo biological activity. J Clin Endocrinol Metab. 2000 Apr;85(4): 1518-1524.

[49] Raman P, Singal AK, Behl A. Effect of insulin-like growth Factor-1 on diabetic retinopathy in pubertal age patients with type 1 diabetes. Asia Pac J Ophthalmol (Phila). 2019 Jul-Aug;8(4):319-323.

[50] Wong CG, Rich KA, Liaw LH, Hsu HT, Berns MW. Intravitreal VEGF and bFGF produce florid retinal neovascularization and hemorrhage in the rabbit. Curr Eye Res. 2001;22: 140-147.

[51] Semeraro F, Cancarini A, dell'Omo R, Rezzola S, Romano MR, Costagliola C. Diabetic Retinopathy: Vascular and Inflammatory Disease. J Diabetes Res. 2015;2015:582060.

[52] Hueber A, Wiedemann P, Esser P, Heimann K. Basic fibroblast growth factor mRNA, bFGF peptide and FGF receptor in epiretinal membranes of intraocular proliferative disorders (PVR and PDR). Int Ophthalmol. 1996-1997;20:345-350.

[53] Abrams GW. Basic fibroblast growth factor and vascular endothelial growth factor are present in epiretinal and choroidal neovascular membranes. Am J Ophthalmol. 1996 Sep;122(3): 393-403.

[54] Sivalingam A, Kenney J, Brown GC, Benson WE, Donoso L. Basic fibroblast growth factor levels in the vitreous of patients with proliferative diabetic retinopathy. Arch Ophthalmol. 1990 Jun;108(6):869-872.

[55] Mitamura Y., Harada C., Harada T. Role of cytokines and trophic factors in the pathogenesis of diabetic retinopathy. Current Diabetes Reviews. 2005;1(1): 73-81.

[56] Kubota N., Terauchi Y., Yamauchi T., et al. Disruption of adiponectin causes insulin resistance and neointimal formation. Journal of Biological Chemistry. 2002;277(29):25863-25866.

[57] Sato Y. Role of aminopeptidase in angiogenesis. Biol Pharm Bull. 2004 Jun;27(6):772-776.

[58] Costagliola C., Daniele A., dell'Omo R., et al. aqueous humor levels of vascular endothelial growth factor and adiponectin in patients with type 2 diabetes before and after intravitreal bevacizumab injection. Experimental Eye Research. 2013;110:50-54.

[59] Ramazani Y, Knops N, Elmonem MA, Nguyen TQ, Arcolino FO, van den Heuvel L, Levtchenko E, Kuypers D, Goldschmeding R. Connective tissue growth factor (CTGF) from basics to clinics. Matrix Biol. 2018 Aug;68-69:44-66.

[60] Abu El-Asrar AM, Van den Steen PE, Al-Amro SA, Missotten L, Opdenakker G, Geboes K. Expression of angiogenic and fibrogenic factors in proliferative vitreoretinal disorders. Int Ophthalmol. 2007 Feb;27(1):11-22.

[61] Kita T., Hata Y., Miura M., Kawahara S., Nakao S., Ishibashi T. Functional characteristics of connective tissue growth factor on vitreoretinal cells. Diabetes. 2007;56(5):1421-1428.

[62] Matsumoto K., Nakamura T. Emerging multipotent aspects of hepatocyte growth factor. Journal of Biochemistry. 1996;119(4):591-600.

[63] Lorenc VE, Lima E Silva R, Hackett SF, Fortmann SD, Liu Y, Campochiaro PA. Hepatocyte growth factor is upregulated in ischemic retina and contributes to retinal vascular leakage and neovascularization. FASEB Bioadv. 2020 Feb 18;2(4):219-233.

[64] Cai W., Rook S. L., Jiang Z. Y., Takahara N., Aiello L. P. Mechanisms of hepatocyte growth factor-induced retinal endothelial cell migration and growth. Investigative Ophthalmology and Visual Science. 2000;41(7): 1885-1893.

[65] Erslev A. J. Erythropoietin. The New England Journal of Medicine. 1991;324(19):1339-1344.

[66] Watanabe D., Suzuma K., Matsui S., et al. Erythropoietin as a retinal angiogenic factor in proliferative diabetic retinopathy. The New England Journal of Medicine. 2005;353(8):782-792.

[67] Chen J., Connor K. M., Aderman C. M., Smith L. E. H. Erythropoietin deficiency decreases vascular stability in mice. Journal of Clinical Investigation. 2008;118(2):526-533. DOI:10.1172/jci33813.

[68] García-Ramírez M., Hernández C., Simó R. Expression of erythropoietin and its receptor in the human retina: A comparative study of diabetic and non-diabetic subjects. Diabetes Care. 2008;31(6):1189-1194.

[69] Becerra SP, Amaral J. Erythropoietin—An endogenous retinal survival factor. The New England Journal of Medicine. 2002;347(24): 1968-1970.

[70] Hernández C, Fonollosa A, García-Ramírez M, et al. Erythropoietin is expressed in the human retina and it is highly elevated in the vitreous fluid of patients with diabetic macular edema. Diabetes Care. 2006;29(9): 2028-2033.

[71] Stockmann C, Fandrey J. Hypoxia-induced erythropoietin production: A paradigm for oxygen-regulated gene expression. Clin Exp Pharmacol Physiol. 2006 Oct;33(10):968-979.

[72] Katsura Y., Okano T., Matsuno K., et al. Erythropoietin is highly elevated in vitreous fluid of patients with proliferative diabetic retinopathy. Diabetes Care. 2005;28(9):2252-2254.

[73] Jelkmann W. Regulation of erythropoietin production. J Physiol. 2011 Mar 15;589(Pt 6):1251-1258

[74] Cancarini A., Costagliola C., dell'Omo R., et al. effect of intravitreal bevacizumab on serum, aqueous, and vitreous humor levels of erythropoietin in patients with proliferative diabetic retinopathy. Minerva Endocrinologica. 2014;39:305-311.

[75] Takagi H., Watanabe D., Suzuma K., et al. Novel role of erythropoietin in proliferative diabetic retinopathy. Diabetes Research and Clinical Practice. 2007;77(3):S62–S64.

[76] Barnes P. J. Nuclear factor-κB. International Journal of Biochemistry and Cell Biology. 1997;29(6):867-870.

[77] Tang J., Kern T. S. Inflammation in diabetic retinopathy. Progress in Retinal and Eye Research. 2011;30(5): 343-358.

[78] Choudhuri S, Chowdhury IH, Das S, Dutta D, Saha A, Sarkar R, Mandal LK, Mukherjee S, Bhattacharya B. Role of NF-κB activation and VEGF gene polymorphisms in VEGF up regulation in non-proliferative and proliferative diabetic retinopathy. Mol Cell Biochem. 2015 Jul;405(1-2):265-279.

[79] Harada C, Harada T, Mitamura Y, Quah HM, Ohtsuka K, Kotake S, Ohno S, Wada K, Takeuchi S, Tanaka K. Diverse NF-kappaB expression in epiretinal membranes after human diabetic retinopathy and proliferative vitreoretinopathy. Mol Vis. 2004 Jan 15;10:31-36.

[80] Ock S, Park S, Lee J, Kim J. RANKL blockade suppresses pathological angiogenesis and vascular leakage in ischemic retinopathy. Biochem Biophys Res Commun. 2019 Aug 20;516(2):350-356.

[81] Kiechl S., Wittmann J., Giaccari A., et al. Blockade of receptor activator of nuclear factor-κB (RANKL) signaling improves hepatic insulin resistance and prevents development of diabetes mellitus. Nature Medicine. 2013;19(3): 358-363.

[82] Ke Q, Costa M. Hypoxia-inducible factor-1 (HIF-1). Mol Pharmacol. 2006 Nov;70(5):1469-1480.

[83] Treins C., Giorgetti-Peraldi S., Murdaca J., Monthouël-Kartmann M.-N., van Obberghen E. Regulation of hypoxia-inducible factor (HIF)-1 activity and expression of HIF hydroxylases in response to insulin-like growth factor I. Molecular Endocrinology. 2005;19(5): 1304-1317.

[84] Poulaki V., Qin W., Joussen A. M., et al. Acute intensive insulin therapy exacerbates diabetic blood-retinal barrier breakdown via hypoxia-inducible factor-1α and VEGF. The Journal of Clinical Investigation. 2002;109(6):805-815.

[85] El-Asrar A. M. A., Missotten L., Geboes K. Expression of hypoxia-inducible factor-1 alpha and the protein products of its target genes in diabetic fibrovascular epiretinal membranes. British Journal of Ophthalmology. 2007;91(6):822-826.

[86] Legendre F., Bogdanowicz P., Boumediene K., Pujol J. P. Role of interleukin 6 (IL6)/IL-6R-induced signal transducesrs and activators of transcription and mitogen-activaded protein kinase/extracellular. The Journal of Rheumatology. 2005;32:1307-1316.

[87] Symeonidis C, Papakonstantinou E, Androudi S, et al. Interleukin-6 and the matrix metalloproteinase response in the vitreous during proliferative vitreoretinopathy. Cytokine. 2011;54: 212-217.

[88] Cohen T., Nahari D., Cerem L. W., Neufeld G., Levin B.-Z. Interleukin 6 induces the expression of vascular endothelial growth factor. The Journal of Biological Chemistry. 1996;271(2): 736-741.

[89] Morohoshi M., Fujisawa K., Uchimura I., Numano F. Glucose-dependent interleukin 6 and tumor necrosis factor production by human peripheral blood monocytes in vitro. Diabetes. 1996;45(3):954-959.

[90] Wu F, Phone A, Lamy R, Ma D, Laotaweerungsawat S, Chen Y, Zhao T, Ma W, Zhang F, Psaras C, Stewart JM. Correlation of aqueous, vitreous, and plasma cytokine levels in patients with proliferative diabetic retinopathy. Invest Ophthalmol Vis Sci. 2020 Feb 7;61(2):26.

[91] Funatsu H., Yamashita H., Noma H., et al. Aqueous humor levels of cytokines are related to vitreous levels and progression of diabetic retinopathy in diabetic patients. Graefe's Archive for Clinical and Experimental Ophthalmology. 2005;243(1):3-8.

[92] Guarda G., So A. Regulation of inflammasome activity. Immunology. 2010;130(3):329-336.

[93] Elner S. G., Elner V. M., Jaffe G. J., Stuart A., Kunkel S. L., Strieter R. M.

Cytokines in proliferative diabetic retinopathy and proliferative vitreoretinopathy. Current Eye Research. 1995;14(11):1045-1053.

[94] Rosenbaum J. T., Samples J. R., Hefeneider S. H., Howes E. L. Ocular inflammatory effects of intravitreal interleukin 1. Archives of Ophthalmology. 1987;105(8):1117-1120.

[95] Weber A, Wasiliew P, Kracht M. Interleukin-1beta (IL-1beta) processing pathway. Sci Signal. 2010 Jan 19;3(105):cm2.

[96] Chaurasia SS, Lim RR, Parikh BH, Wey YS, Tun BB, Wong TY, Luu CD, Agrawal R, Ghosh A, Mortellaro A, Rackoczy E, Mohan RR, Barathi VA. The NLRP3 Inflammasome may contribute to pathologic neovascularization in the advanced stages of diabetic retinopathy. Sci Rep. 2018 Feb 12;8(1):2847.

[97] Oh IK, Kim SW, Oh J, Lee TS, Huh K. Inflammatory and angiogenic factors in the aqueous humor and the relationship to diabetic retinopathy. Curr Eye Res. 2010 Dec;35(12): 1116-1127.

[98] Parameswaran N., Patial S. Tumor necrosis factor-a signaling in macrophages. Critical Reviews in Eukaryotic Gene Expression. 2010;20(2):87-103.

[99] Tezel G., Wax M. B. Increased production of tumor necrosis factor-α by glial cells exposed to simulated ischemia or elevated hydrostatic pressure induces apoptosis in cocultured retinal ganglion cells. Journal of Neuroscience. 2000;20(23):8693-8700.

[100] Aveleira CA, Lin CM, Abcouwer SF, Ambrósio AF, Antonetti DA. TNF-α signals through PKCζ/NF-κB to alter the tight junction complex and increase retinal endothelial cell permeability. Diabetes. 2010;59(11): 2872-2882.

[101] Madigan M. G., Sadun A. A., Rao N. S., Dugel P. U., Tenhula W. N., Gill P. S. Tumor necrosis factor-alpha (TNF-α)-induced optic neuropathy in rabbits. Neurological Research. 1996;18(2):176-184.

[102] Anderson GM, Nakada MT, DeWitte M. Tumor necrosis factor-alpha in the pathogenesis and treatment of cancer. Curr Opin Pharmacol. 2004 Aug;4(4):314-320.

[103] Capitão M, Soares R. Angiogenesis and inflammation crosstalk in diabetic retinopathy. J Cell Biochem. 2016 Nov;117(11):2443-2453.

[104] Patel J. I., Saleh G. M., Hykin P. G., Gregor Z. J., Cree I. A. Concentration of haemodynamic and inflammatory related cytokines in diabetic retinopathy. Eye. 2008;22(2):223-228.

[105] Doganay S, Evereklioglu C, Er H, et al. Comparison of serum NO, TNF-α, IL-1β, sIL-2R, IL-6 and IL-8 levels with grades of retinopathy in patients with diabetes mellitus. Eye. 2002;16(2): 163-170.

[106] Goldberg RB. Cytokine and cytokine-like inflammation markers, endothelial dysfunction, and imbalanced coagulation in development of diabetes and its complications. Journal of Clinical Endocrinology and Metabolism. 2009;94(9):3171-3182.

[107] Armstrong D, Augustin AJ, Spengler R, Al-Jada A, Nickola T, Grus F, Koch F. Detection of vascular endothelial growth factor and tumor necrosis factor alpha in epiretinal membranes of proliferative diabetic retinopathy, proliferative vitreoretinopathy and macular pucker. Ophthalmologica. 1998;212(6):410-414.

[108] Popa C, Netea MG, van Riel PL, van der Meer JW, Stalenhoef AF. The role of TNF-alpha in chronic

inflammatory conditions, intermediary metabolism, and cardiovascular risk. J Lipid Res. 2007 Apr;48(4):751-762.

[109] Arimura N., Ki-I Y., Hashiguchi T., et al. Intraocular expression and release of high-mobility group box 1 protein in retinal detachment. Laboratory Investigation. 2009;89(3):278-289.

[110] Watanabe T., Keino H., Sato Y., Kudo A., Kawakami H., Okada A. A. High mobility group box protein-1 in experimental autoimmune uveoretinitis. Investigative Ophthalmology & Visual Science. 2009;50(5):2283-2290.

[111] Lotze M. T., Tracey K. J. High-mobility group box 1 protein (HMGB1): Nuclear weapon in the immune arsenal. Nature Reviews Immunology. 2005;5(4):331-342.

[112] Dell'Omo R., Semeraro F., Bamonte G., Cifariello F., Romano M. R., Costagliola C. Vitreous mediators in retinal hypoxic diseases. Mediators of Inflammation. 2013;2013:16.

[113] Jakuš V., Rietbrock N. Advanced glycation end-products and the progress of diabetic vascular complications. Physiological Research. 2004;53(2):131-142.

[114] El-Asrar A. M. A., Nawaz M. I., Kangave D., et al. High-mobility group box-1 and biomarkers of inflammation in the vitreous from patients with proliferative diabetic retinopathy. Molecular Vision. 2011;17:1829-1838.

[115] Deshmane SL, Kremlev S, Amini S, Sawaya BE. Monocyte chemoattractant protein-1 (MCP-1): An overview. J Interferon Cytokine Res. 2009 Jun;29(6):313-326.

[116] Hong K. H., Ryu J., Han K. H. Monocyte chemoattractant protein-1-induced angiogenesis is mediated by vascular endothelial growth factor-A. Blood. 2005;105(4):1405-1407.

[117] Mitamura Y., Takeuchi S., Matsuda A., Tagawa Y., Mizue Y., Nishihira J. Monocyte chemotactic protein-1 in the vitreous of patients with proliferative diabetic retinopathy. Ophthalmologica. 2001;215(6):415-418.

[118] Tashimo A., Mitamura Y., Nagai S., et al. Aqueous levels of macrophage migration inhibitory factor and monocyte chemotactic protein-1 in patients with diabetic retinopathy. Diabetic Medicine. 2004;21(12):1292-1297.

[119] Taghavi Y, Hassanshahi G, Kounis NG, Koniari I, Khorramdelazad H. Monocyte chemoattractant protein-1 (MCP-1/CCL2) in diabetic retinopathy: Latest evidence and clinical considerations. J Cell Commun Signal. 2019 Dec;13(4):451-462.

[120] Carmeliet P., Moons L., Luttun A., et al. Synergism between vascular endothelial growth factor and placental growth factor contributes to angiogenesis and plasma extravasation in pathological conditions. Nature Medicine. 2001;7(5):575-583.

[121] Hernàndez C., Segura R. M., Fonollosa A., Carrasco E., Francisco G., Simó R. Interleukin-8, monocyte chemoattractant protein-1 and IL-10 in the vitreous fluid of patients with proliferative diabetic retinopathy. Diabetic Medicine. 2005;22(6):719-722.

[122] Suzuki Y, Nakazawa M, Suzuki K, Yamazaki H, Miyagawa Y. Expression profiles of cytokines and chemokines in vitreous fluid in diabetic retinopathy and central retinal vein occlusion. Jpn J Ophthalmol. 2011 May;55(3):256-263.

[123] Wakabayashi Y., Usui Y., Okunuki Y., et al. Increased levels of monokine induced by interferon-gamma (Mig) in the vitreous of patients with diabetic retinopathy. Diabetic Medicine. 2008;25:875-877.

[124] Kaji Y., Usui T., Ishida S., et al. Inhibition of diabetic leukostasis and blood-retinal barrier breakdown with a soluble form of a receptor for advanced glycation end products. Investigative Ophthalmology and Visual Science. 2007;48(2):858-865.

[125] You JJ, Yang CH, Huang JS, Chen MS, Yang CM. Fractalkine, a CX3C chemokine, as a mediator of ocular angiogenesis. Investigative Ophthalmology and Visual Science. 2007;48(11):5290-5298.

[126] Lai DW, Lin KH, Sheu WH, Lee MR, Chen CY, Lee WJ, Hung YW, Shen CC, Chung TJ, Liu SH, Sheu ML. TPL2 (therapeutic targeting tumor progression Locus-2)/ATF4 (activating transcription Factor-4)/SDF1α (chemokine stromal cell-derived factor-α) Axis suppresses diabetic retinopathy. Circ Res. 2017 Sep 1;121(6):e37-e52.

[127] Lauro C, Catalano M, Trettel F, Limatola C. Fractalkine in the nervous system: Neuroprotective or neurotoxic molecule? Ann N Y Acad Sci. 2015 Sep;1351:141-148.

[128] Mendiola AS, Garza R, Cardona SM, Mythen SA, Lira SA, Akassoglou K, Cardona AE. Fractalkine Signaling attenuates perivascular clustering of microglia and fibrinogen leakage during systemic inflammation in mouse models of diabetic retinopathy. Front Cell Neurosci. 2017 Jan 10;10:303.

[129] Aiello L. P., Avery R. L., Arrigg P. G., et al. Vascular endothelial growth factor in ocular fluid of patients with diabetic retinopathy and other retinal disorders. The New England Journal of Medicine. 1994;331(22):1480-1487.

[130] Mitamura Y, Takeuchi S, Matsuda A, Tagawa Y, Mizue Y, Nishihira J. Macrophage migration inhibitory factor levels in the vitreous of patients with proliferative diabetic retinopathy. Br J Ophthalmol. 2000 Jun;84(6):636-639.

[131] Bui TM, Wiesolek HL, Sumagin R. ICAM-1: A master regulator of cellular responses in inflammation, injury resolution, and tumorigenesis. J Leukoc Biol. 2020 Sep;108(3):787-799.

[132] Frystyk J., Tarnow L., Krarup Hansen T., Parving H.-H., Flyvbjerg A. Increased serum adiponectin levels in type 1 diabetic patients with microvascular complications. Diabetologia. 2005;48(9):1911-1918.

[133] Zheng L, Howell SJ, Hatala DA, Huang K, Kern TS. Salicylate-based anti-inflammatory drugs inhibit the early lesion of diabetic retinopathy. Diabetes. 2007b; 56:337-345

[134] Rodríguez González-Herrero ME, Ruiz M, López Román FJ, Marín Sánchez JM, Domingo JC. Supplementation with a highly concentrated docosahexaenoic acid plus xanthophyll carotenoid multivitamin in nonproliferative diabetic retinopathy: Prospective controlled study of macular function by fundus microperimetry. Clin Ophthalmol. 2018;12:1011-1020.

[135] Kim JH, Yu YS, Cho CS, Kim KW. Blockade of angiotensin II attenuates VEGF-mediated blood-retinal barrier breakdown in diabetic retinopathy. J Cereb Blood Flow Metab. 2009; 29:621-628

[136] Miller AG, Tan G, binger KJ, Pickering RJ, Thomas MC, Nagaraj RH, Cooper ME, Wilkinson-BerkaJL. Candesartan attenuates diabetic retinal vascular pathology by restoring glyoxalase-I function. Diabetes. 2010; 59:3208-3215.

[137] Kang EY, Chen T, Garg SJ, et al. Association of Statin Therapy with Prevention of vision-threatening diabetic retinopathy. JAMA Ophthalmol. 2019;137(4):363-371.

[138] Tuuminen R, Sahanne S, Loukovaara S. Low intravitreal angiopoietin-2 and VEGF levels in vitrectomized diabetic patients with simvastatin treatment. Acta Ophthalmol. 2014;92(7):675-681.

[139] Effects of aspirin treatment on diabetic retinopathy. ETDRS report number 8. Early Treatment Diabetic Retinopathy Study Research Group. Ophthalmology. 1991 May;98 (5 Suppl):757-65.]

[140] Jiang Y, Thakran S, Bheemreddy R, Coppess W, Walker RJ, Steinle JJ. Sodium salicylate reduced insulin resistance in the retina of a type 2 diabetic rat model. PLoS One. 2015 Apr 14;10(4):e0125505.

[141] Joussen AM, Poulaki V, Mitsiades N, Kirchhof B, Koizumi K, Döhmen S, Adamis AP. Nonsteroidal anti-inflammatory drugs prevent early diabetic retinopathy via TNF-alpha suppression. FASEB J. 2002 Mar; 16(3):438-440.

[142] Sfikakis PP, Markomichelakis N, Theodossiadis GP, Grigoropoulos V, Katsilambros N, Theodossiadis PG. Regression of sight-threatening macular edema in type 2 diabetes following treatment with the anti-tumor necrosis factor monoclonal antibody infliximab. Diabetes Care. 2005;28(2):445-447

[143] Rao VR, Prescott E, Shelke NB, et al. Delivery of SAR 1118 to retina via ophthalmic drops and its effectiveness in reduction of retinal Leukostasis and vascular leakiness in rat Streptozotocin (STZ) model of diabetic retinopathy (DR) Invest Ophthalmol Vis Sci. 2010;51(10):5198-5204.

[144] Iliaki E, Poulaki V, Mitsiades N, Mitsiades CS, Miller JW, Gragoudas ES. Role of alpha 4 integrin (CD49d) in the pathogenesis of diabetic retinopathy. Invest Ophthalmol Vis Sci. 2009; 50(10):4898-4904.

[145] Bernardino, A.L.; Kaushal, D.; Philipp, M.T. The antibiotics doxycycline and minocycline inhibit the inflammatory responses to the Lyme disease spirochete borrelia burgdorferi. J. Infect. Dis. 2009, 199, 1379-1388.

[146] Cukras, C.A.; Petrou, P.; Chew, E.Y.; Meyerle, C.B.;Wong,W.T. Oral minocycline for the treatment of diabetic macular edema (DME): Results of a phase I/II clinical study. Investig. Ophthalmol. Vis. Sci. 2012, 53, 3865-3874.

[147] Scott, I.U.; Jackson, G.R.; Quillen, D.A.; Larsen, M.; Klein, R.; Liao, J.; Holfort, S.; Munch, I.C.; Gardner, T.W. Effect of doxycycline vs placebo on retinal function and diabetic retinopathy progression in patients with severe nonproliferative or non-high-risk proliferative diabetic retinopathy: A randomized clinical trial. JAMA Ophthalmol. 2014, 132, 535-543.

[148] Tang, J.; Herda, A.A.; Kern, T.S. Photobiomodulation in the treatment of patients with non-center-involving diabetic macular oedema. Br. J. Ophthalmol. 2014, 98, 1013-1015.

[149] Lachin, J.M.; Genuth, S.; Nathan, D.M.; Zinman, B.; Rutledge, B.N.; Group, D.E.R. Effect of glycemic exposure on the risk of microvascular complications in the diabetes control and complications trial—Revisited. Diabetes 2008, 57, 995-1001.

Chapter 4

Local Inflammatory Biomarkers and Potential Inflammation-Targeting Therapies in Diabetic Retinopathy

Ioana Damian and Simona Delia Nicoară

Abstract

Diabetic retinopathy (DR) is one of the most frequent microvascular complications of diabetes. A large body of evidence supports the role of inflammation in the development and progression of DR. Currently, DR is diagnosed based on the presence of morphological lesions detected on fundus examination. Yet, there are other laboratory or imaging biomarker whose alteration precede DR lesions. This chapter will first briefly explain the role of inflammation in DR pathogenesis and will analyze the molecules involved. Further, it will discuss significant and recent studies that analyzed local laboratory or imaging inflammatory biomarkers in different DR stages. It will then focus on several potential inflammation-targeting therapies which proved to be effective in animal or human studies. Validation of these reviewed biomarkers would allow the identification of patients who do not respond to the current available treatment and could benefit from an adjunctive therapy.

Keywords: diabetic retinopathy, inflammation, biomarker, retinal imaging, anti-inflammatory therapy

1. Introduction

Diabetus mellitus (DM) is an important public health issue, with a constantly growing prevalence from 4.7% in 1980 to 8.5% in 2014 [1]. In 2019, 463 million adults between 20 and 79 years had DM [2]. Diabetic retinopathy (DR) is one of the most frequent microvascular complications of diabetes. Most type 1 DM (T1DM) patients develop DR only after 5 years or even more from the onset of DM, but after 20- year history of disease, 99% present a form of DR [3]. On the contrary, for type 2 DM (T2DM) patients, DR may be present even from the diagnosis, while after 20 years of T2DM, 60% of the patients develop DR [3]. Currently, DR staging is performed depending on the presence of clinical ocular biomarkers, such as microaneurysms, hemorrhages, soft or hard exudates, macular oedema and new vessels. The treatment for DR targets especially the severe non-proliferative diabetic retinopathy (NPDR) or proliferative diabetic retinopathy (PDR) stage and diabetic macular oedema (DME). The therapeutic options are intravitreal injections with anti-VEGF agents, corticosteroids injections, retinal laser or surgery such as pars plana vitrectomy (PPV). A large body of evidence supports the role of inflammation in the development and progression of DR. There is evidence that low-grade subclinical inflammation is responsible for many of the characteristic vascular lesions of DR [4]. In this review we provide an overview of several local inflammatory biomarkers of DR laboratory and retinal imaging together with anti-inflammatory therapeutic options.

2. Inflammation and diabetic retinopathy

Inflammation is defined as the body's mechanism of self-defense against pathogens. In this complex process, mediators such as pro-inflammatory cytokines, chemokines and adhesion molecules are involved. They initiate the interaction between the endothelium and leukocytes and consequently induce the migration of leukocytes towards the injured or infected tissue [5]. Although acute inflammation is considered beneficial, a chronic and dysregulated one produces harmful effects, being known to be involved in diseases such as rheumatoid arthritis, multiple sclerosis and atherosclerosis [5].

Lutty et al. were the first who reported an increased neutrophil number per square millimeter in both retinal and choroidal vessels in DR patients [6]. Moreover, they continued the study of neutrophils in diabetic monkeys and found an association between the accumulation of neutrophils and capillary closure [7]. Further studies found evidence that capillary occlusion and intraretinal neovascularization are associated with the attachment of neutrophils and monocytes [8], while the level of leukocytes adherence to the retinal vasculature, known as leukostasis, is associated with the progression of DR [9]. Recent findings implicate that an increase of ICAM-1 and integrins at the level of endothelial cells and leukocytes is responsible for the increase in leukostasis, while ICAM-1 blocking and CD18 deletion decreases the leukostasis induced by DM [10, 11]. Microglial cell is a resident macrophage distributed throughout the retina, which releases inflammatory cytokines such as TNF-α after being activated [12].

There are several processes in DR pathogenesis in which inflammation is involved:

1. vessel leakage: retinal endothelial permeability is induced by TNF-α, but is successfully prevented by PKCζ inhibitor [13]. After TNF-α was blocked with Etanercept, a soluble TNF-α receptor, the activation of NF-κB was inhibited and blood retinal barrier (BRB) breakdown was prevented [14]. Similarly, VEGF is directly involved in the breakdown of inner BRB, being proved that after blocking ICAM-1, the leukostasis is reduced but also VEGF induced vascular leakage is blocked [15].

2. vessel closure: IL-1β and TNF-α increase caspase 3 activity and induce endothelial cell apoptosis [16, 17].

3. pathological neovascularization: New vessels' formation is induced by leukocytes by interfering in the releasing of pro-angiogenic factors, such as VEGF, angiopoietin 1, basic fibroblast growth factor, transforming growth factor and platelet derived factor. All these agents promote recruitment of endothelial progenitor cells and enhance the migration, proliferation and survival of the pre-existing endothelial cells [17].

4. retinal neuronal death: TNF-α, IL-1β, reactive oxygen species (ROS) and excessive nitric oxide (NO) released by leukocytes during inflammation are involved in retinal neuronal cell death [5].

DM causes increased systemic and local production of numerous inflammatory molecules involved in DR onset and development.

3. Inflammatory biomarkers

A biomarker has been defined as "a biological molecule found in blood, or other bodily fluids, or tissue which represents a sign of a normal or abnormal process of a condition or disease" [18]. Due to the rapid advancement in engineering, methodology and equipment, researchers are able to generate large amounts of data analyzing only small amounts of samples, using mass spectrometry techniques. In DR studies, several kinds of samples were used, such as tear, cornea, aqueous humor (AH), lens, vitreous humor (VH), retina and serum [19]. Although VH is in direct contact with the retina, it requires a highly invasive procedure, whereas the tears can be collected using non-invasive methods but interact indirectly with the retina [19].

3.1 Local laboratory biomarkers

3.1.1 Tears

The tears are composed of an aqueous solution of water, lipids, proteins and salt. The major proteins are lactoferrin, lysozyme, serum albumin, secretory immunoglobin A, lipocalin and lipophilin [20]. One study identified 1526 proteins using protemics approaches, most of them being shown to respond to insults such as cataract surgery or diseases like DM [21, 22]. Mainly because it contains proteins in high concentration (about 8 μg/μl) and it is easy to collect, tears have been a fluid of interest for many studies [21]. Herber et al. was one of the first to demonstrate that DM patients' tear composition is different from control subjects [23]. Azzaralo et al. found increased levels of lactotransferin, also known as lactoferrin, a glycoprotein with immunomodulatory, anti-microbial and anti-tumor effects [24]. Increased levels of monocyte chemoattractant protein-1 (MCP-1) were also identified in DM with or without DR. A previous study demonstrated elevated Interleukin-1 receptor anatagonist (IL-1ra) levels, which represent an anti-inflammatory factor inhibiting pro-inflammatory activity of IL-1beta [25]. A positive correlation between IL-6 levels and DR stage was found. IL-6 is involved in synthesis and the release of acute phase reactants and matrix metalloproteinase 9 (MMP-9), decreased tear production, having also a role in the release of IL-1β [26]. TNF-α is a cytokine able to induce the disruption of BRB by loosening the tight junctions between endothelial cells and between RPE cells, with a role in the leukocytes adhesion to the endothelium [13]. TNF-α level was increased in patients with PDR (13.5 pg./mL) compared to NPDR (2.8 pg./mL) [27]. The tear sample can be obtained using two techniques: the direct one using aspiration with the help of a micropipette or a microcapillary tube placed in the inferior fornix, or the indirect one, with the help of a Schirmer test strip or cellulose sponge.

3.1.2 Aqueous humor

Aqueous humor (AH) is produced by the ciliary body epithelium and represents the fluid in the anterior chamber of the eye. It is involved in the removal of metabolic wastes, in ocular immunity, it supplies oxygen and nutrients, and has a role in refraction. AH is composed of water, electrolytes and proteins, which although are present in relatively low concentrations compared to blood serum, are vital in the maintenance of anterior segment homeostasis. AH is not in direct contact with the retina but proteins released from it can enter AH either through disrupted BRB, cilio-retinal circulation or through diffusion from the VH and the VH-AH barrier [28]. Proteomic analysis studying AH from patients with DR compared to subjects without DM, found several proteins associated with PDR like apolipoprotein A-I (APOA1), apolipoprotein A-II (APOA2), apolipoprotein A-IV (APOA4), and α-1-acid glycoprotein 1 (ORM1) [29] as well as selenoprotein P (SELENOP), and cystathionine β-synthase (CBS) [28].

IL-23 levels were increased in PDR patients, and IL-17 was also higher in NPDR and PDR compared to control subjects as shown by Wang et al. in 625 patients with T2DM [30]. IL-17 is a powerful pro-inflammatory cytokine capable of mobilizing neutrophils and inducing the secretion of IL-6 and IL-8 prostagladin E2 [30]. Regarding IL-23, it stimulates Th17 cells to secrete IL-17, which further increases the cycle of inflammation.

Concerning IL-10, the cytokine with immunosuppresive properties, capable of attenuating the antigen-presenting ability of APC, studies found contradictory results: decreased concentrations in DR compared to NPDR by Cheung et al. and Zhang et al., contrary to Hu et al. who reported increased levels [30]. It was also suggested that IL-10 levels could be correlated with central subfield thickness (CST), one study reporting higher IL-10 concentration in PDR (224,79 pg./mL) that in the control group (160/14 pg./mL) [31]. TGF-beta is involved in the differentiation of activated $CD4^{+}Th_0$ cells into Treg cells, but it is also involved in promoting differentiation of $CD4^{+}Th_0$ cells into Th_{17} cells in combination with IL-23 [32]. Zhang et al. found elevated and stable TGF-beta levels in DM compared to control [30].

Myonectin inhibits the inflammatory response triggered by lipopolysaccharide in macrophages and in myonectin-knockout mices, in which the proinflammatory gene expression was identified. Previous studies demonstrated decreased myonectin concentrations in AH belonging to T2DM especially with PDR but also in NPDR compared to control subjects [33, 34]. In refractory DME, IL-2, IL-8, PIGF and VEGF were found elevated but only IL-8 was correlated with responsiveness, exhibiting higher levels in the refractory group [31]. This result is supported by Jeon et al., who observed that after injecting triamcinolone intravitreally to patients unresponsive to IVB, the effect was positive while the efficacy was associated with IL-8 levels in the AH [35].

IL-6, another proinflammatory cytokine was found elevated in PDR and DME patients. Additionally, it induces VEGF expression, being involved in the breakdown of BRB and thus being involved in the pathogenesis of earlier stages of NPDR [36]. IL-6 is considered as a driving force because it changes the overall cytokine profile in the AH of DM patients. Moreover, the level of VEGF in AH was strongly correlated with VEGF level from the VH [37].

IFN-α is a known angiogenic inhibitor, with a protective role against retinal damage in diabetes. Cheung et al. found reduced IFN-α levels in DM patients compared to control subjects [38].

MCP-1 level in AH is believed to be a predictor for a worse visual acuity outcome of PDR patients after vitrectomy, while there was no significant correlation between VEGF levels and BCVA, as noted by Lei et al. [39]. MCP-1 stimulates the recruitment and activation of monocytes and macrophages which further leads to higher microvascular permeability or ischemia from vessel occlusions. A few studies have investigated the effect of intravitreal triamcinolone [40] or dexamethasone implant [41] on the intraocular inflammatory cytokines and concluded that both drugs could significantly decrease the level of MCP-1 in the AH.

Samples from AH are collected through a paracenthesis from patients undergoing cataract surgery, trabeculectomy or from post-mortem eyes. The volume collected ranges from 100 to 150 μL. The samples from living patients are more useful since the profile from post-mortem eye is different due to the accumulation of metabolic waste [26].

3.1.3 Vitreous humor

The vitreous humor is the gelatinous component of the posterior segment of the eye that gives its spherical shape. In addition to its role in structural support, the transparent nature of the vitreous body aids in light transmission to the retina. Because of its avascular nature, much of the proteins found in VH are derived from the retina itself [28]. Several proteins in the VH have been identified as biomarkers for different stages of DR, like components of the acute phase response, coagulation pathway, complement system and other inflammatory pathways (e.g., VEGF, amyloid-β A4 protein, metalloproteinase inhibitor 1, kininogen-1) [19].

Pigment epithelium-derived factor (PEDF) is a negative regulator of inflammatory processes, with lower levels in VH from DR patients compared to NDR. This finding suggest that beside an increase in proinflammatory cytokines, there is also a decrease in the anti-inflammatory ones [42]. Clusterin, a protein involved in the regulation of complement cascade, was found decreased in DR patients [43]. One of its function consists in an anti-inflammatory protection for the BRB [44]. Kallikrein, a known central component of pro-inflammatory kallikrein-kinin system, was found elevated in the VH from DR patients [45].

Anti-VEGF agents such as bevacizumab did not have a significant effect on VH inflammatory proteins as shown by Loukovaara et al. [46], as opposed to Zou et al. who studied VH proteome from patients treated with anti-VEGF agent ranibizumab and found decreased VEGF levels as well as a decrease in complement activation protein, acute inflammatory response and platelet degranulation [47]. Similarly, photocoagulation reduced the levels of pro-inflammatory protein osteopontin (SPP1), as shown by Wei et al. [48].

When exposed to intravitreal injection of IL-1β, retinal capillary endothelial cells degenerate [49], while co-administration of IL-1β, together with high concentrations of glucose, disrupt the RPE cells [50]. Increased levels of IL-1β were found in the VH collected from diabetic patients compared to control [51], underlining its role it the DR-related inflammatory processes.

IL-8, responsible for activating neutrophils and T Lymphocytes, together with IL-6, a chemokine responsible for increased endothelial cell permeability by rearranging actin filaments and changing the shape of endothelial cells, were both found elevated in VH of PDR patients [52]. Their origin does not seem to be the serum, since higher levels were found in the vitreous, suggesting that macrophages, RPE cells, glial cells or monocytes from the vitreous of PDR patients, could produce citokines [53]. IL-10, another anti-inflammatory cytokine, with the ability of deactivating macrophages, was not found to be increased in PDR patients, the author of the study suggesting the lack of a counter balanced by the anti-inflammatory cytokines [54].

MCP-1, with its known role in promoting leukocyte recruitment and inducer of angiogenesis and fibrosis, was found elevated in DR VH, with levels being higher than in the serum [55]. Hyperglycemia seems to increase the formation of MCP-1 from RPE cells, retinal vascular endothelial cells and Muller's cells [56]. This finding further encouraged that MCP-1 gene polymorphism to be proposed as a potential risk factor for DR [57].

Stromal cell-derived factor-1 (SDF-1) is upregulated in damaged tissues and as a response, it mobilizes progenitor cells to promote repair [58]. Together with VEGF, it promotes endothelial progenitor cells from the bone marrow to the ischemic retina [59]. Butler et al. found increased SDF-1 concentrations in VH from DME or PDR patients, and moreover the increase was correlated with disease severity [60].

Extracellular High-Mobility Group Box-1 Protein (HMGB1) as a proinflammatory cytokine, leads to overexpression of TNF-α, MCP-1, ICAM-1, through activation of NF-β [61]. In addition, El-Asrar reported elevated levels of HMGB1 in VH belonging to PDR patients. They further reported that HMGB1 and its receptor for advanced glycation products (RAGE) are expressed by vascular endothelial cells and stromal cells in PDR fibrovascular epiretinal membranes [61].

Tumor Necrosis Factor-α (TNF-α) was found elevated in VH from DM patients, with a higher vitreous/serum ratio [51]. In addition, TNF-α was also found expressed in vascular endothelial and stromal cells in epiretinal membranes belonging to PDR eyes [62].

ICAM-1 levels in PDR were found increased, especially in active PDR compared to inactive PDR [61]. ICAM-1 was highly expressed in retinal and choroidal blood vessels, as well as in fibrovascular membranes, and its expression seems to correlate with the number of migrated neutrophils in the retina and choroid [6]. When ICAM-1 blocking was obtained, the leukostasis, endothelial cell death and also the vascular leakage in the retinal vessels was diminished.

When retinal capillary endothelial cells were exposed to high concentration of glucose, TNF-α or IL-1β, they produce the membrane-bound form of vascular adhesion protein-1(VAP1) and release the soluble vascular adhesion protein 1 (sVAP-1) [63]. Its role consists in leukostasis and leukocyte entrapment. High levels of sVAP-1 were found in the serum and VH of patients with PDR [64].

Samples from VH are collected through vitreous taps from patients that underwent PPV or after intravitreal injections. Simo et al. raised the problem of confounding factors that could lead to misinterpretation of result. Vitreous hemorrhage could induce a massive influx of serum proteins. Similarly, the disruption of BRB also leads to increased protein levels in VH. The first problem could be solved by rejecting samples with hemoglobin >5 mg/mL, while the second one, by correcting the intravitreal concentration of peptide under study for total vitreal proteins or calculating the vitreous/plasma ratio [56].

3.2 Imaging retinal biomarkers

3.2.1 Hyperreflective retinal foci

These lesions are found under the name of hyperreflective foci, dots or spots. Hyperreflective retinal foci (HRF) have been first described in wet AMD but they were also noted in retinal vein occlusion, MacTel type 2, central serous retinopathy, retinitis pigmentosa, Stargardt disease and Best disease. Different pathogenetic origins were hypothesized: initially they were considered precursor of hard exudates or lipid-laden macrophages [65], representing subclinical features of lipoprotein extravasation that were not observed on clinical examination, fundus photography, or fluorescein angiography, due to their small size [66]. In contrast to the previous studies, Lee et al. proposed that HRF represent activated microglial cells since they determined the presence of increased soluble CD14 in the AH. Soluble CD14 seems to be released by activated microglial cells [67, 68]. Other theories assumed that HRF represent debris of photoreceptors or RPE hyperplasia [65, 66].

HRF are initially present in the inner retinal layers, where resting retinal microglia are normally located and after they are activated, they subsequently migrate to the outer retinal layers [66, 69]. Another argument that HRF are in fact microglia is that both are primarily found in the inner retina in DR without edema and show an extended distribution into the outer retina in DME [68]. By contrast, Bolz et al. described that HRF are distributed throughout all retinal layers in eyes with different types of diabetic macular edema (DME), diffuse or cystoid [70]. Uji et al. reported the presence of HRF in the outer retina in 53.7% cases while in the inner retina in 99.1% cases in eyes with DME [71]. Uji et al. further suggested an origin from degenerated photoreceptors or macrophages engulfing the former, since HRF were found in the outer retina closely associated with disrupted external limiting membrane or IS/OS line [71].

HRF appears on OCT as small discrete, well-circumscribed, dot-shaped hyperreflective intraretinal lesions (**Figure 1**) [69]. Their size is less than 30 μm, and as opposed to hard exudates they do not induce back-shadowing, while their reflectivity is similar to retinal nerve fiber layer and equal or greater than the retinal pigment epithelium (RPE) band [67, 72].

As opposed to HRF, hard exudates are thought to form from microaneurysms, which is the major source of leakage in focal edema [68]. Other theories even suggested that HRF can occur even before DR development, representing a neurodegenerative process [69]. Both the presence and number of HRF was increased in diabetics versus control subjects, especially in those with signs of DR, but interestingly, none of the patients had signs of DME, hard exudates nor subclinical signs of DME on OCT examinations [68].

The size and also the number of HRF seem to decrease after treatment with anti-VEGF or corticosteroids [71]. The decreased microglial activity following anti-VEGF therapy could contribute to the reduced loads of inflammatory cytokines, which further translates into decreased number of HRS and reduced CMT [68]. Moreover, HRS was the first feature to disappear or reduce after anti-VEGF therapy [66]. One study revealed that an initial presence of larger number of HRF responded better to dexamethasone implants than anti-VEGF therapy but a higher number of HRF is associated with early recurrence of DME after steroid implant [67].

One study found that eyes with HRF in the outer retinal layers presented a greater disruption in EZ (IS/OS) lines at baseline but they improved more than the eyes without the foci at 12 months. Taking into account this result, the authors further suggested that greater VA improvement could be partially explained by foveal photoreceptor restoration in eyes with HRF in the outer retinal layers [65].

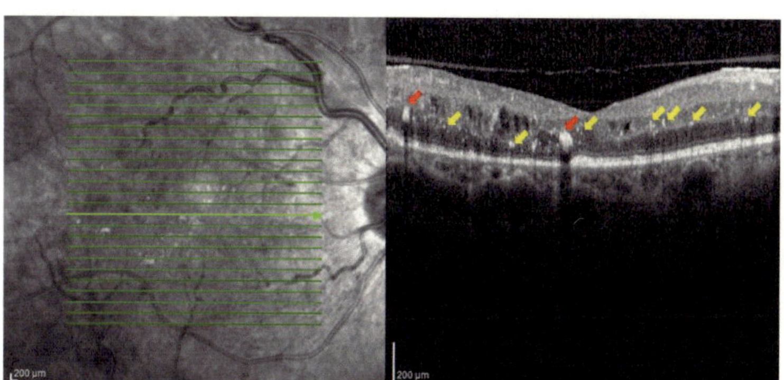

Figure 1.
Spectral domain OCT linear scan in the macula of a diabetic patient with PDR. The yellow arrows indicate HRF while red arrows indicate hard exudates.

3.2.2 Sub-foveal neurosensory detachment

Hypoalbuminemia lowers the intravascular osmotic pressure and together with increased hydrostatic pressure can cause retention of fluid in the subretinal space. The role of subretinal fluid (SRF) in final visual and anatomical outcomes is still unclear. There is a number of studies which have shown that the presence of SRF is associated with good anatomical and functional gains. Contrary to this, there are other studies which have reported the association between the presence of SRF with poor visual gains [73]. Results from RESTORE study [74] and post hoc analysis from RISE/RIDE study [75] proved the protective role of SRF. These studies revealed the correlation between the presence of baseline SRF with better visual gains at the end of 1 year. These studies also showed a positive impact from SRF in response to ranibizumab therapy. Eyes with SRF seem to have increased IL-6 levels, which signifies active inflammation in these eyes, suggesting that inflammation has an important role in the development of this phenotype of DME [76]. Sonoda et al. found that eyes with subretinal detachment (SRD) presented increased intravitreal levels of IL-6, IL-8 and VEGF [77]. Discontinuation of the external limiting membrane in the SRD type of DME induces cellular damage, which further attracts scavenger cells to the retina, producing IL-6 (**Figure 2**) [78]. The migration of activated microglia in the outer segments of the retinal layer could support the production of IL-6 and subsequently the accumulation of SRF. The SRD type of DME is associated with an increased number of HRF and significant functional impairment of the macula [78]. The presence of numerous HRF is also associated with poorer glycemic control in patients without significant DME [79]. The levels of ICAM 1 are associated with the height of SRF, indicating that increased vascular permeability by inflammatory mediators results in SRF [80]. An important finding was that DME eyes with SRF respond significantly better to dexamethasone implants and the authors consequently supported the use of dexamethasone implants in patients with DME with SRF [81]. Interestingly, a recent study assessing the change of parameters in DME with SRD after treatment, reported that intravitreal injection of steroid like dexamethasone implant showed greater decrease in number of RHF compared to anti-VEGF agent such as ranibizumab [82].

3.2.3 Hyperreflective choroidal foci

The analysis of the choroid could be an important tool in the assessment of progressing DR. Choroidal parameters such as luminal area (LA), stromal area (SA) and total choroidal area (TCA) were found decreased in diabetic patients compared to control by a recent study [83]. Hyperreflective choroidal foci (HCF) is a recently described entity in DR. It is postulated that HCF represent HRF migrated from the retina, into the choroidal layers, which was permitted by ELM and EZ disruption (**Figure 3**). The hypothesis that HCF are actually migrated HRF, is supported by the study of Roy and al. where all 59 eyes with HCF had HRF as well and there was no eye which had HCF in the absence of HRF on SD-OCT [84]. Presence of HCF could be used as a biomarker of disease severity in eyes with DR [84]. HCF were found to be present significantly more in PDR eyes than NPDR eyes [67].

3.2.4 Intraretinal cystoid spaces

Inner BRB is affected by elevated levels of VEGF leading to increased vascular permeability, which will result in a decreased osmotic gradient, extracellular fluid accumulation, and cyst formation [67]. VEGF is also responsible for the depletion of the occludin in RPE which will further disrupt the tight junction in the outer

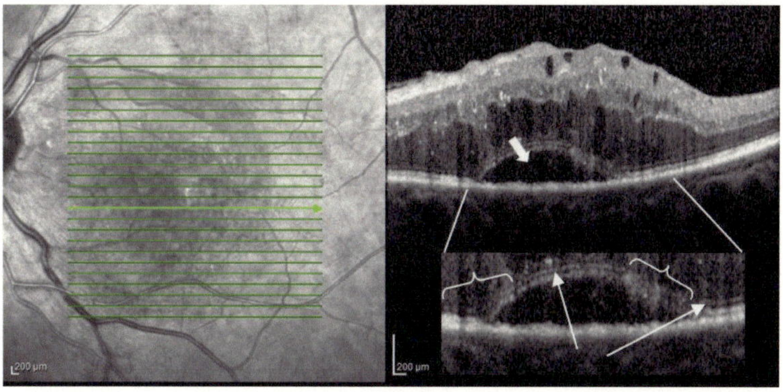

Figure 2.
Spectral domain OCT linear scan in the macula of a diabetic patient with PDR. The small arrow indicates sub-foveal detachment. In the magnified segment of the image, the tall arrows indicate intact external limiting membrane (ELM) while the curly brackets indicate a discontinuous ELM.

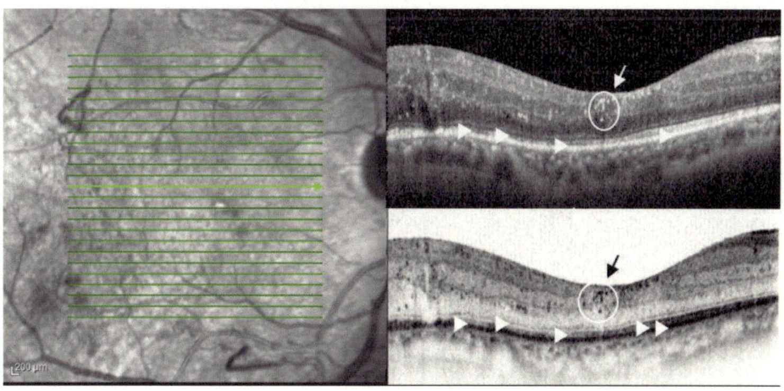

Figure 3.
Spectral domain OCT linear scan in the macula of a diabetic patient with PDR. Right upper image: White-on-black OCT scan. Right lower image: Black-on-white OCT scan. The white arrows head indicate hyperreflective choroidal foci. The white and black arrow highlights a group of hyperreflective retinal foci.

BRB [85]. Damian and al. found decreased RPE thickness in almost all quadrants in the PDR-DMO group as opposed to NPDR-DMO group, where the quadrants number was lower [86]. This finding was explained by a disruption of the RPE-photoreceptors complex due to ischemia and level of inflammation that varies according to the stage of DR. Cysts larger than >200 μm in the outer nuclear layer (ONL) are seen in advanced stages of DME and may cause irreversible damage to visual functions. Due to their location, they damage photoreceptor cells and disrupt inner segment–outer segment (IS/OS) junction (**Figure 4**). Regarding their content, there is paucity of information in the literature. Liang and al. hypothesize that fibrin and other inflammatory cells may fill these spaces [87]. Treatment with anti-VEGF therapy leads to a decrease in the number and size of ONL cysts by decreasing the permeability of the inner BRB. This was associated with improvement in BCVA and microperimetric retinal sensitivity. Hyperreflective signals within the cyst are associated with severe disruption of the BRB [67].

3.2.5 Foveal hyperautofluorescence

Fundus autofluorescence (FAF) is a rapid, noninvasive imaging technique that may give new insights into the evaluation of DME. Short wavelength FAF derives its signal mainly from lipofuscin in the RPE. Long wavelength autofluorescence

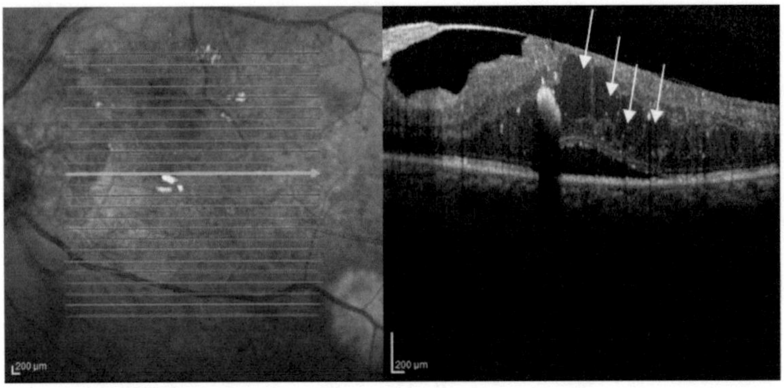

Figure 4.
Spectral domain OCT linear scan in the macula of a diabetic patient with PDR. The white arrows indicate intraretinal cystoid spaces.

or near-infrared (NIR) FAF derives its signal from melanin which is present in RPE and choroid. Melanin accumulates in the apical parts of the RPE cells and is thought to protect the RPE. In DR, local ocular inflammation and oxidative stress lead to increased amount of lipofuscin and decreased amount of lutein and zeaxanthin in the macula. This is responsible for increased FAF signal in subjects with DME. In addition, activation of microglia in DM could cause oxidation of proteins and lipids. Histologic studies have found lipofuscin to accumulate in microglia [67].

4. Potential inflammation-targeting in diabetic retinopathy

Over the years, significant effort has been made to develop new strategies for the treatment of DR by targeting inflammation. Clinical and pre-clinical trials have tested a variety of anti-inflammatory therapeutics.

4.1 Steroids

Intravitreal injection of crystalline cortisone was first reported in 2001 by Jonas et al. [88]. Their mechanism of action consist in repressing pro-inflammatory transcription factors. Several routes of administration were tried but the oral steroids were avoided because of the high risk of DM exacerbation and systemic complications [89]. Tamura et al. found that intravitreal injection of dexamethasone suppresses the leukostasis, the up-regulation of ICAM-1 and also prevents retinal vascular leakage [90]. Since it seems to target different pathways than those targeted by anti-VEGF agents, corticosteroids may improve DME [91]. Especially DME with SRD, no HRF and a continuous ellipsoid zone at the fovea seems to have a better response to injectable dexamethasone implant, as shown by previous studies [92], explained by the increased concentrations of inflammatory cytokines and IL-6 found in the AH and VH of eyes with SRD. In a similar manner, intravitreal triamcinolone has proved to be effective in the resolution of cyst in the CME type of DME [93]. The source of intraretinal cyst is the liquefaction and necrosis of Müller cells which subsequently induces the production of prostaglandins and inflammatory cytokines. The better outcome of steroid might be explained by the reduction of Müller cells' swelling [94]. One study found better results for intravitreal injection of triamcinolone than with anti-VEGF therapy in reducing macular thickness and improving BCVA in patients with SRD but the authors requested cautious interpretation of the results because of the short follow-up (24 weeks) and the increased risk of associated long-term complications like cataract and elevated intraocular pressure [95].

4.2 NSAIDs

Their anti-inflammatory activity is characterized by inhibiting the production of the two isoforms of cyclooxygenase enzyme-mediated eicosanoid (COX): COX-1 and COX-2. While COX-1 is involved in homeostatic processes, COX-2 produces pro-inflammatory Prostaglandins (PGE), like PGE2 and PGF2α [96]. In the retina of diabetic animal models, increased expression of COX-2 and PGE2 was found, and it seems that COX-2 has a pivotal role in DR pathogenesis since the inhibition of COX-2 but not COX-1 reduced the levels of PGE2 [97]. Retinal inflammatory reactions such as ICAM-1 expression and leukostasis were blocked after COX-2 inhibition [98]. Aspirin, sodium salicylate and sulfasalazine prevented capillary cell apoptosis and vessel degeneration while COX-2 inhibitors reduced vessel degeneration, vascular leakage and capillary cell apoptosis [99–101]. Moreover, retinal microaneurysm development was decreased by high doses of aspirin (900 mg/day), as shown by the Early Treatment DR study and the Dipyridamole Aspirin Microangiopathy of Diabetes Study [102, 103]. While COX-2 inhibitors have the potential to increase the incidence of strokes and heart attacks, their use in clinical trial being discouraged [104], local COX-2 inhibitors have shown reduction of DR sigs similar to systemic COX-2 [105].

4.3 SAR 1118

It is a small-molecule antagonist of leukocyte function-associated antigen (LFA)-1 a cell surface adhesion molecule of the β_2 (CD18) family of integrin receptors expressed on leukocytes, and intercellular adhesion molecule (ICAM)-1, expressed by endothelial cells. SAR 1118 inhibits the binding of LFA-1, to ICAM1–1, being capable of preventing leukocytes adhesion to endothelial cells in vivo [106]. Rao et al. found that SAR 1118 eye drops significantly reduced BRB breakdown and leukostasis in a dose dependent manner [106].

4.4 Etanercept, infliximab

Both drugs block TNF-α induced inflammation. High dose of etanercept reduced leukocyte adhesion and suppressed BRB breakdown, reduced ICAM-1 expression but it did not reduced the expression of CD11a, CD11b and CD18, and neither changed the retinal vascular endothelial growth factor levels [14]. After Infliximab administration, BCVA improved and CMT decreased [107]. But caution should be taken since intravitreal use of TNF-α inhibitors has proved to induce intraocular inflammation [56].

4.5 Anti-CD49a neutralizing antibody

Integrin alpha 4 (CD49d), in complex with integrin beta1, forms very late antigen-4 (VLA-4), which interacts with vascular cell adhesion molecule-1, being involved in leukocyte adhesion. Iliaki et al. showed that injection of an anti-alpha 4 integrin/CD49d neutralizing antibody reduced the diabetes induced upregulation of NF- kappaB activation, VEGF, and TNF-alpha protein levels and significantly reduced diabetes-induced leukocyte adhesion and vascular leakage [108].

4.6 Vitamins C and E

Another key mediator in inflammation is oxidative stress. Vitamin C attenuated the development of acellular capillaries [109] and vitamin E reversed some changes in the retinal vessels of diabetic patients [110].

4.7 Soluble RAGE, LR-90

The receptor for advanced glycation end products (AGEs) has been implicated in the pathogenesis of diabetic complications. When soluble RAGE, a competitor of cellular RAGE for its ligands was administered, neuronal dysfunction and reduced development of capillary lesions was proved by Barile et al. in mouse diabetic models [111].

4.8 Apocynin, statin

NAPDH oxidase activity blocking by apocynin reduces oxidative stress. Previous studies showed that by blocking NADPH oxidase, oxidative stress, retinal inflammation, vessel leakage as well as neovascularization are prevented [5].

4.9 Captopril, Telmisartan, Talsartan, Olmesartan, candesartan, Enalapril

The RAS system is involved in different DR pathways, such as oxidative stress and AGEs. Captopril proved to inhibit capillary degeneration in early stages of DR, while Losartan (an AT1R blocker) and Enalapril (angiotensin converting enzyme inhibitor) reduced the progression of DR by 70% and 65% respectively [112]. Retinal adherent leukocyte was significantly suppressed by telmisartan or valsartan [113].

4.10 Plasma kallikrein inhibitors: KVD001 and THR-149

Plasma kallikrein is involved in both VEGF-mediated and VEGF-independent mechanisms of DME. In a Phase 1B study, KVD001, a novel intravitreous plasma kallikrein selective competitive inhibitor was administered in DME eyes [114]. The authors of the previous study reported that KVD001 was safe and well tolerated while a significant number of eyes experienced a reduction of CRT (central retinal thickness) and BCVA improvement. Another recent Phase 2A study evaluated patients who received either a sham, a high dose or a low dose of 4 intravitreal injections of KVD001 at monthly intervals [115]. There were no statistical differences between the number of gained letters, neither regarding the central subfield thickness (CST) nor the diabetic retinopathy severity scale (DRSS) but only 32.5% of patients from the 6 μg dose group experienced a reduction in vision compared to 54.5% of patients from the sham group ($p = 0.042$) [116]. THR-149 is a reversible peptide inhibitor of plasma kallikrein, by inhibiting the release of bradykinin in the vitreous. Since it is VEGF-independent, anti-VEGF nonresponding patients could benefit from its effect. A Phase 1 study in which 12 patients were followed, proved THR-149 is safe and well tolerated while BCVA improved since day 1 and maintained until month 3 [117].

5. Conclusions

In accordance with the presented studies, multiple local laboratory and imaging biomarkers are involved in the onset and progression of DR, which could support and improve the screening, treatment and follow-up of these patients.

The encouraging positive effects of several tested drugs on BCVA but also on anatomical outcomes are likely to provide a background for further research.

Conflict of interest

The authors declare no conflict of interest.

Author details

Ioana Damian* and Simona Delia Nicoară
University of Medicine and Pharmacy "Iuliu Hațieganu", Cluj-Napoca, Romania

*Address all correspondence to: ioana.damian@umfcluj.ro

References

[1] Diagnosis and Management of Type 2 Diabetes. World Health Organization [Internet]2020. Available from: https://www.who.int/publications/i/item/who-ucn-ncd-20.1.[Accessed: 2021-06-10]

[2] International Diabetes Federation. Diabetes Atlas 9th edition 2019. Available at: https://www.diabetesatlas.org/en/.

[3] Jenkins, A.J., Joglekar, M.V., Hardikar, A.A. et al. Biomarkers in Diabetic Retinopathy. Rev Diabet Stud, 12(1-2): 159-195. DOI: 10.1900/RDS.2015.12.159

[4] Joussen, A. M., Poulaki, V., Le, M. L., Koizumi, K., Esser, C., Janicki, H., et al. A central role for inflammation in the pathogenesis of diabetic retinopathy. *FASEB J.* 18, 1450-1452. DOI: 10.1096/fj.03-1476fje.

[5] Zhang W, Liu H, Rojas M, Caldwell RW, Caldwell RB. Anti-inflammatory therapy for diabetic retinopathy. Immunotherapy. 2011 May;3(5):609-628. DOI: 10.2217/imt.11.24

[6] McLeod DS, Lefer DJ, Merges C, Lutty GA. Enhanced expression of intracellular adhesion molecule-1 and P-selectin in the diabetic human retina and choroid. Am J Pathol. 1995 Sep;147(3):642-53. PMID: 7545873; PMCID: PMC1870979.

[7] Kim SY, Johnson MA, McLeod DS, Alexander T, Hansen BC, Lutty GA. Neutrophils are associated with capillary closure in spontaneously diabetic monkey retinas. Diabetes. 2005 May;54(5):1534-1542. DOI: 10.2337/diabetes.54.5.1534.

[8] Schröder S, Palinski W, Schmid-Schönbein GW. Activated monocytes and granulocytes, capillary nonperfusion, and neovascularization in diabetic retinopathy. Am J Pathol. 1991 Jul;139(1):81-100. PMID: 1713023; PMCID: PMC1886150.

[9] Miyamoto K, Khosrof S, Bursell SE, Rohan R, Murata T, Clermont AC, Aiello LP, Ogura Y, Adamis AP. Prevention of leukostasis and vascular leakage in streptozotocin-induced diabetic retinopathy via intercellular adhesion molecule-1 inhibition. Proc Natl Acad Sci U S A. 1999 Sep 14;96(19):10836-10841. DOI: 10.1073/pnas.96.19.10836.

[10] Joussen AM, Poulaki V, Le ML, Koizumi K, Esser C, Janicki H, Schraermeyer U, Kociok N, Fauser S, Kirchhof B, Kern TS, Adamis AP. A central role for inflammation in the pathogenesis of diabetic retinopathy. FASEB J. 2004 Sep;18(12):1450-1452. DOI: 10.1096/fj.03-1476fje.

[11] Barouch FC, Miyamoto K, Allport JR, Fujita K, Bursell SE, Aiello LP, Luscinskas FW, Adamis AP. Integrin-mediated neutrophil adhesion and retinal leukostasis in diabetes. Invest Ophthalmol Vis Sci. 2000 Apr;41(5):1153-1158. PMID: 10752954.

[12] Yang LP, Sun HL, Wu LM, Guo XJ, Dou HL, Tso MO, Zhao L, Li SM. Baicalein reduces inflammatory process in a rodent model of diabetic retinopathy. Invest Ophthalmol Vis Sci. 2009 May;50(5):2319-2327. DOI: 10.1167/iovs.08-2642.

[13] Aveleira CA, Lin CM, Abcouwer SF, Ambrósio AF, Antonetti DA. TNF-α signals through PKCζ/NF-κB to alter the tight junction complex and increase retinal endothelial cell permeability. Diabetes. 2010 Nov;59(11):2872-2882. doi: 10.2337/db09-1606.

[14] Joussen AM, Poulaki V, Mitsiades N, Kirchhof B, Koizumi K, Döhmen S, Adamis AP. Nonsteroidal

anti-inflammatory drugs prevent early diabetic retinopathy via TNF-alpha suppression. FASEB J. 2002 Mar;16(3): 438-440. DOI: 10.1096/fj.01-0707fje

[15] Miyamoto K, Khosrof S, Bursell SE, Moromizato Y, Aiello LP, Ogura Y, Adamis AP. Vascular endothelial growth factor (VEGF)-induced retinal vascular permeability is mediated by intercellular adhesion molecule-1 (ICAM-1). Am J Pathol. 2000 May;156(5):1733-1739. DOI: 10.1016/S0002-9440(10)65044-4.

[16] Kowluru RA, Odenbach S. Role of interleukin-1beta in the pathogenesis of diabetic retinopathy. Br J Ophthalmol. 2004 Oct;88(10):1343-1347. DOI: 10.1136/bjo.2003.038133

[17] Costa C, Incio J, Soares R. Angiogenesis and chronic inflammation: cause or consequence? Angiogenesis. 2007;10(3):149-166. DOI: 10.1007/s10456-007-9074-0

[18] Simo-Servat O., Simo, R., Hernandez, C. Circulating Biomarkers of Diabetic Retinopathy: An Overview Based on Physiopathology. Journal of Diabetes Research. 2016. https://DOI.org/10.1155/2016/5263798

[19] Youngblood H, Robinson R, Sharma A, Sharma S. Proteomic Biomarkers of Retinal Inflammation in Diabetic Retinopathy. Int J Mol Sci. 2019 Sep 25;20(19):4755. DOI: 10.3390/ijms20194755.

[20] Kijlstra A, Kuizenga A. Analysis and function of the human tear proteins. Adv Exp Med Biol. 1994;350:299-308. DOI: 10.1007/978-1-4615-2417-5_51

[21] de Souza GA, Godoy LM, Mann M. Identification of 491 proteins in the tear fluid proteome reveals a large number of proteases and protease inhibitors. Genome Biol. 2006;7(8):R72. DOI: 10.1186/gb-2006-7-8-R72.

[22] Aass C, Norheim I, Eriksen EF, Thorsby PM, Pepaj M. Single unit filter-aided method for fast proteomic analysis of tear fluid. Anal Biochem. 2015 Jul 1;480:1-5. DOI: 10.1016/j.ab.2015.04.002

[23] Herber S, Grus FH, Sabuncuo P, Augustin AJ. Two-dimensional analysis of tear protein patterns of diabetic patients. Electrophoresis. 2001 May;22(9):1838-1844. DOI: 10.1002/1522-2683(200105)22:9<1838::AID-ELPS1838>3.0.CO;2-7.

[24] Azzarolo, AM, Brew, K, Kota, S, Ponomareva, O, Schwartz, J, Zylberberg, C. Presence of tear lipocalin and other major proteins in lacrima fluid of rabits. Comparative biochemistry and physiology Part B: Biochemistry and Molecular Biology. 2004. 138(2): 111-117. https://DOI.org/10.1016/j.cbpc.2004.02.012

[25] Eizirik DL, Tracey DE, Bendtzen K, Sandler S. An interleukin-1 receptor antagonist protein protects insulin-producing beta cells against suppressive effects of interleukin-1 beta. Diabetologia. 1991 Jun;34(6):445-448. DOI: 10.1007/BF00403185.

[26] López-Contreras AK, Martínez-Ruiz MG, Olvera-Montaño C, Robles-Rivera RR, Arévalo-Simental DE, Castellanos-González JA, Hernández-Chávez A, Huerta-Olvera SG, Cardona-Muñoz EG, Rodríguez-Carrizalez AD. Importance of the Use of Oxidative Stress Biomarkers and Inflammatory Profile in Aqueous and Vitreous Humor in Diabetic Retinopathy. Antioxidants (Basel). 2020 Sep 20;9(9):891. DOI: 10.3390/antiox9090891. PMID: 32962301;

[27] Costagliola C, Romano V, De Tollis M, Aceto F, dell'Omo R, Romano MR, Pedicino C, Semeraro F. TNF-alpha levels in tears: a novel biomarker to assess the degree of diabetic retinopathy. Mediators Inflamm. 2013;2013:629529. DOI: 10.1155/2013/629529.

[28] Chiang SY, Tsai ML, Wang CY, Chen A, Chou YC, Hsia CW, Wu YF, Chen HM, Huang TH, Chen PH, Liu HT, Shui HA. Proteomic analysis and identification of aqueous humor proteins with a pathophysiological role in diabetic retinopathy. J Proteomics. 2012 Jun 6;75(10):2950-2959. DOI: 10.1016/j.jprot.2011.12006.

[29] Balaiya S, Zhou Z, Chalam KV. Characterization of Vitreous and Aqueous Proteome in Humans With Proliferative Diabetic Retinopathy and Its Clinical Correlation. Proteomics Insights. 2017 Mar 15;8:117864181 6686078. DOI: 10.1177/11786418166 86078.

[30] Zhang H, Liang L, Huang R, Wu P, He L. Comparison of inflammatory cytokines levels in the aqueous humor with diabetic retinopathy. Int Ophthalmol. 2020 Oct;40(10):2763-2769. DOI: 10.1007/s10792-020-01463-9

[31] Kwon JW, Jee D. Aqueous humor cytokine levels in patients with diabetic macular edema refractory to anti-VEGF treatment. PLoS One. 2018 Sep 11;13(9):e0203408. DOI: 10.1371/journal.pone.0203408

[32] Kajdaniuk D, Marek B, Borgiel-Marek H, Kos-Kudła B. Transforming growth factor β1 (TGFβ1) in physiology and pathology. Endokrynol Pol. 2013;64(5):384-396. DOI: 10.5603/EP.2013.0022.

[33] Sun, H., Li, Z., Hu, W. *et al.* Association of serum and aqueous humor myonectin concentrations with diabetic retinopathy. Sci Rep **11**, 7215 (2021). https://DOI.org/10.1038/s41598-021-86677-2

[34] Zhang J, Hu W, Lin P, Wang R. Decreased serum myonectin concentrations in diabetic nephropathy patients. Clin Exp Med. 2020 Nov;20(4):601-607. DOI: 10.1007/s10238-020-00654-z.

[35] Jeon S, Lee WK. Effect of intravitreal triamcinolone in diabetic macular edema unresponsive to intravitreal bevacizumab. Retina. 2014 Aug;34(8):1606-1611. DOI: 10.1097/IAE.0000000000000109.

[36] Moriarty AP, Spalton DJ, Moriarty BJ, Shilling JS, Ffytche TJ, Bulsara M. Studies of the blood-aqueous barrier in diabetes mellitus. Am J Ophthalmol. 1994 Jun 15;117(6):768-771. DOI: 10.1016/s0002-9394(14) 70320-4.

[37] Funatsu H, Yamashita H, Noma H, Mimura T, Nakamura S, Sakata K, Hori S. Aqueous humor levels of cytokines are related to vitreous levels and progression of diabetic retinopathy in diabetic patients. Graefes Arch Clin Exp Ophthalmol. 2005 Jan;243(1):3-8. DOI: 10.1007/s00417-004-0950-7

[38] Cheung CM, Vania M, Ang M, Chee SP, Li J. Comparison of aqueous humor cytokine and chemokine levels in diabetic patients with and without retinopathy. Mol Vis. 2012;18:830-7. Epub 2012 Apr 4. PMID: 22511846; PMCID: PMC3327438.

[39] Lei J, Ding G, Xie A, Hu Y, Gao N, Fan X. Aqueous humor monocyte chemoattractant protein-1 predicted long-term visual outcome of proliferative diabetic retinopathy undergone intravitreal injection of bevacizumab and vitrectomy. PLoS One. 2021 Mar 5;16(3):e0248235. DOI: 10.1371/journal.pone.0248235.

[40] Sohn HJ, Han DH, Kim IT, Oh IK, Kim KH, Lee DY, Nam DH. Changes in aqueous concentrations of various cytokines after intravitreal triamcinolone versus bevacizumab for diabetic macular edema. Am J Ophthalmol. 2011 Oct;152(4):686-694. DOI: 10.1016/j.ajo.2011.03.033

[41] Podkowinski D, Orlowski-Wimmer E, Zlabinger G, Pollreisz A,

Mursch-Edlmayr AS, Mariacher S, Ring M, Bolz M. Aqueous humour cytokine changes during a loading phase of intravitreal ranibizumab or dexamethasone implant in diabetic macular oedema. Acta Ophthalmol. 2020 Jun;98(4):e407-e415. DOI: 10.1111/aos.14297.

[42] Gao BB, Chen X, Timothy N, Aiello LP, Feener EP. Characterization of the vitreous proteome in diabetes without diabetic retinopathy and diabetes with proliferative diabetic retinopathy. J Proteome Res. 2008 Jun;7(6):2516-2525. DOI: 10.1021/pr800112g

[43] Hernández C, Garcia-Ramírez M, Simó R. Overexpression of hemopexin in the diabetic eye: a new pathogenic candidate for diabetic macular edema. Diabetes Care. 2013 Sep;36(9):2815-2821. DOI: 10.2337/dc12-2634.

[44] Kim JH, Kim JH, Jun HO, Yu YS, Min BH, Park KH, Kim KW. Protective effect of clusterin from oxidative stress-induced apoptosis in human retinal pigment epithelial cells. Invest Ophthalmol Vis Sci. 2010 Jan;51(1):561-566. DOI: 10.1167/iovs.09-3774

[45] Kita T, Clermont AC, Murugesan N, Zhou Q, Fujisawa K, Ishibashi T, Aiello LP, Feener EP. Plasma Kallikrein Kinin System as a VEGF-Independent Mediator of Diabetic Macular Edema. Diabetes. 2015 Oct;64(10):3588-3599. DOI: 10.2337/db15-0317

[46] Loukovaara S, Nurkkala H, Tamene F, Gucciardo E, Liu X, Repo P, Lehti K, Varjosalo M. Quantitative Proteomics Analysis of Vitreous Humor from Diabetic Retinopathy Patients. J Proteome Res. 2015 Dec 4;14(12):5131-5143. DOI: 10.1021/acs.jproteome.5b00900

[47] Zou C, Han C, Zhao M, Yu J, Bai L, Yao Y, Gao S, Cao H, Zheng Z. Change of ranibizumab-induced human vitreous protein profile in patients with proliferative diabetic retinopathy based on proteomics analysis. Clin Proteomics. 2018 Mar 9;15:12. DOI: 10.1186/s12014-018-9187-z.

[48] Wei Q, Zhang T, Jiang R, Chang Q, Zhang Y, Huang X, Gao X, Jin H, Xu G. Vitreous Fibronectin and Fibrinogen Expression Increased in Eyes With Proliferative Diabetic Retinopathy After Intravitreal Anti-VEGF Therapy. Invest Ophthalmol Vis Sci. 2017 Nov 1;58(13):5783-5791. DOI: 10.1167/iovs.17-22345.

[49] Kowluru RA, Odenbach S. Role of interleukin-1β in the pathogenesis of diabetic retinopathy British Journal of Ophthalmology 2004;**88:**1343-1347. http://dx.DOI.org/10.1136/bjo.2003.038133

[50] Ludwig W, Strunk O, Westram R, Richter L, Meier H, Yadhukumar, Buchner A, Lai T, Steppi S, Jobb G, Förster W, Brettske I, Gerber S, Ginhart AW, Gross O, Grumann S, Hermann S, Jost R, König A, Liss T, Lüssmann R, May M, Nonhoff B, Reichel B, Strehlow R, Stamatakis A, Stuckmann N, Vilbig A, Lenke M, Ludwig T, Bode A, Schleifer KH. ARB: a software environment for sequence data. Nucleic Acids Res. 2004 Feb 25;32(4):1363-1371. DOI: 10.1093/nar/gkh293

[51] Demircan N, Safran BG, Soylu M, Ozcan AA, Sizmaz S. Determination of vitreous interleukin-1 (IL-1) and tumour necrosis factor (TNF) levels in proliferative diabetic retinopathy. Eye (Lond). 2006 Dec;20(12):1366-1369. DOI: 10.1038/sj.eye.6702138

[52] Murugeswari P, Shukla D, Kim R, Namperumalsamy P, Stitt AW, Muthukkaruppan V. Angiogenic potential of vitreous from Proliferative Diabetic Retinopathy and Eales' Disease patients. PLoS One. 2014 Oct 13;9(10):e107551. DOI: 10.1371/journal.pone.0107551

[53] El-Ghrably IA, Dua HS, Orr GM, Fischer D, Tighe PJ. Intravitreal invading cells contribute to vitreal cytokine milieu in proliferative vitreoretinopathy. Br J Ophthalmol. 2001 Apr;85(4):461-70. DOI: 10.1136/bjo.85.4.461. PMID: 11264138; PMCID: PMC1723908.

[54] Hernández C, Segura RM, Fonollosa A, Carrasco E, Francisco G, Simó R. Interleukin-8, monocyte chemoattractant protein-1 and IL-10 in the vitreous fluid of patients with proliferative diabetic retinopathy. Diabet Med. 2005 Jun;22(6):719-722. DOI: 10.1111/j.1464-5491.2005.01538.x

[55] Abu El-Asrar AM, Struyf S, Kangave D, Geboes K, Van Damme J. Chemokines in proliferative diabetic retinopathy and proliferative vitreoretinopathy. Eur Cytokine Netw. 2006 Sep;17(3):155-165. PMID: 17194635.

[56] Simó-Servat O, Hernández C, Simó R. Usefulness of the vitreous fluid analysis in the translational research of diabetic retinopathy. Mediators Inflamm. 2012;2012:872978. DOI: 10.1155/2012/872978. Epub 2012 Sep 17. PMID: 23028204; PMCID: PMC3457631

[57] Rangasamy S, McGuire PG, Das A. Diabetic retinopathy and inflammation: novel therapeutic targets. Middle East Afr J Ophthalmol. 2012 Jan;19(1):52-59. DOI: 10.4103/0974-9233.92116

[58] Heather M. Hatch, Donghang Zheng, Marda L. Jorgensen, and Bryon E. Petersen.Cloning and Stem Cells.Dec 2002.339-351.http://DOI.org/10.1089/153623002321025014

[59] Grant MB, Afzal A, Spoerri P, Pan H, Shaw LC, Mames RN. The role of growth factors in the pathogenesis of diabetic retinopathy. Expert Opin Investig Drugs. 2004 Oct;13(10):1275-1293. DOI: 10.1517/13543784.13.10.1275.

[60] Butler JM, Guthrie SM, Koc M, Afzal A, Caballero S, Brooks HL, Mames RN, Segal MS, Grant MB, Scott EW. SDF-1 is both necessary and sufficient to promote proliferative retinopathy. J Clin Invest. 2005 Jan;115(1):86-93. DOI: 10.1172/JCI22869.

[61] El-Asrar AM, Nawaz MI, Kangave D, Geboes K, Ola MS, Ahmad S, Al-Shabrawey M. High-mobility group box-1 and biomarkers of inflammation in the vitreous from patients with proliferative diabetic retinopathy. Mol Vis. 2011;17:1829-38. Epub 2011 Jul 6. PMID: 21850157; PMCID: PMC3137555.

[62] El-Asrar AM. Role of inflammation in the pathogenesis of diabetic retinopathy. Middle East Afr J Ophthalmol. 2012 Jan;19(1):70-74. DOI: 10.4103/0974-9233.92118.

[63] Noda K, Nakao S, Ishida S, Ishibashi T. Leukocyte adhesion molecules in diabetic retinopathy. J Ophthalmol. 2012;2012:279037. DOI: 10.1155/2012/279037. Epub 2011 Nov 2. PMID: 22132315; PMCID: PMC3216271.

[64] Murata M, Noda K, Fukuhara J, Kanda A, Kase S, Saito W, Ozawa Y, Mochizuki S, Kimura S, Mashima Y, Okada Y, Ishida S. Soluble vascular adhesion protein-1 accumulates in proliferative diabetic retinopathy. Invest Ophthalmol Vis Sci. 2012 Jun 26;53(7):4055-4062. DOI: 10.1167/iovs.12-9857.

[65] Yoshitake, T., Murakami, T., Suzuma, K. *et al.* Hyperreflective Foci in the Outer Retinal Layers as a Predictor of the Functional Efficacy of Ranibizumab for Diabetic Macular Edema. Sci Rep **10**, 873 (2020). https://DOI.org/10.1038/s41598-020-57646-y

[66] Vujosevic, S., Bini, S., Midena, G., Berton, M., Pilotto, E, Midena, E. Hyperreflective Intraretinal Spots in Diabetics without and with Nonproliferative Diabetic Retinopathy:

An *In Vivo* Study Using Spectral Domain OCT. Journal of Diabetes research. 2013. https://DOI.org/10.1155/2013/491835

[67] Markan A, Agarwal A, Arora A, Bazgain K, Rana V, Gupta V. Novel imaging biomarkers in diabetic retinopathy and diabetic macular edema. Ther Adv Ophthalmol. 2020 Sep 4;12:2515841420950513. DOI: 10.1177/2515841420950513. PMID: 32954207; PMCID: PMC7475787.

[68] Lee H, Jang H, Choi YA, Kim HC, Chung H. Association Between Soluble CD14 in the Aqueous Humor and Hyperreflective Foci on Optical Coherence Tomography in Patients With Diabetic Macular Edema. Invest Ophthalmol Vis Sci. 2018 Feb 1;59(2):715-721. DOI: 10.1167/iovs.17-23042.

[69] Liu S, Wang D, Chen F, Zhang X. Hyperreflective foci in OCT image as a biomarker of poor prognosis in diabetic macular edema patients treating with Conbercept in China. BMC Ophthalmol. 2019 Jul 23;19(1):157. DOI: 10.1186/s12886-019-1168-0.

[70] Bolz M, Schmidt-Erfurth U, Deak G, Mylonas G, Kriechbaum K, Scholda C; Diabetic Retinopathy Research Group Vienna. Optical coherence tomographic hyperreflective foci: a morphologic sign of lipid extravasation in diabetic macular edema. Ophthalmology. 2009 May;116(5):914-920. DOI: 10.1016/j.ophtha.2008.12.039.

[71] Uji A, Murakami T, Nishijima K, Akagi T, Horii T, Arakawa N, Muraoka Y, Ellabban AA, Yoshimura N. Association between hyperreflective foci in the outer retina, status of photoreceptor layer, and visual acuity in diabetic macular edema. Am J Ophthalmol. 2012 Apr;153(4):710-7, 717.e1. DOI: 10.1016/j.ajo.2011.08.041.

[72] Midena E, Pilotto E, Bini S. Hyperreflective Intraretinal Foci as an OCT Biomarker of Retinal Inflammation in Diabetic Macular Edema. Invest Ophthalmol Vis Sci. 2018 Nov 1;59(13):5366. DOI: 10.1167/iovs.18-25611.

[73] Giocanti-Aurégan A, Hrarat L, Qu LM, Sarda V, Boubaya M, Levy V, Chaine G, Fajnkuchen F. Functional and Anatomical Outcomes in Patients With Serous Retinal Detachment in Diabetic Macular Edema Treated With Ranibizumab. Invest Ophthalmol Vis Sci. 2017 Feb 1;58(2):797-800. DOI: 10.1167/iovs.16-20855.

[74] Bianca Gerendas, Christian Simader, Gabor Gy Deak, Sonja Gudrun Prager, Jan Lammer, Sebastian M Waldstein, Michael Kundi, Ursula Schmidt-Erfurth; Morphological parameters relevant for visual and anatomic outcomes during anti-VEGF therapy of diabetic macular edema in the RESTORE trial. Invest. Ophthalmol. Vis. Sci. 2014;55(13):1791

[75] Sophie R, Lu N, Campochiaro PA. Predictors of Functional and Anatomic Outcomes in Patients with Diabetic Macular Edema Treated with Ranibizumab. Ophthalmology. 2015 Jul;122(7):1395-1401. DOI: 10.1016/j.ophtha.2015.02.036.

[76] Sonoda S, Sakamoto T, Yamashita T, Shirasawa M, Otsuka H, Sonoda Y. Retinal morphologic changes and concentrations of cytokines in eyes with diabetic macular edema. Retina. 2014;34(4):741-748. DOI: 10.1097/IAE.0b013e3182a48917.

[77] Sonoda S, Sakamoto T, Shirasawa M, Yamashita T, Otsuka H, Terasaki H. Correlation between reflectivity of subretinal fluid in OCT images and concentration of intravitreal VEGF in eyes with diabetic macular edema. Invest Ophthalmol Vis Sci. 2013 Aug 9;54(8):5367-5374. DOI: 10.1167/iovs.13-12382.

[78] Vujosevic S, Torresin T, Berton M, Bini S, Convento E, Midena E. Diabetic

Macular Edema With and Without Subfoveal Neuroretinal Detachment: Two Different Morphologic and Functional Entities. Am J Ophthalmol. 2017 Sep;181:149-155. DOI: 10.1016/j.ajo.2017.06.026.

[79] De Benedetto U, Sacconi R, Pierro L, Lattanzio R, Bandello F. Optical coherence tomographic hyperreflective foci in early stages of diabetic retinopathy. Retina. 2015 Mar;35(3):449-453. DOI: 10.1097/IAE.0000000000000336

[80] Zhu D, Zhu H, Wang C, Yang D. Intraocular soluble intracellular adhesion molecule-1 correlates with subretinal fluid height of diabetic macular edema. Indian J Ophthalmol. 2014 Mar;62(3):295-298. DOI: 10.4103/0301-4738.111184.

[81] Moon BG, Lee JY, Yu HG, Song JH, Park YH, Kim HW, Ji YS, Chang W, Lee JE, Oh J, Chung I. Efficacy and Safety of a Dexamethasone Implant in Patients with Diabetic Macular Edema at Tertiary Centers in Korea. J Ophthalmol. 2016;2016:9810270. DOI: 10.1155/2016/9810270

[82] Vujosevic S, Toma C, Villani E, Muraca A, Torti E, Florimbi G, Leporati F, Brambilla M, Nucci P, De Cilla' S. Diabetic macular edema with neuroretinal detachment: OCT and OCT-angiography biomarkers of treatment response to anti-VEGF and steroids. Acta Diabetol. 2020 Mar;57(3):287-296. DOI: 10.1007/s00592-019-01424-4.

[83] Damian I, Nicoara, SD. Optical coherence tomography biomarkers of the outer blood-retina barrier in patients with diabetic macular oedema. Journal of Diabetes research. 2020; article ID 8880586. DOI: 10.1155/2020/8880586.

[84] Roy R, Saurabh K, Shah D, Chowdhury M, Goel S. Choroidal Hyperreflective Foci: A Novel Spectral Domain Optical Coherence Tomography Biomarker in Eyes With Diabetic Macular Edema. Asia Pac J Ophthalmol (Phila). 2019 Jul-Aug;8(4):314-318. DOI: 10.1097/APO.0000000000000249

[85] E. M. Hartnett, A. Lappas, D. Darland, J. R. McColm, S. Lovejoy, and P. A. D'Amore, "Retinal pigment epithelium and endothelial cell interaction causes retinal pigment epithelial barrier dysfunction via a soluble VEGF-dependent mechanism," Experimental Eye Research, vol. 77, no. 5, pp. 593-599,2003.)

[86] Damian I, Roman G, Nicoara, SD. Analysis of the choroid and its relationship with the outer retina in patients with diabetes mellitus using binarization techniques based on spectral-domain optical coherence tomography. J. Clin. Med. 2021: 10,210. DOI: 10.3390/jcm10020210.

[87] Liang MC, Vora RA, Duker JS, Reichel E. Solid-appearing retinal cysts in diabetic macular edema: a novel optical coherence tomography finding. Retin Cases Brief Rep. 2013 Summer;7(3):255-258. DOI: 10.1097/ICB.0b013e31828eef49

[88] Jonas JB, Hayler JK, Söfker A, Panda-Jonas S. Intravitreal injection of crystalline cortisone as adjunctive treatment of proliferative diabetic retinopathy. Am J Ophthalmol. 2001 Apr;131(4):468-471. DOI: 10.1016/s0002-9394(00)00882-5.

[89] Cunningham MA, Edelman JL, Kaushal S. Intravitreal steroids for macular edema: the past, the present, and the future. Surv Ophthalmol. 2008 Mar-Apr;53(2):139-149. DOI: 10.1016/j.survophthal.2007.12.005

[90] Tamura H, Miyamoto K, Kiryu J, Miyahara S, Katsuta H, Hirose F, Musashi K, Yoshimura N. Intravitreal injection of corticosteroid attenuates leukostasis and vascular leakage in

experimental diabetic retina. Invest Ophthalmol Vis Sci. 2005 Apr;46(4):1440-4. DOI: 10.1167/iovs.04-0905.

[91] Amoaku WM, Saker S, Stewart EA. A review of therapies for diabetic macular oedema and rationale for combination therapy. Eye (Lond). 2015 Sep;29(9):1115-1130. DOI: 10.1038/eye.2015.110

[92] Zur D, Iglicki M, Busch C, Invernizzi A, Mariussi M, Loewenstein A; International Retina Group. OCT Biomarkers as Functional Outcome Predictors in Diabetic Macular Edema Treated with Dexamethasone Implant. Ophthalmology. 2018 Feb;125(2):267-275. DOI: 10.1016/j.ophtha.2017.08.031

[93] Shimura M, Yasuda K, Nakazawa T, Hirano Y, Sakamoto T, Ogura Y, Shiono T. Visual outcome after intravitreal triamcinolone acetonide depends on optical coherence tomographic patterns in patients with diffuse diabetic macular edema. Retina. 2011 Apr;31(4):748-754. DOI: 10.1097/IAE.0b013e3181f04991.

[94] Reichenbach A, Wurm A, Pannicke T, Iandiev I, Wiedemann P, Bringmann A. Müller cells as players in retinal degeneration and edema. Graefes Arch Clin Exp Ophthalmol. 2007 May;245(5):627-636. DOI: 10.1007/s00417-006-0516-y

[95] Liu Q, Hu Y, Yu H, Yuan L, Hu J, Atik A, Guan M, Li D, Li X, Tang S. Comparison of intravitreal triamcinolone acetonide versus intravitreal bevacizumab as the primary treatment of clinically significant macular edema. Retina. 2015 Feb;35(2):272-279. DOI: 10.1097/IAE.0000000000000300.

[96] Wang D, DuBois RN. Pro-inflammatory prostaglandins and progression of colorectal cancer. Cancer Lett. 2008 Aug 28;267(2):197-203. DOI: 10.1016/j.canlet.2008.03.004. Epub 2008 Apr 11. PMID: 18406516; PMCID: PMC2553688.

[97] Ayalasomayajula SP, Amrite AC, Kompella UB. Inhibition of cyclooxygenase-2, but not cyclooxygenase-1, reduces prostaglandin E2 secretion from diabetic rat retinas. Eur J Pharmacol. 2004 Sep 13;498(1-3):275-278. DOI: 10.1016/j.ejphar.2004.07.046.

[98] Ayalasomayajula SP, Kompella UB. Celecoxib, a selective cyclooxygenase-2 inhibitor, inhibits retinal vascular endothelial growth factor expression and vascular leakage in a streptozotocin-induced diabetic rat model. Eur J Pharmacol. 2003 Jan 5;458(3):283-289. DOI: 10.1016/s0014-2999(02)02793-0

[99] Sun W, Gerhardinger C, Dagher Z, Hoehn T, Lorenzi M. Aspirin at low-intermediate concentrations protects retinal vessels in experimental diabetic retinopathy through non-platelet-mediated effects. Diabetes. 2005 Dec;54(12):3418-3426. DOI: 10.2337/diabetes.54.12.3418

[100] Zheng L, Howell SJ, Hatala DA, Huang K, Kern TS. Salicylate-based anti-inflammatory drugs inhibit the early lesion of diabetic retinopathy. Diabetes. 2007 Feb;56(2):337-345. DOI: 10.2337/db06-0789.

[101] Amrite AC, Ayalasomayajula SP, Cheruvu NP, Kompella UB. Single periocular injection of celecoxib-PLGA microparticles inhibits diabetes-induced elevations in retinal PGE2, VEGF, and vascular leakage. Invest Ophthalmol Vis Sci. 2006 Mar;47(3):1149-1160. DOI: 10.1167/iovs.05-0531

[102] Effects of aspirin treatment on diabetic retinopathy. ETDRS report number 8. Early Treatment Diabetic Retinopathy Study Research Group. Ophthalmology. 1991 May;98(5 Suppl):757-65. PMID: 2062511

[103] Effect of aspirin alone and aspirin plus dipyridamole in early diabetic retinopathy. A multicenter randomized controlled clinical trial. The DAMAD Study Group. Diabetes. 1989 Apr;38(4):491-8. PMID: 2647556.

[104] Kim SJ, Flach AJ, Jampol LM. Nonsteroidal anti-inflammatory drugs in ophthalmology. Surv Ophthalmol. 2010 Mar-Apr;55(2):108-133. DOI: 10.1016/j.survophthal.2009.07.005

[105] Kern TS, Miller CM, Du Y, Zheng L, Mohr S, Ball SL, Kim M, Jamison JA, Bingaman DP. Topical administration of nepafenac inhibits diabetes-induced retinal microvascular disease and underlying abnormalities of retinal metabolism and physiology. Diabetes. 2007 Feb;56(2):373-379. DOI: 10.2337/db05-1621.

[106] Rao VR, Prescott E, Shelke NB, Trivedi R, Thomas P, Struble C, Gadek T, O'Neill CA, Kompella UB. Delivery of SAR 1118 to the retina via ophthalmic drops and its effectiveness in a rat streptozotocin (STZ) model of diabetic retinopathy (DR). Invest Ophthalmol Vis Sci. 2010 Oct;51(10):5198-204. DOI: 10.1167/iovs.09-5144. Epub 2010 May 5. PMID: 20445119; PMCID: PMC3066602.

[107] Sfikakis PP, Markomichelakis N, Theodossiadis GP, Grigoropoulos V, Katsilambros N, Theodossiadis PG. Regression of sight-threatening macular edema in type 2 diabetes following treatment with the anti-tumor necrosis factor monoclonal antibody infliximab. Diabetes Care. 2005 Feb;28(2):445-447. DOI: 10.2337/diacare.28.2.445.

[108] Iliaki E, Poulaki V, Mitsiades N, Mitsiades CS, Miller JW, Gragoudas ES. Role of alpha 4 integrin (CD49d) in the pathogenesis of diabetic retinopathy. Invest Ophthalmol Vis Sci. 2009 Oct;50(10):4898-4904. DOI: 10.1167/iovs.08-2013.

[109] Kowluru RA, Tang J, Kern TS. Abnormalities of retinal metabolism in diabetes and experimental galactosemia. VII. Effect of long-term administration of antioxidants on the development of retinopathy. Diabetes. 2001 Aug;50(8):1938-1942. DOI: 10.2337/diabetes.50.8.1938

[110] Bursell SE, King GL. Can protein kinase C inhibition and vitamin E prevent the development of diabetic vascular complications? Diabetes Res Clin Pract. 1999 Sep;45(2-3):169-182. DOI: 10.1016/s0168-8227(99)00047-9.

[111] Barile GR, Pachydaki SI, Tari SR, Lee SE, Donmoyer CM, Ma W, Rong LL, Buciarelli LG, Wendt T, Hörig H, Hudson BI, Qu W, Weinberg AD, Yan SF, Schmidt AM. The RAGE axis in early diabetic retinopathy. Invest Ophthalmol Vis Sci. 2005 Aug;46(8):2916-2924. DOI: 10.1167/iovs.04-1409

[112] Mauer M, Zinman B, Gardiner R, Suissa S, Sinaiko A, Strand T, Drummond K, Donnelly S, Goodyer P, Gubler MC, Klein R. Renal and retinal effects of enalapril and losartan in type 1 diabetes. N Engl J Med. 2009 Jul 2;361(1):40-51. DOI: 10.1056/NEJMoa0808400.

[113] Nagai N, Izumi-Nagai K, Oike Y, Koto T, Satofuka S, Ozawa Y, Yamashiro K, Inoue M, Tsubota K, Umezawa K, Ishida S. Suppression of diabetes-induced retinal inflammation by blocking the angiotensin II type 1 receptor or its downstream nuclear factor-kappaB pathway. Invest Ophthalmol Vis Sci. 2007 Sep;48(9):4342-4350. DOI: 10.1167/iovs.06-1473. PMID: 17724226.

[114] Sun JK, Maturi RK, Boyer DS, Wells JA, Gonzalez VH, Tansley R, Hernandez H, Maetzel A, Feener EP, Aiello LP. One-Time Intravitreal Injection of KVD001, a Plasma Kallikrein Inhibitor, in Patients with

Central-Involved Diabetic Macular Edema and Reduced Vision: An Open-Label Phase 1B Study. Ophthalmol Retina. 2019 Dec;3(12):1107-1109. DOI: 10.1016/j.oret.2019.07.006

[115] Study of the Intravitreal Plasma Kallikrein Inhibitor, KVD001, in Subjects With Center-involving Diabetic Macular Edema (ciDME). [Internet]. 2020. Available from: https://clinicaltrials.gov/ct2/show/results/NCT03466099. [Accessed: 2021-07-27]

[116] KalVista for DME. [Internet] Available from: https://www.kalvista.com/products-pipeline/kalvista-dme [Accessed: 2021-07-27

[117] Results of a Phase 1, Open-Label, Dose-Escalation Study of THR-149 for the Treatment of DME. [Internet]. 2019. Available from: https://www.oxurion.com/sites/default/files/THR-149-001_%20Retina%20Society%20PDugel_15Sep2019.pdf[Accessed: 2021-07-27]

Chapter 5

Role of Lipid, Protein-Derived Toxic Molecules, and Deficiency of Antioxidants behind the Pathogenesis of Diabetic Retinopathy (DR) in Type 2 Diabetes Mellitus

Subhasish Pramanik, Lakshmi Kanta Mondal, Subhankar Chowdhury, Chiranjit Bose, Debgopal Bera and Koena Bhattacharjee

Abstract

To determine the role of NADPH-oxidase mediated formation of different lipid, protein-derived molecules, and depletion of vitamin-C level in vitreous behind the endothelial dysfunction-induced vascular endothelial growth factor secretion and pathogenesis of diabetic retinopathy (DR) in type 2 diabetes mellitus (T2DM). Fourteen T2DM patients with mild non-proliferative diabetic retinopathy (MNPDR), 11 patients without diabetic retinopathy (DNR), 17 T2 DM subjects with high-risk proliferative diabetic retinopathy (HRPDR), and 5 healthy individuals without DM underwent vitreous analysis for estimation NADPH oxidase, lipid peroxide like malondialdehyde (MDA), 4-Hydroxy-noneal (HNE) and advanced lipoxidation end product (ALE) like Hexanoyl-lysine (HLY), protein carbonyl compound (PCC), Vitamin-C and concentration of vascular endothelial growth factor (VEGF) secretion following standard spectrophotometric methods and enzyme-linked immunosorbent assay (ELISA). Vitreous concentration of NADPH-oxidase, different protein and lipid-derived molecule, and VEGF were found to be significantly elevated among DNR and of DR subjects with different grades compared to HC subjects whereasthe vitamin-C level was found to be decreased among different DR subjects and DNR subjects in comparison to healthy individuals. Oxidative stress-mediated lipid and protein-derived biomolecules not only add important mediators in the pathogenesis of DR, but also accelerate the progression and severity of microangiopathy.

Keywords: Diabetic retinopathy, NADPH-oxidase, Lipid peroxide, advanced lipoxidation end product, protein carbonyl compound

1. Introduction

Despite remarkable advances in diagnosis and treatment, diabetic retinopathy (DR), the most frequently occurring complication causing vision loss in working population, is becoming the burning social problem. Two landmark studies have established that hyperglycemia is the principal contributing factor to the development of the disease, though a reasonable portion of diabetic subjects develops this complication in spite of good control of blood sugar [1–3]. In a large densely populated country like India, where strict control of hyperglycemia is far from reality due to lack of clinic adherence, bad economy and illiteracy. Here, principal diet is carbohydrate since childhood. Enormous intracellular glucose in tissues including retina where glucose transport is insulin independent, overwhelms the glycolysis and citric acid cycle owing to gradual deficiency of oxidized cofactors i.e. nicotinamide adenine dinucleotide (NAD), flavin adenine dinucleotide (FAD), thiamine pyrophosphate (TPP), Coenzyme A and lipoate. The essential vitamins, the precursors of these factors could not be provided with only carbohydrates [4]. Unutilized glucose is diverted to anomalous biochemical pathways like sorbitol pathway, and advanced glycation end products formation [5]. Hexose monophosphate shunt (HMP-shunt) or pentose phosphate pathway (PPP) take-up glucose-6-phosphate for its catabolism and produces specialized products like pentose ribose 5-phosphate to make RNA, DNA, and NADPH for reductive synthesis e.g. reduced glutathione peroxidase and fatty acids, the building blocks of lipid structure.

Beside reductive biosynthesis, NADPH carries life-saving roles to counter the damaging effects of oxygen radicals on erythrocytes, cells of lens, cornea and retina. Retina is a tissue where renewal of outer segment of photoreceptors is continuously going on in one side and other side shows light and oxygen induced death of cells as an inevitable phenomenon caused by oxidative stress.

Poorly controlled glycemia and lack of proper metabolism of glucose mainly result in formation and accumulation of advanced glycation end products (AGEs) and reactive oxygen species (ROS) which in turn cause microvascular endothelial cell dysfunction by oxidative modifications of membrane proteins and lipids [6]. Production of advanced lipoxidation end products (ALEs) during peroxidative damage of lipids may be the important source of protein modification by covalent bonding with catalytic site. Circulating AGEs and ALEs exert their detrimental effects through interactions with their cell surface receptor for AGE (RAGE) leading to post receptor activation of reduced nicotinamide adenine dinucleotide phosphate (NADPH) oxidase in endothelial cells, mesangial cells and macrophases [7]. Activation and subsequent uncoupling of NADPH oxidase is coupled with increased formation of intracellular reactive oxygen species. Activation of this system also follows the other pathways which suggest increased production of intermediate of faster glycolysis e.g. glycerol 3-phosphate derived inositol triphosphate and diacylglycerol. Inositol triphosphate mediates a transient increase in the level of cytosolic Ca^{++} which is essential for activation of NADPH oxidase and induction respiratoy burst e.g. generation of large amounts of superoxide anion, hydroxyl anion, and hydrogen peroxide [8].

Diacylglycerol (DAG) induces the translocation of protein kinase C (PKC) into plasma membrane from cytosol, where it catalyzes the phosphorylation of various proteins including the components of NADPH oxidase, and thus activates this system [9].

Beside structural modifications of retinal membrane, AGEs and ALEs invite up regulation of inflammatory mediators and adhesion molecules in capillary beds which cause apoptosis of endothelial cell and breakdown of tight junctions of blood-retinal barrier [10]. Active vitamin C is ascorbic acid and acts as a donor of reducing equivalents which is capable of reducing compounds as molecular oxygen, nitrate and cytochromes a and c. This ascorbic acid acts as a water soluble antioxidant reduce oxidized tocopherol in lipid membranes [11]. Such vitamin is also required for hydroxylation of amino acids, proline and lysine in the synthesis of collagen [12]. So, deficiency of vitamin C leading to defective collagen synthesis and accumulation of reactive carbonyl compounds due to oxidative stress results in fragility of retinal capillary membranes and enhancement of break-down of inner blood-retinal barrier. In this study we attempted to determine the accompanying role of different lipid derived toxic molecules and deficiency of antioxidant in the pathogenesis of an inflammatory disease, DR.

2. Methodology

A number of 17 subjects with high-risk proliferative diabetic retinopathy (HRPDR), 14 subjects with mild non-proliferative DR (MNPDR), 11 age and gender-matched diabetic subjects without clinically evident retinopathy (DNR), and 5 healthy controls (HCs), whose clinical condition independently indicated for vitrectomy were enrolled in the present cross-sectional study. Subjects with hypertension (systolic BP > 140 mm Hg and or diastolic BP > 90 mm Hg), cardiovascular diseases, neuropathy (assessed by Michigan Neuropathy Screening Instrument), nephropathy (serum creatinine level > 1.5 mg/dl and or urinary albumin creatinine ratio 300 μg/mg), deficiency of B vitamins, any other ocular diseases (glaucoma, optic neuropathy, cataract, branch retinal vein occlusion, and Eales disease) were excluded from the study. The subjects were chosen consecutively from the 'Outdoor Patient Department' of 'Regional Institute of Ophthalmology, Calcutta Medical College, West Bengal, and Kolkata, India. The institutional ethical committee was approved the study and informed consent was collected from all the study subjects according to the Helsinki guideline.

Subjects with type 2 DM were diagnosed according to the guideline of the American Diabetes Association (2010). The fasting plasma glucose (FPG), postprandial plasma glucose (PPG), and glycated hemoglobin (HbA1c %) levels were used for the assessment of the glycaemic status of each subject. None of the study subjects were taking insulin or lipid-lowering drugs during the study period.

2.1 Comprehensive ophthalmological examinations

The subjects enrolled in the study had undergone different ophthalmological examinations which included slit-lamp biomicroscopy (by ±90 diopters and Goldman 3 mirror lens), seven fields of digital fundus photography with fluorescein angiography, and spectral-domain optical coherence tomography (SD-OCT). Visual functions were evaluated by measuring VA. The subjects with different grades of DR were diagnosed according to the modified guideline of 'Early Treatment of Diabetic Retinopathy Study' [13].

2.2 Collection of vitreous sample

Vitreous samples from study subjects were drawn by 3-port parsplana vitrectomy during surgery of vitreous hemorrhage, of idiopathic macular hole or removal of a dropped nucleus which occurred accidentally after blunt trauma. Vitreous was also collected during management of preoperative complication of phacoemulsification. Undiluted vitreous gel (500 μL) was excised from midvitreous by vitreous cutter and carefully aspirated into the hand-held sterile syringe attached to the suction port of the vitrectomy probe. Immediately after collection, the vitreous samples were taken in micro centrifuged tube and centrifuged at 3000 rpm for 5 minutes. The clear solution without any precipitate was then collected in another tube and preserved in - 80° C for farther use.

2.3 Measurement of NADPH oxidase activity

NADPH oxidase activity was measured in vitreous using Nitrobluetetrazolium (NBT) as the substrate. Briefly, 100 μl plasma/ vitreous was mixed with NBT (4 mg/ml in water) and incubated for 20 minutes at 37°C. 1 M HCl was used to terminate the reaction. Then the samples were centrifuged at 3500 rpm for 5 minutes. 400 μl Dimethylsulfoxide (DMSO) was added to form a stable triphenylmethyl ester whose absorbance was measured at 550 nm using a microplate reader (MerilyzerEiaquant, Meril Diagnostics Pvt. Ltd., Vapi, Gujarat). OD 550 is directly proportional to NADPH oxidase activity [14].

2.4 Measurement of vitamin C level

Vitamin C level was measured by the protocol of Kyaw et al. [15]. Briefly, the colored reagent was prepared using Sodium Tungstate, DisodiumHydrogen Phosphate, H_2SO_4 and distilled water. Plasma/vitreous sample (1 ml) was thoroughlymixed with 2 ml colored reagent. After 30 minutes incubation at room temperature (RT) the tubes were centrifuged at 3000 pm for 10 minutes. The absorbance was measured at 700 nm from the supernatant, without disturbing the precipitate. Standard curve was prepared using oxalic acid and distilled water is used as substrate blank in the experiment. The vitamin C concentration in samples was expressed in mg/dl.

2.5 Measurement of protein carbonylation (PCC)

Protein carbonylation was measured from vitreous by spectrophotometric method by protein derivatization with 2, 4-dinitrophenyl-hydrazine (DNPH). Briefly, protein lysates from vitreous (50 μl) were incubated in dark for 30 minutes with DNPH (10 mM in 2 N HCl, 100 μl). After that TCA (20%, 100 μl) was used to precipitate proteins and free DNPH was removed by washing with ethanol-ethyl acetate (1:1). The resultant pellet was dissolved in 350 μl of sodium dodecyl sulfate (2% SDS) and protein-hydrazone complex's absorbance was measured at 370 nm using spectrophotometer. The carbonyl concentration was calculated using the extinction coefficient of the protein-hydrazone complex (22,000 M^{-1} cm^{-1}) from the specific absorption (relative to the reagent blank). The final concentration was expressed as nanomoles of carbonyl groups per milligram protein [16–18].

2.6 Estimation of malondialdehyde (MDA)

The MDA level in vitreous was measured by thiobarbituric acid (TBA) assay method. In the assay procedure, the plasma samples were first reacted with trichloroacetic acid (TCA) to remove proteins. Then chromogenic adducts of MDA was precipitated using TBA. Finally the precipitated MDA was extracted using n-butyl alcohol, by vigorous shaking. Then the chromogenic adduct was measured spectrophotometrically at 532 nm; the results were expressed as mM/L [19].

2.7 Measurement of HNE

Human vitreous HNE was estimated by competitive inhibition enzyme immunoassay technique (ELISA) using research kit from CUSABIO (cat no: CSB-E16214h). In the assay, an antibody specific for human HNE was coated on the well plate. A series of standards ranging from 39 pg/ml to 2500 pg/ml and samples (vitreous samples were run in 5 fold diluted form respectively) were added into the wells with Horseradish Peroxide (HRP) conjugated HNE. The competitive inhibition reaction was launched between HRP conjugated HNE and HNE in the samples. Then a substrate solution was added to the wells and the color developed is inversely proportional to the amount of HNE in the sample. The color development was stopped using stop solution and the intensity of the color was measured colorimetrically by using 450 nm filter in an ELISA plate reader MerilyzerEiaquant (Meril Diagnostics Pvt. Ltd., Vapi, Gujarat).

2.8 Measurement of HLY

Human vitreous HLY was estimated also by competitive enzyme immunoassay technique using commercial kits (MyBiosource, Catalog no: MBS753480) and utilizing a polyclonal anti-HLY antibody and an HLY-HRP conjugate. At first the assay sample and buffer were incubated together with HLY-HRP conjugate in pre-coated plate for one hour. After the incubation period, the wells were decanted and washed five times. The wells were then incubated with a substrate for HRP enzyme. The product of the enzyme-substrate reaction forms a blue colored complex. Then, a stop solution was added to stop the reaction, which will then turn the solution yellow. The intensity of color was measured spectrophotometrically at 450 nm in a microplate reader. The intensity of the color was inversely proportional to the HLY concentration present in the sample. A standard curve was also plotted relating the intensity of the color (or O.D.) to the concentration of standards. The HLY concentration in each sample was interpolated from this standard curve.

2.9 Measurement of VEGF

Human vitreous VEGF was estimated by sandwich enzyme-linked immune sorbent assay (ELISA) method using Ray Biotech kit (cat no: ELH-VEGF-001, Norcross USA). In the assay, an antibody specific for human VEGF was coated on the well plate. A series of standards ranging from 8.23 pg/ml to 6000 pg/ml and samples (vitreous samples were run in a half diluted form respectively) were added into the wells. VEGF protein present in the sample was bound to the wells by the immobilized antibody. The wells were washed and a biotinylated anti-human VEGF antibody was added. After buffer washing, HRP –conjugated streptavidin was pipette to wash and TMB substrate solution was added into the wells and was placed in incubation at room temperature for 30 minutes. The intensity of the final color product was proportional to the concentration of VEGF protein present in the samples and absorbance of the color product was measured colorimetrically by using 450 nm filter in an ELISA plate reader MerilyzerEiaquant (Meril Diagnostics Pvt. Ltd., Vapi, Gujarat). The concentration of VEGF was determined by a standard curve and the assay detects less than 10 pg/ml of VEGF from the sample.

3. Results

As shown in the **Table 1**, different study groups enrolled in the present study showed no statistically significant differences for age, gender distributions, body

Parameters		HC (N = 5)	DNR (N = 11)	MNPDR (N=14)	HRPDR (N = 17)	p value
Age (years)		52.00 ± 7.48	51.29 ± 5.46	52.64 ± 2.853	50.94 ± 7.45	0.905
Gender	M	3(60%)	6(54.54%)	7(50%)	8(47.05%)	0.954
	F	2(40%)	5(45.45%)	7(50%)	9(52.94%)	
BMI (kg/m^2)		23.30 ± 3.54	25.15 ± 2.183	26.61 ± 4.349	23.15 ± 6.54	0.439
Duration of DM (years)		------	10.14 ± 5.16	11.19 ± 4.35	11.27 ± 3.80	0.484
Glycaemic Status	FPG (mg/dl)	80.46 ± 8.48	153.5 ± 9.55*	159.3 ± 28.50††	154.9 ± 16.11$^{!!!!}$	0.0001
	PPG (mg/dl)	118.2 ± 11.19	182.0 ± 33.00*	193.5 ± 62.14††	218.4 ± 32.16$^{!!}$	0.005
	HbA1C (%)	4.81 ± 0.290	7.61 ± 0.476*	8.43 ± 1.117†††	7.78 ± 1.102$^{!}$	0.002

HC, healthy control; DNR, diabetic subjects without clinically evident retinopathy, MNPDR, early non-proliferative diabetic retinopathy; HRPDR, high-risk proliferative diabetic retinopathy; BMI, body mass index; FPG, fasting plasma glucose, PPG, postprandial plasma glucose; HbA1C, glycated haemoglobin. The Kruskal Wallis nonparametric ANOVA followed by Dunn's multiple comparisons test was administrated to find out significant differences between the groups. A value of p < 0.05 was considered as statistically significant.
*HC vs DNR, p < 0.05.
†††HC vs MNPDR, p < 001.
††HC vs MNPDR, p < 0.01.
$^{!!!!}$HC vs HRPDR, p < 0001.
$^{!!}$HC vs HRPDR, p < 0.01.
$^{!}$, HC vs HRPDR, p < 0.05.

Table 1.
Demographic and clinical characteristics of study subjects.

mass index (BMI), and duration of diabetes, systolic and diastolic blood pressure. Glycaemic parameters like FPG level were found to be increased significantly in the DNR ($p < 0.05$), MNPDR ($p < 0.01$), and HRPDR ($p < 0.01$) subjects compared to the HCs. Similarly, the PPG level were found to be increased significantly in the DNR ($p < 0.05$), MNPDR ($p < 0.01$), and HRPDR ($p < 0.0001$) subjects compared to the HCs. Regarding, HbA1C DNR ($p < 0.05$), MNPDR ($p < 0.001$), and HRPDR ($p < 0.05$) subjects showed significantly higher values of HbA1c compared to HCs. However, statistical analysis showed no significant differences in FPG, PPG, and HbA1C levels between DNR, MNPDR, and HRPDR subjects.

Vitreous NADPH oxidase activity was found to be increased significantly among DNR (0.217 ± 0.031 OD_{550}/100 μL, vitreous, $p < 0.0001$), MNPDR (0.286 ± 0.033 OD_{550}/100 μL, vitreous, $p < 0.0001$), and HRPDR (0.365 ± 0.032 OD_{550}/100 μL, vitreous, $p < 0.0001$) subjects compared to HC (0.121 ± 0.018 OD_{550}/100 μL, vitreous) subjects. Again, both the MNPDR ($p < 0.01$) and HRPDR subjects ($p < 0.0001$) showed significantly higher level of NADPH oxidase than DNRs. Further, the HRPDR subjects showed a higher NADPH oxidase level ($p < 0.0001$) than the former (**Figure 1A**).

Regarding vitamin-C concentration in vitreous, the DNR (0.807 ± 0.043 mg/dl, $p < 0.01$), MNPDR (0.874 ± 0.061 mg/dl, $p < 0.0001$), and HRPDR (0.970 ± 0.110 mg/dl, $p < 0.0001$) subjects showed lower vitamin-C level compared to HC (0.682 ± 0.038 mg/dl) subjects. Again, both the MNPDR ($p < 0.05$) and HRPDR subjects ($p < 0.0001$) showed significantly lower level of vitamin-C than DNRs. HRPDR subjects showed a lower vitamin-C level ($p < 0.01$) than the MNPDR ones (**Figure 1B**).

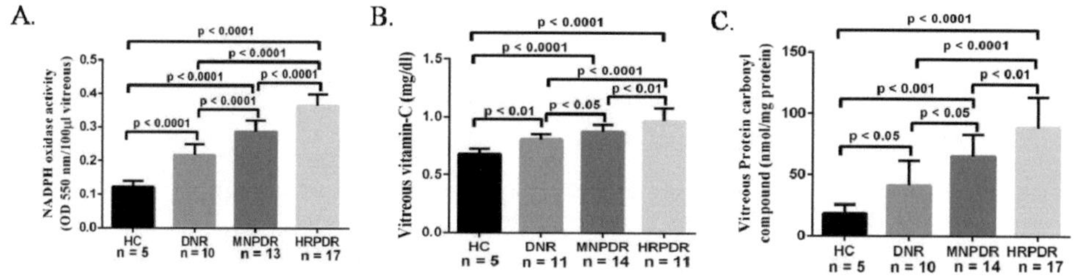

Figure 1.
Comparison of vitreous level NADPH oxidase, vitamin-C and protein carbonyl compound among study groups. [A] Comparison of vitreous level NADPH oxidase, [B] Comparison of vitreous level vitamin-C, [C] Comparison of vitreous level protein carbonyl compound. The one way ANOVA followed by Tuky's comparisons test was administrated to find out significant differences between the groups. A value of p < 0.05 was considered as statistically significant.

Vitreous PCC concentration was found to be increased significantly among DNR (41.57 ± 19.96 nmol/mg protein, $p < 0.05$), MNPDR (65.43 ± 17.31 nmol/mg protein, $p < 0.001$), and HRPDR (88.65 ± 24.93 nmol/mg protein, $p < 0.0001$) subjects compared to HC (18.46 ± 7.18 nmol/mg protein) subjects. Again, both the MNPDR ($p < 0.05$) and HRPDR subjects ($p < 0.0001$) showed significantly higher level of PCC than DNRs. Further, the HRPDR subjects showed a higher PCC level ($p < 0.01$) than the former (**Figure 1C**).

Vitreous MDA level was found to be increased significantly among DNR (2.814 ± 0.482 µM/L, $p < 0.01$), MNPDR (4.58 ± 0.655 µM/L, $p < 0.0001$), and HRPDR (8.51 ± 1.23 µM/L, $p < 0.0001$) subjects compared to HC (1.129 ± 0.579 µM/L) subjects. Again, both the MNPDR ($p < 0.0001$) and HRPDR subjects ($p < 0.0001$) showed significantly higher level of MDA than DNRs. Further, the HRPDR subjects showed a higher MDA level ($p < 0.0001$) than MNPDR subjects (**Figure 2A**).

Regarding HNE concentration in vitreous, the DNR (3936 ± 457.2 pg/ml, $p < 0.0001$), MNPDR (8643 ± 771.8 pg/ml, $p < 0.0001$), and HRPDR (7407 ± 622.3 pg/ml, $p < 0.0001$) subjects showed higher HNE level compared to HC (2092 ± 1201 pg/ml) subjects. Again, both the MNPDR ($p < 0.0001$) and HRPDR subjects ($p < 0.0001$) showed significantly higher level of HNE than DNRs. HRPDR subjects showed a higher HNE level ($p < 0.0001$) than the MNPDR ones (**Figure 2B**).

Vitreous HLY level was found to be increased significantly among DNR (70.93 ± 16.29 nmol/L, $p < 0.0001$), MNPDR (113.0 ± 10.56 nmol/L, $p < 0.0001$), and HRPDR (132.1 ± 16.22 nmol/L, $p < 0.0001$) subjects compared to HC (30.68 ± 7.29 nmol/L) subjects. Again, both the MNPDR ($p < 0.01$) and HRPDR subjects ($p < 0.0001$) showed significantly higher level of HLY than DNRs. Further, the HRPDR subjects showed a higher HLY level ($p < 0.01$) than MNPDR subjects (**Figure 2C**).

Vitreous VEGF level was found to be increased significantly among DNR (90.53 ± 5.611 pg/ml, $p < 0.05$), MNPDR (117.0 ± 17.09 pg/ml, $p < 0.0001$), and HRPDR (131.3 ± 12.21 pg/ml, $p < 0.0001$) subjects compared to HC (72.06 ± 5.109 pg/ml) subjects. Again, both the MNPDR ($p < 0.0001$) and HRPDR subjects ($p < 0.0001$) showed significantly higher level of VEGF than DNRs. Further, the HRPDR subjects showed a higher VEGF level ($p < 0.05$) than MNPDR subjects (**Figure 2D**).

In the DNR and DR group, vitreous NADPH activity showed significant positive correlations with PCC, MDA, HNE, and HLY respectively. However, the study showed no significant correlation with the same in the HC group (**Table 2**).

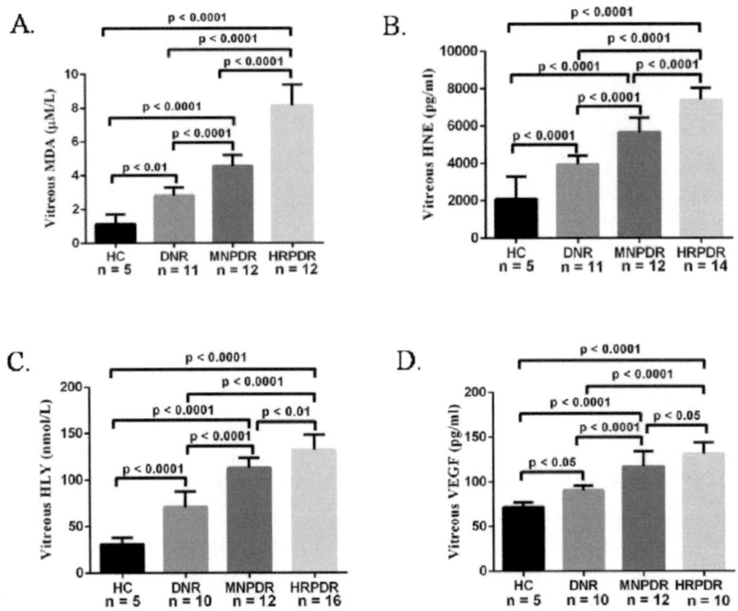

Figure 2.
Comparison of vitreous level MDA, HNE, HLY and VEGF among study groups. [A] Comparison of vitreous level MDA, [B] Comparison of vitreous level HNE, [C] Comparison of vitreous level HLY, [D] Comparison of vitreous level VEGF. The one way ANOVA followed by Tuky's comparisons test was administrated to find out significant differences between the groups. A value of p < 0.05 was considered as statistically significant.

Study groups	PCC	MDA	HNE	HLY
HC	r = 0.300, p = 0.491	r = 0.205, p = 0.741	r = 0.200, p = 0.825	r = 0.100, p = 0.100
DNR	r = 0.833, p = 0.005	r = 0.673, p = 0.033	r = 0.632, p = 0.040	r = 0.733, p = 0.040
DR	r = 0.667, p < 0.0001	r = 0.768, p < 0.0001	r = 0.891, p < 0.0001	r = 0.726, p < 0.0001

A Pearson or spearman correlation coefficient (r) was used and p < 0.05 was considered statistically significant.

Table 2.
Correlation of vitreous NADPH oxidase activity with PCC, MDA, HNE and HLY in HC, DNR and DR (MNPDR+HRPDR) group.

The VEGF level of vitreous showed a significant negative correlation with vitamin-C and positive correlations with PCC, MDA, HNE, and HLY levels respectively in both DNR and DR groups. However, the study showed no significant correlation with the same in the HC group (**Table 3**).

Parameters	HC group	DNR group	DR group
Vitamin-C	r = 0.16, p = 0.722	r = -0.755, p = .007	r = -.451, p = 0.035
PCC	r = 0.235, p = 0.684	r = 0.774, p = 0.009	r = .748, p < 0.0001
MDA	r = 0.285, p = 0.691	r = 0.810, p = 0.003	r = .660, p = 0.003
HNE	r = 0.085, p = 0.875	r = 0.871, p < 0.0001	r = .807, p < 0.0001
HLY	r = 0.145, p = 0.802	r = 0.783, p = 0.007	r = .655, p = 0.002

A Pearson or Spearman correlation coefficient (r) was used and p < 0.05 was considered statistically significant.

Table 3.
Correlation of vitamin-C, PCC, MDA, HNE and ALE with VEGF in different study groups.

4. Discussion

Our study showed that a gradual increment of NADPH Oxidase activity with the pathogenesis and severity of DR (HC < DNR < MNPDR< HRPDR). However there is no direct evidence regarding gradual increment and association of NADPH Oxiadse activity with different graded of DR. An in-Vitro study, Meng et al. [20] demonstrated that NADPH Oxidase augment insulin-induced VEGF expression and angiogenesis. In another study by Ushio-Fukai, [21] also showed that VEGF expression is augmented through ROS, produced by NADPH Oxidase.

Vitreous level of vitamin C was also found to be declined with pathogenesis and severity of DR (HC > DNR > MNPDR > HRPDR). However there is lack of evidence between vitreous level of Vitamin C and different stages of DR. Vitamin C suppress the VEGF gene expression through HIF-1α pathway [22].

Vitreous PCC level was found to be increase gradually with progression of DR (HC < DNR < MNPDR< HRPDR). Nevertheless there is no such evidence of vitreous level of PCC and different stages of DR. Loukovaara et al. [23] shown that amount of protein carbonylation and HIF-1α elevated in vitreous of PDR subjects.

The present study showed a gradual increment of LPO products like MDA and HNE and ALE like HLY both in plasma and vitreous sample towards the development and progression of DR. The studies by Chatziralli et al. [24], Mondal et al., [4] also showed plasma MDA level increases towards the DR pathogenesis and progression. Another study by Mancino et al. [25] showed that vitreous MDA level increases among NPDR and PDR subjects compared to nondiabetic HC subjects. Researchers have demonstrated that the MDA compound is associated with protein modification in a pH-dependent fashion. At the physiological pH, it rapidly forms enolates, which are of lower reactivity and do not react as avidly with nucleophilic species as other aldehydes [26]. However, at a lower pH, MDA exists as b-hydroxyacrolein form, exhibiting a higher reactivity, readily reacting with Lys residues of proteins to form the enaminal type MDA adduct, Nϵ -(2-propenal) lysine, and the fluorescent product, dihydropyridine (DHP) lysine and thereby alters proteins structure and functions [27]. On the other hand, the role of HNE in diabetes and its complications is not well understood [28]. Clinical studies have reported elevated levels of HNE in the blood of diabetic patients with retinopathy compared to those without retinopathy and healthy controls [29]. There is also evidence showing that HNE and HNE-derived ALEs increase in the retinas of rats rendered diabetic for 4-6 weeks [30]. Another study confirmed these findings and showed that HNE may contribute to the pathogenesis of DR by activating the WNT signaling pathway through stabilization of the WNT co-receptor LRP6 [31]. Other animal studies have linked HNE to retinal hemodynamics changes during DR. Retinal perfusion deficits during early diabetes are thought to be mediated, at least in part, through the reduced activity of large-conductance $Ca2+$ −activated $K+$ (BK) channels on the retinal vascular smooth muscle cells, causing vasoconstriction [32, 33]. HNE impairs BK channel function in rat retinal arterioles, as demonstrated by reduced vasodilatory responses to the BK channel opener, BMS-191011 [34]. HNE exposure is reported to result in endoplasmic reticulum stress, mitochondrial dysfunction, and apoptosis in cultures of human retinal capillary pericytes and Müller glia [35].

The ALE component like HLY also found to be increased with the pathogenesis and severity of DR in the present study. A previous study by [36] reported a significant elevation of ALE levels among DNR and MNPDR subjects compared to HCs. Moreover, significant elevation of HLY in the vitreous and serum of patients with PDR was also observed by Izuta et al. [37], which is following our findings.

The study showed a significant negative correlation of VEGF with Vitamin-C level and positive correlations with PCC, MDA, HNE, and HLY. Decrease vitamin C level with increased NADPH oxidase activity may turn oxidative stress, which further damages protein and lipids subsequently causes endothelial dysfunction induced VEGF secretion.

5. Conclusion

Oxidative stress-mediated lipid and protein-derived biomolecules not only add important mediators in the pathogenesis of DR, but also accelerate the progression and severity of microangiopathy.

Acknowledgements

Chinmay Saha, Faculty, Genome Science, School of Interdisciplinary Studies, University of Kalyani, for his encouragement and support towards the fulfillment of this work. We also want to acknowledge the “Multidisciplinary Research Unit” (MRU) of IPGME&R and SSKM Hospital for providing us some reagents to perform the biochemical experiments.

Author details

Subhasish Pramanik[1†], Lakshmi Kanta Mondal[2*†], Subhankar Chowdhury[1], Chiranjit Bose[1], Debgopal Bera[1] and Koena Bhattacharjee[2]

1 Department of Endocrinology and Metabolism, Institute of Post Graduate Medical Education and Research and SSKM Hospital, Kolkata, West Bengal, India

2 Department of Ophthalmology, Regional Institute of Ophthalmology, Kolkata, West Bengal, India

*Address all correspondence to: lakshmi.mondal62@gmail.com

† These authors contributed equally to this work.

References

[1] Diabetes Control and Complications Trial (DCCT) Research Group. The effect of intensive treatment of diabetes on the development and progression of long-term complications in insulindependent diabetes mellitus. N Eng J Med 1993; 329: 977-986.

[2] Engerman RL, Kern TS. Progression of incipient diabetic retinopathy during good glycemic control. Diabetes 1987; 36: 808-812.

[3] United Kingdom Prospective Diabetes Study (UKPDS). Intensive blood glucose control with sulphonylureas or insulin compared with conventional treatment and risk of complications in patients with type 2 diabetes (UKPDS 33). Lancet 1998;352: 837-853.

[4] Mondal LK, Pramanik S, De S, Paine SK, Bhaduri G. Modification of biochemical derangements and VEGF secretion may prevent diabetic retinopathy (DR). Journal of Clinical & Experimental Ophthalmology 2019; 10: 803-812.

[5] Mondal LK, Bhaduri G, Bhattacharya B. Biochemical scenario behind initiation of diabetic retinopathy in type 2 diabetes mellitus. Indian J Ophthalmol 2018; 66: 535-540.

[6] Choudhuri S, Dutta D, Chowdhury IH, Mitra B, Sen Aet al. Association of hyperglycemia mediated increased advanced glycation and erythrocyte antioxidant enzyme activity in different stages of diabetic retinopathy. Diabetes Research and Clinical Practice 2013; 100(3): 376-384.

[7] Stitt A. AGEs and Diabetic retinopathy. Investigative Ophthalmology & Visual Science 2010;51(10): 4867-4874

[8] Belambri SA, Rolas L, Raad H, Hurtado-Nedelec M, Dang PM, El-Benna J. NADPH oxidase activation in neutrophils: Role of the phosphorylation of its subunits. Eur J Clin Invest 2018; Nov (48) Suppl 2:e12951.

[9] Xie S., Naslavsky N, Caplan S. Diacylglycerol kinases in membrane trafficking. Cellular Logistics 2015;5(2): 1-9.

[10] Vistoli G, Maddis DD, Cipak A, Zarkovic N, Carni M, et al. Advanced glycation and lipoxidation end products (AGEs and ALEs): an overview of their mechanisms of formation. Free radical research 2013; 47 (suppl. 1): 3-27.

[11] Kurutus EB. The importance of antioxidants which play the role in cellular response against oxidative/nitrosative stress: current state. Kurutas Nutrition Journal 2016; 15(71): 1-22.

[12] Boyera N, Galey I, Bernard BA. Effect of vitamin C and its derivatives on collagen synthesis and cross-linking by normal human fibroblasts. Int J Cosmet Sci 1998; 20(3):151-159.

[13] ETDRS, 1991 ETDRS report number 10. Early Treatment Diabetic Retinopathy Study Research Group Grading diabetic retinopathy from stereoscopic color fundus photographs–an extension of the modified Airlie House classification. Ophthalmology 1991; 98 (Supplement 5): 786-806.

[14] KunduS, Ghosh P, DattaS, Ghosh A, ChattopadhyayS, Chatterjee M. Oxidative stress as a potential biomarker for determining disease activity in patients with Rheumatoid Arthritis. Free Radical Research 2012: 1-8.

[15] Kyaw A. A simple colorimetric method for ascorbic acid determination in blood plasma. ClinChimActa. 1978.86(2): 153-157.

[16] Firuzi O, Fuksa L, Spadaro C, Bousová I, Riccieri V, Spadaro A, et al. Oxidative stress parameters in different systemic rheumatic diseases. J Pharm Pharmacol 2006; 58: 951– 957.

[17] Levine RL, Garland D, Oliver CN, Amici A, Climent I, et al. Determination of carbonyl content in oxidatively modified proteins. Methods Enzymol1990; 186:464-478.

[18] Mantle D, Falkous G, Walker D. Quantification of protease activities in synovial fluid from rheumatoid and osteoarthritis cases: comparison with antioxidant and free radical damage markers. ClinChimActa. 1999; 284(1): 45-58.

[19] Satoh K. Serum lipid peroxide in cerebrovascular disorders determined by a new colorimetric method. ClinChimActa. 1978 ; 90(1): 37-43.

[20] Meng D, Mei A, Liu J, Kang X, Shi X, et al. NADPH oxidase 4 mediates insulin-stimulated HIF-1α and VEGF expression, and angiogenesis in vitro. PLoS One. 2012 ; 7(10).

[21] Ushio-Fukai M. VEGF signaling through NADPH oxidase-derived ROS. Antioxid Redox Signal. 2007; 9(6):731-773.

[22] Zhao L, Wang J, Zhang Y, Wang L, Yu M, et al. Vitamin C decreases VEGF expression levels via hypoxia-inducible factor-1α dependent and independent pathways in lens epithelial cells. Mol Med Rep. 2020;22(1):436-444.

[23] Loukovaara S, Koivunen P, Inglés M, Escobar J, Vento M, et al. Elevated protein carbonyl and HIF-1α levels in eyes with proliferative diabetic retinopathy. Acta Ophthalmol. 2014; 92(4): 323-330.

[24] Chatziralli IP, Theodossiadis G, Dimitriadis P, Charalambidis M, Agorastos A, et. al. The Effect of Vitamin E on Oxidative Stress Indicated by Serum Malondialdehyde in Insulindependent Type 2 Diabetes Mellitus Patients with Retinopathy. The open ophthalmology journal. 2017; 11: 51-58.

[25] Mancino R, Di Pierro D, Varesi C, Cerulli A, Feraco A, et al. Lipid peroxidation and total antioxidant capacity in vitreous, aqueous humor, and blood samples from patients with diabetic retinopathy. Mol Vis. 2011;17:1298-1304.

[26] Esterbauer H, Schaur RJ, & Zollner H. Chemistry and biochemistry of 4-hydroxynonenal, malonaldehyde and related aldehydes. Free Radical Biology & Medicine 1991;11: 81-128.

[27] Ishii T, Kumazawa S, Sakurai T, Nakayama T, & Uchida K. Mass spectroscopic characterization of protein modification by malondialdehyde. Chemical Research in Toxicology 2006;19: 122-129.

[28] Sasson S. 4-Hydroxyalkena-lactivated PPARδ mediates hormetic interactions in diabetes. Biochimie 2017;136: 85-89.

[29] Polak M, Zagórski Z. Lipid peroxidation in diabetic retinopathy. Ann Univ Mariae Curie Sklodowska Med. 2004;59(1):434-441.

[30] Ali TK, Matragoon S, Pillai BA, Liou GI, El-Remessy AB. Peroxynitrite mediates retinal neurodegeneration by inhibiting nerve growth factor survival signaling in experimental and human diabetes.Diabetes 2008; 57: 889-898.

[31] Zhou T, Zhou KK, Lee K, Gao G, Lyons TJ, et. al. The role of lipid peroxidation products and oxidative stress in activation of the canonical winglesstype MMTV integration site (WNT) pathway in a rat model of diabetic retinopathy. Diabetologia 2011; 54: 459-468.

[32] McGahon MK, Dash DP, Arora A, Wall N, Dawicki J, et. al. Diabetes downregulates largeconductance Ca2+-activated potassium beta 1 channel subunit in retinal arteriolar smooth muscle. Circulation Research 2007;100: 703-711.

[33] Nicoletti R, Venza I, Ceci G, Visalli M, Teti D, et. al. Vitreous polyamines spermidine, putrescine, and spermine in human proliferative disorders of the retina. The British Journal of Ophthalmology 2003; 87: 1038-1042.

[34] Mori A, Suzuki S, Sakamoto K, Nakahara T, Ishii K. BMS-191011, an opener of large-conductance Ca2+-activated potassium channels, dilates rat retinal arterioles in vivo. Biol Pharm Bull. 2011;34(1):150-152.

[35] Wu M, Yang S, Elliott MH, Fu D, Wilson K, et al. Oxidative and endoplasmic reticulum stresses mediate apoptosis induced by modified LDL in human retinal Müller cells. Invest Ophthalmol Vis Sci. 2012; 53(8):4595-4604.

[36] Chowdhuri S, Roy PK, Mitra B, Sen S, Sarkar R, et al. Hyperlipidemia-Mediated Increased Advanced Lipoxidation End Products Formation, an Important Factor Associated with Decreased Erythrocyte Glucose-6-Phosphate Dehydrogenase Activity in Mild Nonproliferative Diabetic Retinopathy. canadian Journal of Diabetes 2017; 41(1): 82-89.

[37] Izuta H, Matsunaga N, Shimazawa M, Sugiyama T, Ikeda T, et al. Proliferative diabetic retinopathy and relations among antioxidant activity, oxidative stress, and VEGF in the vitreous body. Mol Vis. 2010;16:130-136.

Section 2

Clinical Diagnostic Methodologies

Chapter 6

Optical Coherence Tomography in Diabetic Retinopathy

Surabhi Ruia and Koushik Tripathy

Abstract

Optical coherence tomography (OCT) has become an indispensable modality of investigation in the assessment of diabetic retinopathy. It is a non-invasive and reliable imaging tool that provides a comprehensive analysis of the retina. The images are obtained very fast. It is useful for quantitative as well as qualitative assessment of structural changes that occur in diabetic retinopathy. It also enables the detection of subclinical diabetic macular edema. Various imaging biomarkers have been identified on OCT imaging. These markers help prognosticate the case and determine treatment response. The follow-up imaging helps assess the response to treatment and detect recurrence of disease or need for further treatment.

Keywords: spectral-domain optical coherence tomography, swept-source optical coherence tomography, diabetic macular edema, optical coherence tomography angiography, imaging biomarkers

1. Introduction

Diabetes Mellitus (DM) is a disease characterized by elevated blood glucose levels due to its impaired metabolism. It is principally classified into Type 1 DM and Type 2 DM, the former being defined by the absence of insulin secretion whereas resistance to insulin defines the latter. According to the figures analyzed at the global level, diabetes is expected to affect 629 million people by 2045 in the age category of 20 to 79 years [1]. Long-term uncontrolled DM leads to both macrovascular and microvascular complications. Diabetic Retinopathy (DR), a microvascular complication, affects one-third of the population suffering from diabetes [2, 3]. The pathology of DR involves capillary endothelial cell proliferation, thickening of the basement membrane, and loss of pericytes, leading to the formation of microaneurysms, increase in vessel permeability, and the destruction of the blood-retinal barrier. This leads to the accumulation of fluid within and beneath the layers of the retina, causing diabetic macular edema (DME). Diabetic retinopathy is the leading cause of blindness in individuals of the working-age group [4]. In more advanced cases, capillary blockage and ischemia result in the formation of new blood vessels, resulting in proliferative diabetic retinopathy (PDR).

The definition of clinically significant macular edema in diabetes was given by the Early Treatment Diabetic Retinopathy Study (ETDRS) where slit-lamp biomicroscopy or stereoscopic fundus photography was used to identify retinal thickening and hard exudates [5]. However, the use of slit-lamp biomicroscopy or color fundus photography for examining macular edema is subjective and may fail to detect mild changes in retinal thickness. Biomicroscopy does not provide information regarding the exact retinal layer involved. Fundus fluorescein angiography

(FA) is an investigation modality that is used to classify DME into focal and diffuse based on the leakage pattern. This classification helps in guiding focal laser treatment to leaking microaneurysms or grid laser to the leaking capillaries. Ischemic areas and macular ischemia are also well identified on FA. Though FA offers useful information, it is also a subjective test and retinal thickness or morphology cannot be assessed on FA. The advent of optical coherence tomography (OCT), has improved the understanding of DME.

OCT has rapidly grown to become a routine tool of investigation in ophthalmology. Its various advantages lie in the fact that it provides an objective, non-invasive, high resolution, reproducible, and cross-sectional image of the retina [6]. It does not require a highly skilled person for its operation, or pharmacological dilation of the pupil. It is sensitive to identify even mild changes in retinal morphology that are often not visible to the naked eye on clinical examination.

2. Principle and technique

In simple terms, OCT is similar to ultrasound in that a beam of sound or light directed onto a tissue is differentially reflected from structures with different acoustic or optical properties. The time it takes for the sound or light to reflect from the

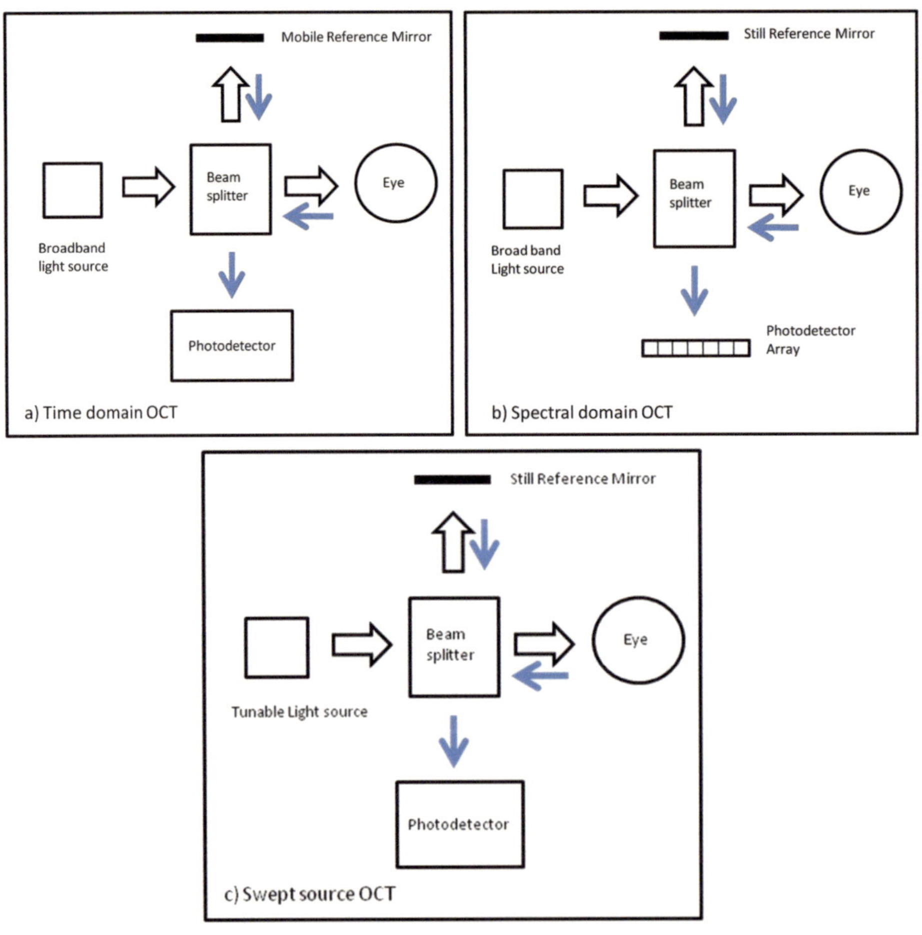

Figure 1.
a) Principle of time domain OCT. b) Principle of spectral domain OCT. c) Principle of swept source OCT.

different structures determines the dimensions of the structures. This provides an image similar to the A-scan or depth scan of ultrasound. Imaging of laterally adjacent depth scans provides a two-dimensional or B-scan image. The time delay involved when using light is in femtoseconds requiring interferometry to do the calculations [7].

The first generation OCT machine or Time-Domain OCT (TD-OCT) uses low time-coherence interferometry to obtain depth scans (**Figure 1a**). A beam splitter splits the light coming from a broadband light source, one directed to the eye and the other to the reference mirror. The position of the reference mirror is changed to mirror the depth of the various layers of tissue being scanned. Light reflected from the two sources is collected and the interferogram is analyzed to give a complete depth scan. TD-OCT involves two scans, one for depth scan and one for lateral scan, thus, resulting in a lesser number of scans acquired per second.

With the use of spectrometer and Fourier-domain technique in the next generation OCT, called Spectral-domain OCT (SD-OCT), the disadvantage of performing a depth scan was avoided. SD-OCT uses an array of photo-detectors to capture the depth scan without having to move the reference mirror (**Figure 1b**). Therefore, only a lateral scan has to be performed [7]. This increased the scan speed enormously. Further refinement of technology led to the change of the broadband near-infrared superluminescent diode light source of wavelength 840 nm in SD-OCT to a tunable swept laser source with a center wavelength of 1050 nm [8]. In conjunction, the array of photodetectors in SD-OCT was replaced with a single photodetector [8]. This led to the evolution of Swept-source OCT (SS-OCT) (**Figure 1c**). SS-OCT provides increased scan speed and denser scans with greater resolution as more A-scan and B scans are acquired per second. The scan area is also increased along with scan depth due to the use of a longer wavelength light source which allows better penetration through retinal pigment epithelium (RPE).

3. Normal retinal morphology on optical coherence tomography

The rapid technological evolution of SD-OCT led to the visualization of different hyperreflective and hyporeflective layers of retina commencing from the innermost vitreoretinal interface to the outermost choroid-scleral interface (**Figure 2**) [9]. The innermost layer visualized is the posterior cortical vitreous which is hyperreflective followed by a hyporeflective preretinal space [10]. The innermost layer of the retina is the hyperreflective internal limiting membrane which overlies the retinal nerve fiber layer (RNFL). The next layer is the ganglion cell layer which is less reflective than the RNFL [11]. Outer to the ganglion cell layer is the hyperreflective inner plexiform layer followed by hyporeflective inner nuclear layer. The outer plexiform layer is hyperreflective. OCT has greatly improved the understanding of human anatomy with the identification of Henle's layer as a component of outer half of the outer plexiform layer [12]. Outer to the outer plexiform layer lies the hyporeflective outer nuclear layer. This is followed by the external limiting membrane (ELM), another hyperreflective layer. Latest OCT machines have also made possible, the identification of outer retinal layers that are anatomic correlates of the myoid and ellipsoid (EZ) zones of the inner segment of the photoreceptors [13]. The myoid zone is hyporeflective and lies next to the ELM followed by EZ layer which is hyperreflective. This is followed by the hyporeflective layer of outer segments of photoreceptor and then a hyperreflective interdigitation zone is noted between cone outer segments and apical processes of RPE [13]. The next layer or the outermost layer of the retina is the hyperreflective RPE-Bruch's membrane complex which can be sometimes visualized as separate layers. OCT also helps visualize the components of the choroid [14]. The innermost layer in the choroid is formed by the choriocapillaris. The Sattler's layer

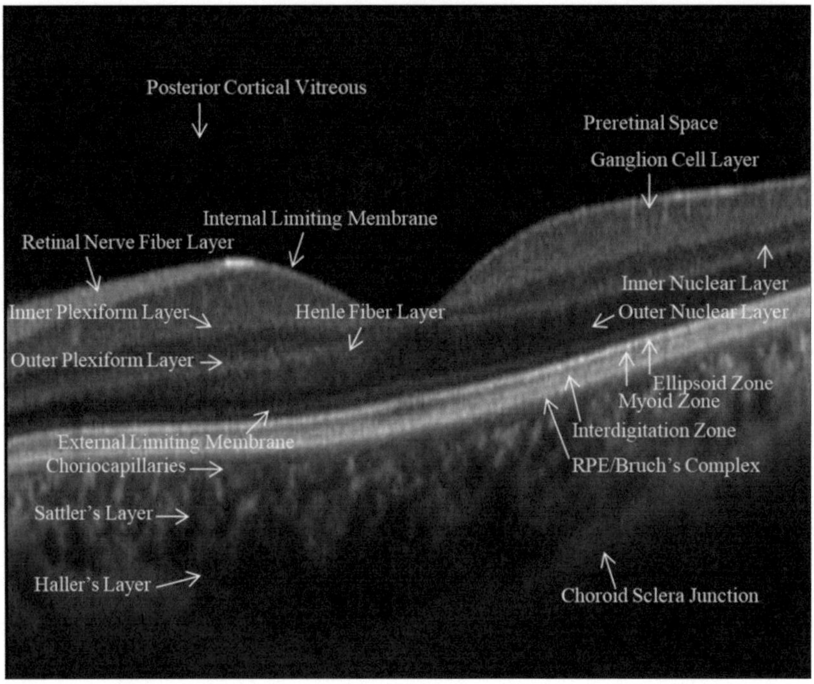

Figure 2.
Normal anatomical landmarks as seen on swept source OCT image.

forms the mid choroid and the Haller's layer forms the outer choroid. The outer boundary of the choroid is the choroidal-scleral junction [14].

Clinically visualized changes of diabetic retinopathy are well delineated on OCT. Hard exudates, cotton wool spots, and epiretinal membrane show hyperreflectivity, edema exhibits hyporeflectivity, and hemorrhages demonstrate backshadowing. Other than these, various discerning features and biomarkers have been identified on OCT which has been discussed later in this chapter.

4. Optical coherence tomography based classification of macular edema

OCT is a sensitive tool to diagnose, quantify, and classify diabetic macular edema. The first OCT-based classification for DME was given by Otani et al [15]. They were the first to identify 3 patterns of fluid accumulation, including sponge-like retinal swelling, cystoid macular edema, and serous retinal detachment (**Figure 3**). They further described that early changes of macular edema were confined to the outer retinal layer mainly the outer plexiform layer when compared to histopathology [15]. With the further accumulation of fluid, the inner retinal layers were involved. The presence of serous retinal detachment in patients with DME is a finding which may not be easily distinguished on biomicroscopy or FA.

In 2004, Panozzo proposed a classification system based on five parameters: retinal thickness, volume, morphology, diffusion, and presence or absence of vitreoretinal traction [16]. They quantified the retinal thickness and volume in three different zones around the fovea. The types of macular edema observed were in agreement with that described by Otani et al., [15] with the only difference being that the size of the cyst was measured to subclassify the grade of the cystoid variety of macular edema. The presence of epiretinal traction and its pattern (tangential or

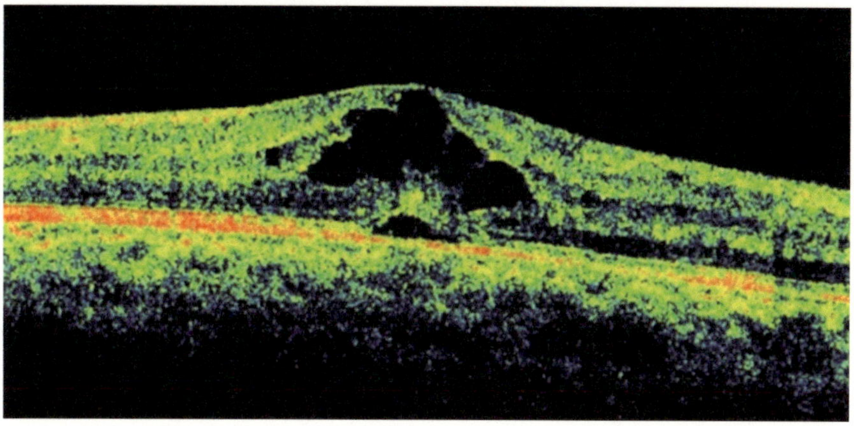

Figure 3.
Cystoid macular edema with presence of serous retinal detachment (spectral-domain OCT).

anteroposterior) were also described. This distinguished cases with an additional component of retinal distortion (**Figure 4**). In 2006, Kim et al. demonstrated similar findings of macular edema and posterior hyaloid traction. In addition, they described tractional retinal detachment as a peak-shaped detachment of the retina [17]. These 3 previous classifications used TD-OCT (**Table 1**).

With the advent of SD-OCT, Murakami et al. for the first time showed that in addition to the morphology of edema, the photoreceptor status played a significant role in the prognosis of visual acuity [18]. They classified edema into serous retinal detachment, cystoid macular edema, and Diffuse type (absence of either cystoid macular edema or serous retinal detachment) with the latter term being used for cases that had retinal thickening but an absence of cysts or serous fluid [18]. Later in 2012, Koleva-Georgieva proposed a classification in which the term early subclinical macular edema was introduced, to describe cases with macular edema which were previously being missed on clinical examination [19]. In addition, they also included the integrity of both the outer retinal layers, the IS/OS (inner segment-outer segment junction, now identified as the EZ layer), and the ELM. Retinal morphology, topography, and presence of traction at macula were also a part of the classification and were similar to the other classifications [19]. In 2013, Helmy et al. further subclassified cystoid macular edema based on the proportion of the largest cyst to the maximum retinal thickness(CME Grade I-IV). The integrity of IS/OS

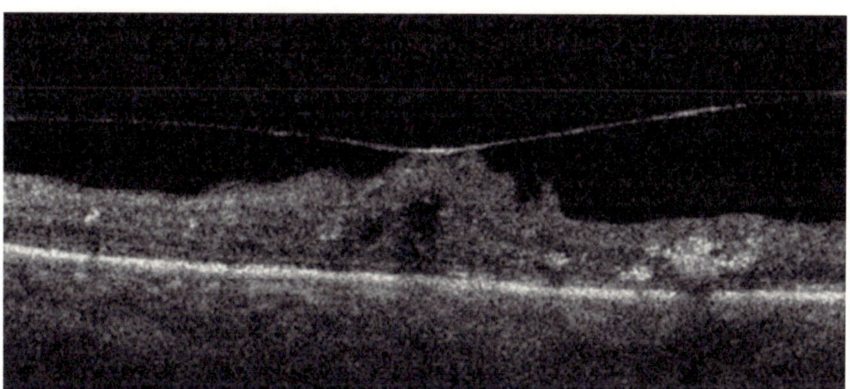

Figure 4.
Vitreomacular traction in a case of diabetic macular edema (captured with SD-OCT).

Classifications based on Time Domain OCT
Otani et al. [15] 1. Sponge-like retinal swelling 2. Cystoid macular edema 3. Serous retinal detachment
Panozzo et al. [16] 1. Retinal thickness 2. Retinal volume 3. Retinal morphology 4. Diffusion 5. Presence of vitreous traction
Kim et al. [17] 1. Diffuse retinal thickening 2. Cystoid macular edema 3. Posterior hyaloidal traction 4. Serous retinal detachment 5. Traction retinal detachment
Classifications based on Spectral Domain OCT
Murakami et al. [18] 1. Serous retinal detachment type 2. Cystoid macular edema type 3. Diffuse type (absence of either cystoid macular edema or serous retinal detachment)
Koleva-Georgieva [19] 1. Retinal thickness 2. Retinal morphology 3. Retinal topography 4. Presence and severity of macular traction 5. Retinal outer layers' integrity (IS/OS and ELM)
Helmy et al. [20] 1. Cystoid macular edema based on the vertical size of the largest macular cyst in proportion to the total macular thickness (CME Grade I-IV) 2. Integrity of External limiting membrane layer and Ellipsoid zone layer (Sub-classification as A-D) [Presence of hyperreflective foci (associated finding)] [Associated neurosensory detachment or vitreomacular traction (associated finding)]
Aiello et al. [21] 1. Center-involved diabetic macular edema 2. Non-center-involved diabetic macular edema

Table 1.
Time domain-OCT and Spectral domain-OCT based classification of Diabetic macular edema.

junction and ELM, presence or absence of neurosensory detachment, or vitreoretinal traction were also included. They extended their classification to include the presence of hyperreflective foci in the outer retina from the ELM to the RPE [20].

5. Role of OCT in treatment of diabetic macular edema

The introduction of intravitreal anti-vascular endothelial growth factor (anti-VEGF) agents significantly changed the treatment of DME a few years ago [22, 23]. Though laser treatment prescribed by the ETDRS study reduced the risk of vision loss significantly, only 20% of laser-treated eyes experienced a gain in visual acuity of at least 3 lines (15 letters) at 2 years [24]. A study by DRCR.net compared the efficacy of anti-VEGF treatment with laser treatment in eyes with DME [25, 26]. Results showed that anti-VEGF therapy was more effective in preventing the loss of visual acuity. In addition, a significant percentage of eyes showed an improvement in mean visual acuity [25, 26].

Monthly injections and follow-up with OCT imaging of the macula have been recommended in various guidelines [27–30]. Monthly treatment till there is no edema on follow-up OCT scan and reinitiating treatment when edema recurs or vision deteriorates is the preferred clinical practice for the management of DME [30, 31].

However, according to the FDA label of Eylea® (aflibercept), 'the recommended dose for eylea (for DME) is 2 mg (0.05 mL) administered by intravitreal injection every 4 weeks (approximately every 28 days, monthly) for the first 5 injections followed by 2 mg (0.05 mL) via intravitreal injection once every 8 weeks (2 months)' [32].

Cases that do not show a response after 3 monthly injections are termed non-responders [31]. Some authorities, however, term a patient nonresponder after the failure of 6 injections [29].

However, other definition of non-responder includes no or minimal reduction in retinal thickness on OCT or no improvement in visual acuity. The study by DRCR.net defined less than 10% decrease in central subfield thickness on OCT and < 5 letter increase in visual acuity as no response to anti-VEGF treatment [21]. Options to treat such cases include other anti-VEGF agents, intravitreal triamcinolone, implantable steroid injection, macular laser, and targeted retinal photocoagulation (TRP) of peripheral capillary nonperfusion areas [30, 31, 33].

Center-involved diabetic macular edema is defined as retinal thickening involving the central subfield zone of the macula that is 1 mm in diameter [34]. The management of center-involved macular edema causing visual decline (visual acuity worse than 20/30) is relatively straightforward and such cases need treatment [28, 35]. The preferred therapy includes intravitreal anti-VEGF agents, steroids, steroid implants, or a combination of these. Cases with center-involved macular edema and good visual function pose a challenge to the treating Ophthalmologist. The dilemma in such cases is whether to start intravitreal therapy or to observe [30, 34]. Such cases have been reported to improve with good control of blood sugar levels alone [31]. The role of anti-VEGF agents in such cases is being explored [36]. These cases have to be monitored at regular intervals to detect deterioration in vision which is an indication to begin anti-VEGF therapy [31, 34].

Non-center involved diabetic macular edema is defined as a retinal thickening in the macula that does not involve the central subfield zone of diameter 1 mm [34]. Laser photocoagulation is still the standard of care for the treatment of cases with non-center involving macular edema [37]. For cases with macular edema with vitreomacular traction, induction of posterior vitreous detachment during pars plana vitrectomy with or without ILM peeling is the recommended choice for treatment [38–40].

6. Biomarkers of DR on OCT

Biomarkers are markers used externally to assess a medical state reliably and accurately [41]. Biomarkers may be physical, chemical, or biological. They are used to assess a physiological state, pathological process, or response to any pharmacological intervention [41]. Imaging biomarkers have the advantage of being non-invasive, reliable, and accurate. Several OCT-based biomarkers have been reported in DME which help in the management of the disease as well as in prognostication [42].

6.1 Disorganization of the retinal inner layers (DRIL)

Earlier studies showed a variable correlation between central retinal thickness measured on OCT and visual acuity achieved post-treatment of DME [43, 44]. A study by DRCR.net revealed that this correlation is modest. They also documented cases with a paradoxical decrease in visual acuity with a decrease in retinal thickening [45]. Further studies documented the role of OCT-based markers other than the central retinal thickness that affect visual acuity.

These include bridging retinal processes, the integrity of ELM and EZ, the reflectivity of cone outer segment tips, presence of hyperreflective foci, and subretinal fluid [46–49].

Long-standing cystoid macular edema with disturbance in ELM and EZ may suggest a poor visual outcome after treatment (**Figure 5**).

Sun and colleagues evaluated a novel marker in OCT, called disorganization of the retinal inner layers (DRIL), within the central 1 mm area of the fovea [50]. They studied the inner retinal layers in cases with existing DME or resolved DME. DRIL is 'defined as the horizontal extent in microns for which any boundaries between the ganglion cell–inner plexiform layer complex, inner nuclear layer, and outer plexiform layer could not be identified.' [50]. DRIL was found to have a substantial association with visual acuity. The presence of DRIL explained the paradoxical decrease in visual acuity in cases with resolved DME [50]. Later, Joltikov et al. reported the presence of DRIL in diabetics even before the presence of DR, DME, or PDR [51]. Further, Pelosini et al. proposed a theory to explain the negative correlation between retinal volume and visual acuity [52]. They suggested that the accumulation of fluid within the inner retinal layers causes the bipolar cells to stretch. Bipolar cells connect the photoreceptors to the ganglion cells. Fluid exceeding the limit of elasticity of these bipolar cell axons, may break the continuity of these axons and affect the transmission of signals between ganglion cells and photoreceptors. The irreversible destruction of bipolar cells provides a plausible explanation for cases with no improvement in visual acuity even after the resolution of DME [52]. In another study, the presence of retinal tissue between the cystic cavities in cases with DME was found to predict improvement in visual acuity after anti-VEGF therapy. These retinal tissues comprise of Müller and bipolar cells that transmit impulses between inner and outer retinal layers. The absence of these retinal bridging tissues at baseline explains the foveal thinning after the resolution of edema [53].

6.2 Hyperreflective retinal foci

SD-OCT imaging of diabetic retinopathy identified an additional intraretinal pathology which was visualized as hyperreflective dot or foci (HF) in few cases of DME [47]. Bolz et al. reported that the location of these HF on OCT was variable

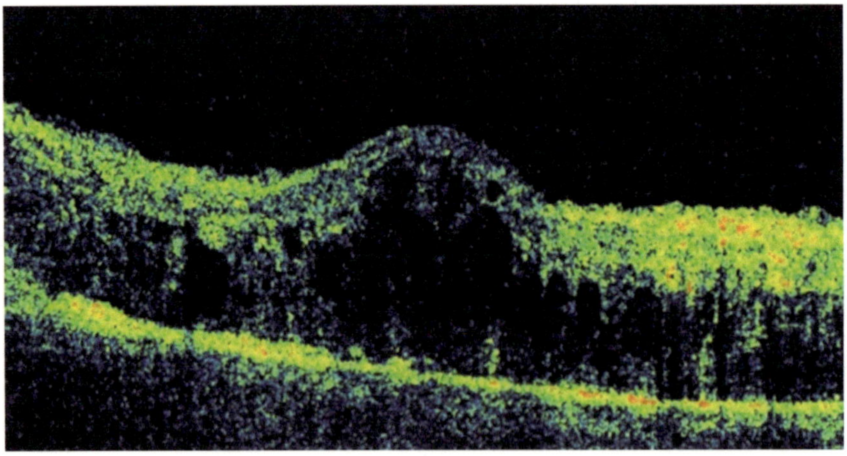

Figure 5.
Long standing cystoid macular edema.

[47]. In some cases, they were noted to be dispersed all through the retinal layers. In other cases, they were observed in the walls of microaneurysms or as confluent plaques at the level of the outer plexiform layer [47]. Bolz et al. hypothesized that the HF represented lipid deposits or precursors of hard exudates [47]. The similarity in the reflective property of HF and hard exudates supported their theory. In contrast, Lee and colleagues proposed that HF corresponded to activated microglial cells [54]. They observed a positive correlation between levels of the cytokine CD14 in the aqueous humor and the number of HF on SD-OCT in patients with DME. Cytokine CD14 is derived from activated microglial cells [55]. Microglial cells are the immune cells in the retina that undergo an inflammatory change in DR [56]. However, further studies are required to establish the origin of HF. Midena et al., described HF as dots with a size less than 30 microns, absence of back shadowing, and reflectivity similar to that of the retinal nerve fiber layer [57]. Their description allowed the distinction of HF from other hyperreflective spots on OCT such as intraretinal hemorrhage and microaneurysm. Intraretinal hemorrhage on OCT has a backshadowing effect such that retinal layers beneath the hemorrhage are not visualized. The microaneurysms on OCT have an external diameter of more than 70 microns in size [58]. Several studies reported a negative correlation between the presence of HF and visual acuity [59–62]. Uji et al. suggested a pathologic association between the presence of HF in the outer retinal layers and disruption of ELM and EZ resulting in photoreceptor dysfunction in cases with DME [59]. The presence of HF has been documented to indicate inflammatory activity or active disease status with studies reporting a significant reduction in HF after treatment with anti-VEGF and steroid implants [60, 61]. HF has also been identified as a predictor of early recurrence of DME after steroid (dexamethasone) implant [62]. HF has also been reported in DME cases that are refractory to anti-VEGF agents [63].

A characteristic arrangement of hyperreflective dots termed as pearl necklace sign in cases of DME was recently reported (**Figure 6**) [64]. It was originally described as HF surrounding the wall of a cyst located in the outer plexiform layer [64]. However, a similar appearance has recently also been described in cystoid spaces in the outer plexiform-outer nuclear layer and the inner wall of the neurosensory detachment [65]. Treatment with anti-VEGF agents in these cases led to the accumulation of hard exudates in the location of HF. A correlation of pearl necklace sign and visual acuity was only described in cases where the cyst or neurosensory detachment involved the fovea [65].

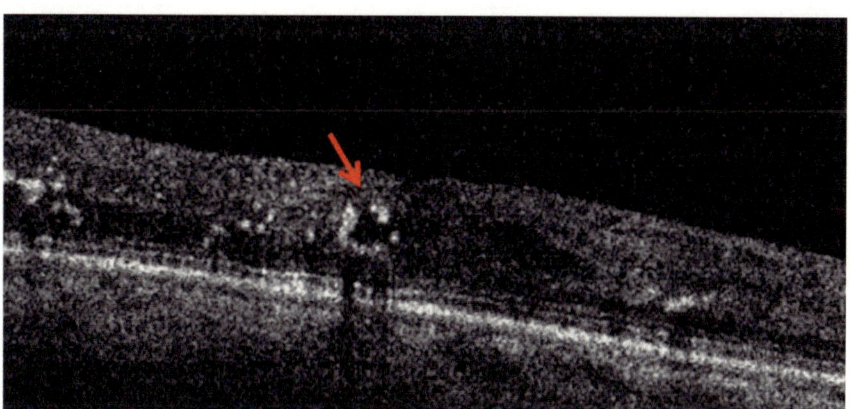

Figure 6.
Pearl necklace sign in a case of diabetic macular edema.

6.3 Hyperreflective material within intraretinal cystoid spaceSolid

Solid appearing cysts with hyper-reflective material within the cyst have been documented in DME (**Figure 7**) [66]. The content of these cysts has been hypothesized to be fibrin or of inflammatory origin [66]. However, no alteration to response to anti-VEGF treatment was reported [66].

Another novel OCT finding that has been recently reported in a patient with DME is a subretinal pseudocyst [67]. Contrary to what has been earlier documented, a cyst-like appearance was observed in the subretinal space and not within the retinal layers. The migration of Müller cells into the subretinal space has been proposed to be the reason for the development of the pseudocyst in that location [67].

6.4 Thickness of photoreceptor outer segment (PROS)

Advancement in technology has allowed the measurement of the thickness of the photoreceptor layer with SD-OCT in patients with diabetes. Patients with DR, DME, or diabetes but no retinopathy, have reported a thin photoreceptor layer in comparison to healthy individuals [46, 68]. Variation in visual acuity has been correlated to the thickness of the outer segment of the photoreceptor (PROS) in eyes with DME. This thickness of PROS is measured from the inner boundary of IS/OS junction to the inner boundary of the RPE layer [69]. The correlation of thickness of PROS with visual acuity is significant particularly when measuring it at the fovea [49].

6.5 Hyperreflective foci within the choroid

Hyperreflective foci within the choroid (HCF) have been recently reported in diabetic eyes [70]. Roy et al. hypothesized that these are intraretinal HF that migrate to the choroid with disruption of ELM and EZ. They documented a negative correlation between visual acuity and the presence of HF in the choroid. The presence of HCF was also observed to have an association with the severity of DR [70].

6.6 Thickness of the choroid

Studies using enhanced depth OCT imaging have evaluated choroidal thickness in eyes with DME and PDR. These studies have reported contradictory results. Kim and associates documented an increase in choroidal thickness with the increase in

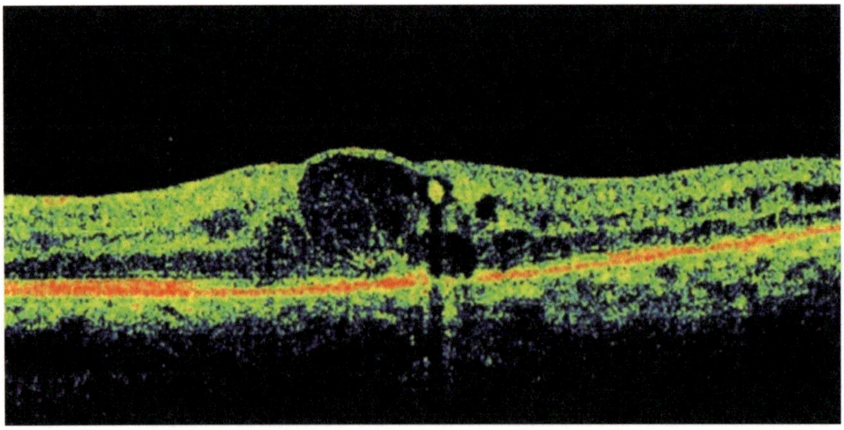

Figure 7.
Hyper reflective material within the cyst in a case of diabetic macular edema.

severity of DR and cases with DME [71]. They also reported a decrease in choroidal thickness in eyes treated with panretinal photocoagulation (PRP) [71]. In contrast, Querques et al. documented thin choroid in diabetic eyes when compared to control [72]. Rayess et al. documented that eyes with thicker choroid at baseline responded better to anti-VEGF treatment [73].

A recent study using swept-source OCT showed that choroidal thickness increased in the early stages of DR and then decreased as the severity of DR progressed [74]. The study proposed several mechanisms to explain choroidal thickening in early DR. Diabetic choroidopathy resulting in dysfunction of RPE and increased vascular permeability was implied as one of the mechanisms. Inflammation and oxidative stress-induced increase in cytokines was also suspected to be associated with choroidal thickening. In contrast, a decrease in blood flow and hypoxia was probably associated with thinning of the choroid with the progression of DR. However, whether choroidal thinning is primary or secondary to retinal ischemia remains to be established [74].

6.7 Choroidal vascularity index (CVI)

Choroidal vascularity index (CVI), another OCT-based marker enables the assessment of vascularity of the choroid [75]. Unlike choroidal thickness, this marker does not vary with physiological factors [75]. The choroid has two main components, the stroma, and the vascular layer. CVI is the proportion of the vascular component to the total choroidal area. A positive correlation has been documented between CVI and the status of choroidal blood supply [75]. Studies evaluating the CVI in diabetes have suggested that reduction in choroidal blood flow occurs as an early manifestation in diabetes even before retinopathy developed [76]. The thickening of choroid noted in the early stages of DR is probably explained by an increase in the stromal component of the choroid. As retinopathy progresses, the choroidal blood vessel further reduces in density [76]. However, further studies are required to confirm these theories.

7. Role of OCT in PDR

7.1 Neovascularization on OCT

High-resolution OCT imaging allows the evaluation of details of neovascularization in patients with PDR [77, 78].

Neovascularization of the retina was observed to breach the internal limiting membrane and protrude into the vitreous cavity [77]. The posterior hyaloid was attached or partially detached around the neovascularization [77]. Neovascular loops were seen as hyperreflective loops protruding into the vitreous with back-shadowing obscuring the retina at the points of attachment [77].

Thick neovascularization of the disc (NVD) was noted to grow along the posterior hyaloid which serves as a scaffold [77]. NVD appeared as hyperreflective tissue over the disc protruding into the vitreous cavity in cases with detached posterior hyaloid, which is uncommon in eyes with NVD [77]. Vaz-Pereira et al. in their study identified SD-OCT-based features that can distinguish active neovascularization from quiescent neovascularization [79]. They observed the presence of hyperreflective dots in the vitreous cavity in cases with active neovascularization. These hyperreflective dots were theorized to represent increased vascular permeability. Features such as the presence of epiretinal membrane, inner retinal tissue contracture, vitreous invasion, and protrusion towards the vitreous were found in cases of quiescent or inactive neovascularization [79]. Another finding in PDR that is observed on OCT is vitreoschisis [80]. This is defined as the splitting of the posterior vitreous which leaves a layer of vitreous attached to the retina when vitreous detachment occurs. These can cause traction on the neovascular vessels and complicate surgery in PDR [80].

In contrast, intraretinal microvascular abnormalities (IRMA) are intraretinal, hyperreflective areas that were observed to distort the inner retinal layers. They do not breach the overlying ILM or vitreous. There is no thickening of the posterior hyaloid [77].

7.2 Wide-field OCT imaging in PDR

Mishra et al. have recently described a novel technique to facilitate wide-field imaging of the retina beyond the posterior pole. These images provide a better assessment of the vitreoretinal interface and therefore help in surgical planning in eyes with PDR [81].

8. Optical coherence tomography angiography (OCTA)

OCT angiography (OCTA) provides non-invasive imaging of the retinal vasculature parallel to images provided by FA [82]. The advantage over FA is that it circumvents the need for dye injection and therefore forestalls the risk of incidents like anaphylaxis. With the help of OCTA, people with contraindications to FA, can also undergo imaging of the retinal vasculature. OCTA uses the split-spectrum amplitude decorrelation algorithm [82]. In simple terms, it analyzes the light signals reflected from various tissues on repeated B scan imaging of a particular location. The mobile blood cells of the retinal or choroidal vasculature are the only structures responsible for providing a signal of different intensity or phases on repeated B scans [82]. The other tissues being stationary will not show any difference. It provides high-resolution images of both superficial and deep capillary plexus [83]. It provides better visualization of retinal capillary non-perfusion areas including capillary drop-out areas and foveal avascular zone [84]. Swept source-OCTA systems provide better imaging of the choroidal vasculature compared to SD-OCTA [85]. OCTA enables delineation of the morphology of microaneurysm into saccular or fusiform swelling [86]. Unlike FA, OCTA does not evaluate hyperpermeable pathological vessels. It does not show leakage (as seen on fundus fluorescein angiography) to indicate retinal edema or neovascularization [87]. OCTA also helps to estimate the activity status of the neovascularization [86]. Various quantitative measures have also been described using OCTA [88, 89]. Further details of OCTA are beyond the scope of this chapter.

9. Newer modalities in OCT

Adaptive optics OCT improves the transverse resolution of OCT images. Adaptive optics OCT provides microscopic images of the vasculature. It has been used to quantitatively analyze the lumen of retinal capillaries and microaneurysms in diabetic retinopathy [90, 91]. Based on the Doppler principle, Doppler OCT is a functional imaging technique that allows for visualization and measurement of blood flow [92]. Studies have observed reduced retinal blood flow in patients with DR compared to healthy individuals [93].

10. Conclusion

OCT has become a very valuable tool in the imaging of diabetic retinopathy. It is useful in the diagnosis of DME as well as decision-making regarding the treatment of DME. It is also helpful in following up the cases with DME after treatment with anti-VEGF therapy. It helps in diagnosing non-responders to treatment. It also provides information regarding the vitreoretinal interface and therefore helps decide the need for surgical intervention. It provides reliable qualitative information regarding retinal thickness. Various OCT-based classifications of DME have helped in better understanding of the disease pathogenesis. The evaluation of retinal layers on OCT explains the correlation between the retinal thickness at baseline and the final visual acuity achieved after treatment. The arrival of OCTA has further enhanced the imaging process. It adds to the information provided by SD-OCT or SS-OCT. It gives information regarding the blood supply of the retina, the density of the vessels, changes in the foveal avascular zone and helps to identify neovascular networks. It precludes the use of the invasive fundus fluorescein angiography and hence can be used in people with contraindications to fundus fluorescein angiography.

Thus, OCT has become a vital tool to diagnose and monitor the response of DME to various intravitreal pharmacotherapies including anti-VEGF agents.

Author details

Surabhi Ruia[1]* and Koushik Tripathy[2]

1 Vitreoretina, Private Practice, Kolkata, West Bengal, India

2 Department of Vitreoretinal Services, ASG Eye Hospital, Kolkata, West Bengal, India

*Address all correspondence to: surabhi.ruia@gmail.com

References

[1] Hou Y, Cai Y, Jia Z, et al. Risk factors and prevalence of diabetic retinopathy. Medicine (Baltimore). 2020 Oct 16;99(42):e22695.

[2] Thapa R, Bajimaya S, Sharma S, et al. Systemic association of newly diagnosed proliferative diabetic retinopathy among type 2 diabetes patients presented at a tertiary eye hospital of Nepal. Nepalese Journal of Ophthalmology. 2015 Sep 17;7(1):26-32.

[3] Wong TY, Sabanayagam C. Strategies to tackle the global burden of diabetic retinopathy: from epidemiology to artificial intelligence. Ophthalmologica. 2020;243(1):9-20.

[4] Klein R, Klein BE, Moss SE, et al. The Wisconsin epidemiologic study of diabetic retinopathy. III. Prevalence and risk of diabetic retinopathy when age at diagnosis is 30 or more years. Archives of Ophthalmology 1984;102(4):527-532.

[5] Early Treatment Diabetic Retinopathy Study Research Group. Grading diabetic retinopathy from stereoscopic color fundus photographs—an extension of the modified Airlie House classification: ETDRS report number 10. Ophthalmology. 1991 May 1;98(5):786-806.

[6] Diabetic Retinopathy Clinical Research Network. Reproducibility of macular thickness and volume using zeiss optical coherence tomography in patients with diabetic macular edema. Ophthalmology. 2007 Aug 1;114(8):1520-1525.

[7] Aumann S, Donner S, Fischer J, et al. Optical coherence tomography (OCT): Principle and technical realization. High Resolution Imaging in Microscopy and Ophthalmology. 2019:59-85.

[8] Chinn SR, Swanson EA, Fujimoto JG. Optical coherence tomography using a frequency-tunable optical source. Optics letters. 1997 Mar 1;22(5):340-342.

[9] Staurenghi G, Sadda S, Chakravarthy U, et al. Proposed lexicon for anatomic landmarks in normal posterior segment spectral-domain optical coherence tomography: the IN•OCT consensus. Ophthalmology. 2014 Aug 1;121(8):1572-1578.

[10] Liu JJ, Witkin AJ, Adhi M, Grulkowski I, Kraus MF, Dhalla AH, Lu CD, Hornegger J, Duker JS, Fujimoto JG. Enhanced vitreous imaging in healthy eyes using swept source optical coherence tomography. PLoS One. 2014 Jul 18;9(7):e102950.

[11] Ishikawa H, Stein DM, Wollstein G, Beaton S, Fujimoto JG, Schuman JS. Macular segmentation with optical coherence tomography. Investigative ophthalmology & visual science. 2005 Jun 1;46(6):2012-2017.

[12] Otani T, Yamaguchi Y, Kishi S. Improved visualization of Henle fiber layer by changing the measurement beam angle on optical coherence tomography. Retina. 2011 Mar 1;31(3):497-501.

[13] Spaide RF, Curcio CA. Anatomical correlates to the bands seen in the outer retina by optical coherence tomography: literature review and model. Retina (Philadelphia, Pa.). 2011 Sep;31(8):1609.

[14] Spaide RF, Koizumi H, Pozonni MC. Enhanced depth imaging spectral-domain optical coherence tomography. American journal of ophthalmology. 2008 Oct 1;146(4):496-500.

[15] Otani T, Kishi S, Maruyama Y. Patterns of diabetic macular edema with optical coherence tomography. American journal of ophthalmology. 1999 Jun 1;127(6):688-693.

[16] Panozzo G, Parolini B, Gusson E, et al. Diabetic macular edema: an OCT-based classification. InSeminars inophthalmology 2004 Jan 1(Vol.19, No. 1-2, pp. 13-20). Taylor & Francis.

[17] Kim BY, Smith SD, Kaiser PK. Optical coherence tomographic patterns of diabetic macular edema. American journal of ophthalmology. 2006 Sep 1;142(3):405-412.

[18] Murakami T, Nishijima K, Sakamoto A, et al. Association of pathomorphology, photoreceptor status, and retinal thickness with visual acuity in diabetic retinopathy. American journal of ophthalmology. 2011 Feb 1;151(2): 310-317.

[19] Desislava Koleva-Georgieva. Optical Coherence Tomography Findings in Diabetic Macular Edema | IntechOpen [Internet]. 2021. Available from: https://www.intechopen.com/books/diabetic-retinopathy/optical-coherence-tomography-findings-in-diabetic-macular-edema

[20] Helmy YM, Allah HRA. Optical coherence tomography classification of diabetic cystoid macular edema. Clinical Ophthalmology(Auckland, NZ). 2013;7: 1731.

[21] Aiello LP, Beck RW, Bressler NM, et al. Rationale for the diabetic retinopathy clinical research network treatment protocol for center-involved diabetic macular edema. Ophthalmology. 2011 Dec 1;118(12):e5-14.

[22] Nguyen QD, Shah SM, Heier JS, et al. Primary end point (six months) results of the ranibizumab for edema of the macula in diabetes (READ-2) study. Ophthalmology. 2009 Nov 1;116(11): 2175-2181.

[23] Shah SM, Nguyen QD, Sy JP, et al. The RIDE and RISE studies of the efficacy and safety of intravitreal ranibizumab (LUCENTIS®) in clinically significant macular edema with center involvement secondary to diabetes mellitus. Investigative ophthalmology & visual science. 2008 May 14;49(13):1562–.

[24] Diabetic Retinopathy Clinical Research Network. A randomized trial comparing intravitreal triamcinolone acetonide and focal/grid photocoagulation for diabetic macular edema. Ophthalmology. 2008 Sep 1;115(9): 1447-1459.

[25] Elman MJ, Qin H, Aiello LP, et al. Intravitreal ranibizumab for diabetic macular edema with prompt versus deferred laser treatment: three-year randomized trial results. Ophthalmology. 2012 Nov 1;119(11):2312-2318.

[26] Elman MJ, Ayala A, Bressler NM, et al. Intravitreal ranibizumab for diabetic macular edema with prompt vs. Deferred laser treatment: 5-year randomized trial results. Ophthalmology. 2015 Feb 1;122(2):375-381.

[27] Bakri SJ, Wolfe JD, Regillo CD, et al. Evidence-based guidelines for management of diabetic macular edema. Journal of VitreoRetinal Diseases. 2019 May;3(3):145-152.

[28] Chhablani J, Wong K, Tan GS, et al. Diabetic macular edema management in asian population: expert panel consensus guidelines. Asia-Pacific Journal of Ophthalmology. 2020 Sep 1;9(5):426-434.

[29] Schmidt-Erfurth U, Garcia-Arumi J, Bandello F, et al. Guidelines for the management of diabetic macular edema by the european society of retina specialists (EURETINA). Ophthalmologica. 2017;237(4):185-222.

[30] Hooper P, Boucher MC, Colleaux K, et al. Contemporary management of diabetic retinopathy in Canada: from guidelines to algorithm guidance. Ophthalmologica. 2014;231(1):2-15.

[31] Das T, Aurora A, Chhablani J, et al. Evidence-based review of diabetic macular edema management: Consensus statement on Indian treatment guidelines. Indian journal ofophthalmology. 2016 Jan;64(1):14.

[32] Eylea. Prescribing information. Regeneron Pharmaceuticals, Inc.; March 2021. Accessed April 21, 2021. https://www.regeneron.com/downloads/eylea_fpi.pdf.

[33] Takamura Y, Tomomatsu T, Matsumura T, Arimura S, Gozawa M, Takihara Y, Inatani M. The effect of photocoagulation in ischemic areas to prevent recurrence of diabetic macular edema after intravitreal bevacizumab injection. Investigative ophthalmology & visual science. 2014 Aug 1;55(8): 4741-4746.

[34] Wong TY, Sun J, Kawasaki R, et al. Guidelines on diabetic eye care: the international council of ophthalmology recommendations for screening, follow-up, referral, and treatment based on resource settings. Ophthalmology. 2018 Oct 1;125(10):1608-1622.

[35] Tripathy K, Raj Sharma Y, Chawla R, et al. Recent advances in management of diabetic macular edema. Current diabetes reviews. 2015 Jun 1;11(2):79-97.

[36] Baker CW, Glassman AR, Beaulieu WT, et al. Effect of initial management with aflibercept vs. laser photocoagulation vs. observation on vision loss among patients with diabetic macular edema involving the center of the macula and good visual acuity: a randomized clinical trial. Jama. 2019 May 21;321(19):1880-1894.

[37] Scott IU, Danis RP, Bressler SB, et al. Effect of focal/grid photocoagulation on visual acuity and retinal thickening in eyes with non-center involved clinically significant diabetic macular edema. Retina (Philadelphia Pa.). 2009 May;29(5):613.

[38] Diabetic Retinopathy Clinical Research Network. Vitrectomy outcomes in eyes with diabetic macular edema and vitreomacular traction. Ophthalmology. 2010 Jun;117(6):1087.

[39] Pendergast SD, Hassan TS, Williams GA, et al. Vitrectomy for diffuse diabetic macular edema associated with a taut premacular posterior hyaloid. American journal of ophthalmology. 2000 Aug 1;130(2):178-186.

[40] Yamamoto T, Akabane N, Takeuchi S. Vitrectomy for diabetic macular edema: the role of posterior vitreous detachment and epimacular membrane. American journal of ophthalmology. 2001 Sep 1;132(3):369-377.

[41] Biomarkers Definitions Working Group, Atkinson Jr. AJ, Colburn WA, DeGruttola VG, DeMets DL, Downing GJ, Hoth DF, Oates JA, Peck CC, Schooley RT, Spilker BA. Biomarkers and surrogate endpoints: preferred definitions and conceptual framework. Clinical pharmacology & therapeutics. 2001 Mar;69(3):89-95.

[42] Markan A, Agarwal A, Arora A, et al. Novel imaging biomarkers in diabetic retinopathy and diabetic macular edema. Therapeutic Advances in Ophthalmology. 2020 Sep;12:2515841420950513.

[43] Bandello F, Polito A, Borrello MD, et al. "Light" versus "classic" laser treatment for clinically significant diabetic macular oedema. British Journal of Ophthalmology. 2005 Jul 1;89(7): 864-870.

[44] Ozdemir H, Karacorlu M, Karacorlu SA. Regression of serous macular detachment after intravitreal triamcinolone acetonide in patients with diabetic macular edema. American journal of ophthalmology. 2005 Aug 1;140(2):251-2e1.

[45] Diabetic Retinopathy Clinical Research Network. Relationship between optical coherence tomography-measured central retinal thickness and visual acuity in diabetic macular edema. Ophthalmology. 2007 Mar 1;114(3): 525-536.

[46] Alasil T, Keane PA, Updike JF, et al. Relationship between optical coherence tomography retinal parameters and visual acuityin diabetic macular edema. Ophthalmology. 2010 Dec 1;117(12): 2379-2386.

[47] Bolz M, Schmidt-Erfurth U, Deak G, et al. Optical coherence tomographic hyperreflective foci. Ophthalmology. 2009 May 1;116(5):914-920.

[48] Deák GG, Bolz M, Ritter M, et al. A systematic correlation between morphology and functional alterations in diabetic macular edema. Investigative ophthalmology & visual science. 2010 Dec 1;51(12):6710-6714.

[49] Forooghian F, Stetson PF, Meyer SA, et al. Relationship between photoreceptor outer segment length and visual acuity in diabetic macular edema. Retina (Philadelphia Pa.). 2010 Jan;30(1):63-70.

[50] Sun JK, Lin MM, Lammer J, et al. Disorganization of the retinal inner layers as a predictor of visual acuity in eyes with center-involved diabetic macular edema. JAMA ophthalmology. 2014 Nov 1;132(11):1309-1316.

[51] Joltikov KA, Sesi CA, de Castro VM, et al. Disorganization of retinal inner layers (DRIL) and neuroretinal dysfunction in early diabetic retinopathy. Investigative ophthalmology & visual science. 2018 Nov 1;59(13):5481-5486.

[52] Pelosini L, Hull CC, Boyce JF, et al. Optical coherence tomography may be used to predict visual acuity in patients with macular edema. Investigative ophthalmology & visual science. 2011 Apr 1;52(5):2741-2748.

[53] Al Faran A, Mousa A, Al Shamsi H, et al. Spectral domain optical coherence tomography predictors of visual outcome in diabetic cystoid macular edema after bevacizumab injection. Retina. 2014 Jun 1;34(6):1208-1215.

[54] Lee H, Jang H, Choi YA, et al. Association between soluble cd14 in the aqueous humor and hyperreflective foci on optical coherence tomography in patients with diabetic macular edema. Investigative ophthalmology & visual science. 2018 Feb 1;59(2):715-721.

[55] Landmann R, Müller B, Zimmerli W. CD14, new aspects of ligand and signal diversity. Microbes and infection. 2000 Mar 1;2(3):295-304.

[56] Zeng HY, Green WR, Tso MO. Microglial activation in human diabetic retinopathy. Archives of ophthalmology. 2008 Feb 1;126(2):227-232.

[57] Midena E, Pilotto E, Bini S. Hyperreflective intraretinal foci as an oct biomarker of retinal inflammation in diabetic macular edema. Investigative ophthalmology & visual science. 2018 Nov 1;59(13):5366.

[58] Wang H, Chhablani J, Freeman WR, et al. Characterization of diabetic microaneurysms by simultaneous fluorescein angiography and spectral-domain optical coherence tomography. American journal of ophthalmology. 2012 May 1;153(5):861-867.

[59] Uji A, Murakami T, Nishijima K, et al. Association between hyperreflective foci in the outer retina, status of photoreceptor layer, and visual acuity in diabetic macular edema. American journal of ophthalmology. 2012 Apr 1;153(4):710-717.

[60] Vujosevic S, Berton M, Bini S, et al. Hyperreflective retinal spots and visual function after anti-vascular endothelial growth factor treatment in center-involving diabetic macular edema. Retina. 2016 Jul 1;36(7):1298-1308.

[61] Vujosevic S, Torresin T, Bini S, et al. Imaging retinal inflammatory biomarkers after intravitreal steroid and anti-VEGF treatment in diabetic macular oedema. Acta Ophthalmologica. 2017 Aug;95(5):464-471.

[62] Kim KT, Kim DY, Chae JB. Association between Hyperreflective Foci on Spectral-Domain Optical Coherence Tomography and Early Recurrence of Diabetic Macular Edema after Intravitreal Dexamethasone Implantation. Journal ofophthalmology. 2019 Nov 19;2019.

[63] Hwang HS, Chae JB, Kim JY, Kim DY. Association between hyperreflective dots on spectral-domain optical coherence tomography in macular edema and response to treatment. Investigative ophthalmology & visual science. 2017 Nov 1;58(13):5958-5967.

[64] Gelman SK, Freund KB, Shah VP, Sarraf D. The pearl necklace sign: a novel spectral domain optical coherence tomography finding in exudative macular disease. Retina. 2014 Oct 1;34(10): 2088-2095.

[65] Ajay K, Mason F, Gonglore B, et al. Pearl necklace sign in diabetic macular edema: Evaluation and significance. Indian journal of ophthalmology. 2016 Nov;64(11):829.

[66] Liang MC, Vora RA, Duker JS, et al. Solid-appearing retinal cysts in diabetic macular edema: a novel optical coherence tomography finding. Retinal Cases and Brief Reports. 2013 July 1;7(3):255-258.

[67] Sacconi R, Lutty GA, Mullins RF, et al. Subretinal pseudocysts: A novel OCT finding in diabetic macular edema. American journal of ophthalmologycase reports. 2019 Dec 1;16:100567.

[68] Özkaya A, Alkin Z, Karatas G, et al. Photoreceptor outer segment layer thickness measured manually on images from spectral domain optical coherence tomography in healthy volunteers. Journal français d'ophtalmologie. 2014 Jun 1;37(6):475-479.

[69] Ozkaya A, Alkin Z, Karakucuk Y, et al. Thickness of the retinal photoreceptor outer segment layer in healthy volunteers and in patients with diabetes mellitus without retinopathy, diabetic retinopathy, or diabetic macular edema. Saudi Journal of Ophthalmology. 2017 Apr 1;31(2):69-75.

[70] Roy R, Saurabh K, Shah D, et al. Choroidal hyperreflective foci: a novel spectral domain optical coherence tomography biomarker in eyes with diabetic macular edema. Asia-Pacific journal of ophthalmology (Philadelphia, Pa.). 2019 Jul;8(4):314.

[71] Kim JT, Lee DH, Joe SG, et al. Changes in Choroidal Thickness in Relation to the Severity of Retinopathy and Macular Edema in Type 2 Diabetic Patients. Investigative ophthalmology & visual science. 2013 May 1;54(5): 3378-3384.

[72] Querques G, Lattanzio R, Querques L, et al. Enhanced depth imaging optical coherence tomography in type 2 diabetes. Investigative ophthalmology & visual science. 2012 Sep 1;53(10):6017-6024.

[73] Rayess N, Rahimy E, Ying G, et al. Baseline choroidal thickness as a predictor for response to anti–vascular endothelial growth factor therapy in diabetic macular edema. American journal of ophthalmology. 2015 Jan 1;159(1):85-91.

[74] Wang W, Liu S, Qiu Z, et al. Choroidal thickness in diabetes and diabetic retinopathy: a swept source OCT study. Investigativeophthalmology &visual science. 2020 Apr 9;61(4):29-29.

[75] Agrawal R, Gupta P, Tan K-A, et al. Choroidal vascularity index as a measure of vascular status of the choroid: Measurements in healthy eyes from a population-based study. Scientific Reports. 2016 Feb 12;6(1):1-9.

[76] Kim M, Ha MJ, Choi SY, et al. Choroidal vascularity index in type-2 diabetes analyzed by swept-source optical coherence tomography. Scientific Reports. 2018 Jan 8;8(1):70.

[77] Cho H, Alwassia AA, Regiatieri CV, et al. Retinal neovascularization secondary to proliferative diabetic retinopathy characterized by spectral domain optical coherence tomography. Retina (Philadelphia, Pa.). 2013 Mar;33(3):542-7.

[78] Pan J, Chen D, Yang X, et al. Characteristics of neovascularization in early stages of proliferative diabetic retinopathy by optical coherence tomography angiography. American journal ofophthalmology. 2018 Aug 1;192:146-156.

[79] Vaz-Pereira S, Zarranz-Ventura J, Sim DA, et al. Optical Coherence Tomography Features of Active And Inactive Retinal Neovascularization In Proliferative Diabetic Retinopathy. Retina. 2016 Jun 1;36(6):1132-1142.

[80] Vaz-Pereira S, Dansingani KK, Chen KC, et al. Tomographic relationships between retinal neovascularization and the posterior vitreous in proliferative diabetic retinopathy. Retina. 2017 Jul 1;37(7): 1287-1296.

[81] Mishra DK, Shanmugam MP, Ramanjulu R, et al. Comparison of standard and "innovative wide-field" optical coherence tomography images in assessment of vitreoretinal interface in proliferative diabetic retinopathy: A pilot study. Indian Journal of Ophthalmology. 2021 Jan;69(1):99.

[82] Spaide RF, Fujimoto JG, Waheed NK, et al. Optical coherence tomography angiography. Progress in retinal and eye research. 2018 May 1;64:1-55.

[83] Couturier A, Mané V, Bonnin S, et al. Capillary plexus anomalies in diabetic retinopathy on optical coherence tomography angiography. Retina. 2015 Nov 1;35(11):2384-2391.

[84] Soares M, Neves C, Marques IP, et al. Comparison of diabetic retinopathy classification using fluorescein angiography and optical coherence tomography angiography. British Journal of Ophthalmology. 2017 Jan 1;101(1):62-68.

[85] Choi W, Waheed NK, Molt EM, et al. Ultrahigh speed swept source optical coherence tomography angiography of retinal and choriocapillaris alterations in diabetic patients with and without retinopathy. Retina. 2017 Jan 1;37(1): 11-21.

[86] Ishibazawa A, Nagaoka T, Takahashi A, et al. Optical coherence tomography angiography in diabetic retinopathy: a prospective pilot study. American journal of ophthalmology. 2015 Jul 1;160(1):35-44.

[87] Hwang TS, Jia Y, Gao SS, et al. Optical coherence tomography angiography features of diabetic retinopathy. Retina (Philadelphia, Pa.). 2015 Nov;35(11):2371.

[88] Kim AY, Chu Z, Shahidzadeh A, et al. Quantifying microvascular density and morphology in diabetic retinopathy using spectral-domain optical coherence tomography angiography. Investigative ophthalmology & visual science. 2016 Jul 1;57(9):OCT362–OCT370.

[89] Chua J, Sim R, Tan B, et al. Optical Coherence Tomography Angiography in Diabetes and Diabetic Retinopathy. Journal of Clinical Medicine. 2020 Jun;9(6):1723.

[90] Jonnal RS, Kocaoglu OP, Zawadzki RJ, et al. A review of adaptive optics optical coherence tomography: technical advances, scientific applications, and the future. Investigative ophthalmology & visual science. 2016 Jul 1;57(9):OCT51–OCT68.

[91] Benesty J, Ayello-Scheer S, Sahel J, et al. Adaptive optics imaging of diabetic retinopathy. Investigative Ophthalmology & Visual Science. 2013 Jun 16;54(15):203.

[92] Tan O, Jia Y, Wei E, Huang D. Clinical applications of Doppler OCT and OCT angiography. InOptical Coherence Tomography: Technology and Applications, Second Edition 2015 Jan 1 (pp. 1413-1428). Springer International Publishing.

[93] Srinivas S, Tan O, Nittala MG, et al. Assessment of retinal blood flow in diabetic retinopathy using Doppler Fourier-domain optical coherence tomography. Retina (Philadelphia, Pa.). 2017 Nov;37(11):2001.

Chapter 7

Adaptive Optics Imaging Technique in Diabetic Retinopathy

Florian Baltă, Irina Elena Cristescu and Ioana Teodora Tofolean

Abstract

Adaptive optics ophthalmoscopy opened a new era in the medical retina field. The possibility of obtaining high-resolution retinal images of photoreceptors and retinal vessels addresses new perspectives in retinal physiology and pathophysiology. The overwhelming incidence of diabetes in the global population justifies the need to develop and refine methods of diagnosing early retinal changes, in order to preserve vision and avoid complications. The current grading of diabetic retinopathy is based on clinical changes only. Nevertheless, imaging tools such as optical coherence tomography and optical coherence tomography angiography are also used for screening of this pathology. The corroboration of the information provided by these imaging methods may lay the foundations for a new approach to the definition and diagnosis of diabetic retinopathy.

Keywords: diabetic retinopathy, retinal imaging, adaptive optics ophthalmoscopy, wall-to-lumen ratio, cone mosaic, rtx1™

1. Introduction: Adaptive optics in retinal imaging

The principle of adaptive optics (AO) belongs to Babcock since 1953. Fifteen years afterward, the technique started to be used in military setups. Its main purpose was obtaining good satellite surveillance images, even in unfavorable meteorological situations. In 1970, the Soviet and American military managed the real-time correction of atmospheric turbulences when studying laser sources and stars [1, 2]. In 1996, the first AO ophthalmoscope allowed *in vivo* imaging of the human retina, compensating for static and dynamic aberrations of the optical system of the human eye. AO technology has three main components: a Hartmann-Shack sensor, to measure distortion, a deformable mirror to compensate for the distortion, and a control system to calculate the required compensation.

AO has been allowing *in vivo* studies of human retinal photoreceptors mosaic and vessels at a two-micron transversal resolution. As it is lessening the effect of optical aberrations on any measurement, it can be combined with almost any imaging device. AO imaging at histological resolution of the retina opened new perspectives toward early detection, monitoring, and treatment of retinal diseases. The devices above are allowing noninvasive *in vivo* imaging of retinal structures:

- retinal nerve fiber layers; axons of ganglion cells can be studied with AO scanning laser ophthalmoscopy (AOSLO) [3, 4], AO optical coherence tomography (AOOCT) [5], and with AO flood illumination ophthalmoscopy [6];

- ganglion cells, although large in size, they have a low signal-to-noise ratio and a low intrinsic contrast. They were visualized in monkeys using intrinsic two-photon excitation fluorescence and AOSLO [7] and in humans using AOOCT [8];

- bipolar cells could not be visualized using any AO system, as they lack intrinsic contrast and scatter to be seen by reflectance;

- Henle fibers were visible with AOSLO, but in pathological cases only. In a study that included four family members with Best vitelliform macular dystrophy, the inner retinal layers changed their orientation because of the large subretinal lesions, thus producing sufficient scatter to reveal their structure;

- photoreceptors have been the most studied microscopic retinal structures, being the first neuron of the human visual pathway. Both cones and rods could be assessed using AO imaging techniques [9]. Advances in AO ophthalmoscopy led to substantial refinement in the ability to assess these cells, to the point where recording and analyzing clear mosaics of photoreceptors across of the macular region become possible;

- retinal pigment epithelium (RPE) was visualized in patients with age-related degeneration, in which RPE was obvious due to the photoreceptors degeneration, fact confirmed by optical coherence tomography (OCT) scans as well [10]. Moreover, AOSLO dark field showed RPE cell mosaic in a subject with no eye disease [11];

- lamina cribrosa—morphological changes were noticed in glaucomatous patients using flood illumination AO retinal camera [12], AOOCT [13], and AOSLO [10];

- retinal vasculature.

The following section focuses on an overview of AO retinal imaging methods, namely AO flood illumination imaging, adaptive optics scanning laser ophthalmoscopy, and adaptive optics optical coherence tomography.

1.1 AO flood illumination imaging

AO flood illumination imaging was obtained by coupling a wave front sensor and a deformable mirror to a high-magnification fundus camera, thus providing some of the first organized studies of retinal photoreceptors [14]. This is the principle of the AO rtx1 camera (Imagine Eyes, Orsay, France), which has been extensively used in the study of retinal photoreceptors [15–17] and vasculature [18, 19]. Compared with the other two devices, its axial resolution is smaller (~300 μm) [10]. However, an important advantage of this type of imaging is the speed at which the entire retinal image is acquired (a few milliseconds). Thus, with a CCD camera, 40 retinal images are taken in 4 s, which are to be further processed by specialized software in order to deliver a final image [20]. One single image is minimally influenced by eye movement, and the system is capable of providing very high frame rates with high sensitivity [21].

1.2 AO scanning laser ophthalmoscopy

AO scanning laser ophthalmoscope provides a higher contrast relative to AO flood illumination by recording scattered light from a focused beam across the retinal surface through confocality. A pinhole conjugated to the focal retinal plane removes beams of light whose origin is outside the point spread function. By modifying the pinhole size, different transversal and axial resolutions of the system can be obtained, allowing imaging of the retinal structures (nerve fiber layers, photoreceptors, blood vessels). Its accuracy is increased by the AO constituent. In addition to this, continuous scanning allows the study of larger areas at a superior rate relative to conventional fundus imaging [22]. AOSLO is being used in high-resolution imaging, eye-tracking, laser modulations setups, psychophysics and electrophysiology studies [23].

1.3 AO optical coherence tomography

OCT started to be used as a retinal imaging tool in 1991, while the association of AO technology with the OCT was first introduced more than 10 years ago [24]. An advantage of the AOOCT its ability to adjust images in all three coordinates (both axial and lateral) and to offer great visualization of individual cells because of its outstanding axial resolution. Axial resolution increases with the bandwidth of the imaging coherent light source [23]. Time-domain OCT might reach an axial resolution of 2–3 μm, whereas spectral-domain OCT an axial resolution between 2.1 and 2.5 μm [25]. Nevertheless, individual cells cannot be visualized because of low acquisition speed and low lateral resolution (>15 μm). Swept source OCT has a higher acquisition speed, but with an axial resolution of 5.3 μm and a lateral one of 20 μm. Lateral resolution is influenced by the eye's aberrations effect on focal spot size. After coupling AO with OCT imaging, the lateral resolution of the system reached 2–3 μm [26], and 3D imaging of retinal structures (RPE, ganglion cells, lamina cribrosa, nerve fiber layer) was achieved [27].

2. Diabetic retinopathy and adaptive optics

Diabetic retinopathy (DR) is a microvascular complication of diabetes mellitus (DM), representing one of the leading causes of vision loss and blindness worldwide [28]. Its early diagnosis is necessary to preserve vision and avoid its complications.

Staging of diabetic retinopathy is currently performed according to clinical changes only. Given the fact that patients with DR can be asymptomatic for a very long period of time, even in very advanced stages of the disease, regular screening of diabetic patients and appropriate treatment are strongly recommended [29]. Besides clinical examination, the new emerging imaging methods provide valuable information and lay the foundations of a new approach in the definition and diagnosis of diabetic retinopathy.

The accepted pathophysiological mechanisms of vision loss entail both retinal microvascular and neuronal damage [30–34]. Therefore, some authors [35] suggest diabetic retinal disease to be a more appropriate term for retinal changes in diabetes mellitus than diabetic retinopathy, as it encompasses both retinal vasculopathy and neuropathy. Moreover, it appears that retinal diabetic neuropathy (neuronal degeneration of the internal retinal layers) precedes retinal vasculopathy [36].

Diabetic patients without DR are proven by full-field electroretinography (ERG) and multifocal ERG studies to have retinal functional alterations [37], as well as ionic transport changes at photoreceptors' level [38, 39]. In addition to this, given that the retina and the cerebral cortex have the same embryological origin, it can be speculated that the retinal functional alterations may be connected with neurocognitive deficits in diabetic patients [40]. In this context, the study of photoreceptors and retinal vessels can lead to the identification of new biomarkers that are able to mirror retinal alterations induced by DM.

Adaptive optics retinal camera is able to detect early diabetes-induced retinal changes, often before any documentable sign can be traced using other retinal imaging techniques, thus shedding new light on the pathophysiology of microvascular and neuronal changes in DR.

Microaneurysms are considered to be the first visible clinical signs, while the loss of pericytes seems to be the first histological microvascular alteration [41]. Microvascular clinical findings in DR encompass intraretinal hemorrhages, microaneurysms, venous caliber abnormalities, intraretinal microvascular abnormalities (IRMA), lipid exudates, cotton-wool spots, and retinal neovascularization [42]. Among these, microaneurysms [43], microscopic hemorrhages [43–45], hard exudates [46, 47], edematous cyst walls [45], and modified arteriolar structures [48–50] were already morphologically characterized using adaptive optics images (**Figures 1** and 2). Offering a fine documentation of retinal lesions, AO imaging technique might become an important instrument for early diagnosis and progression monitorization of DR [51].

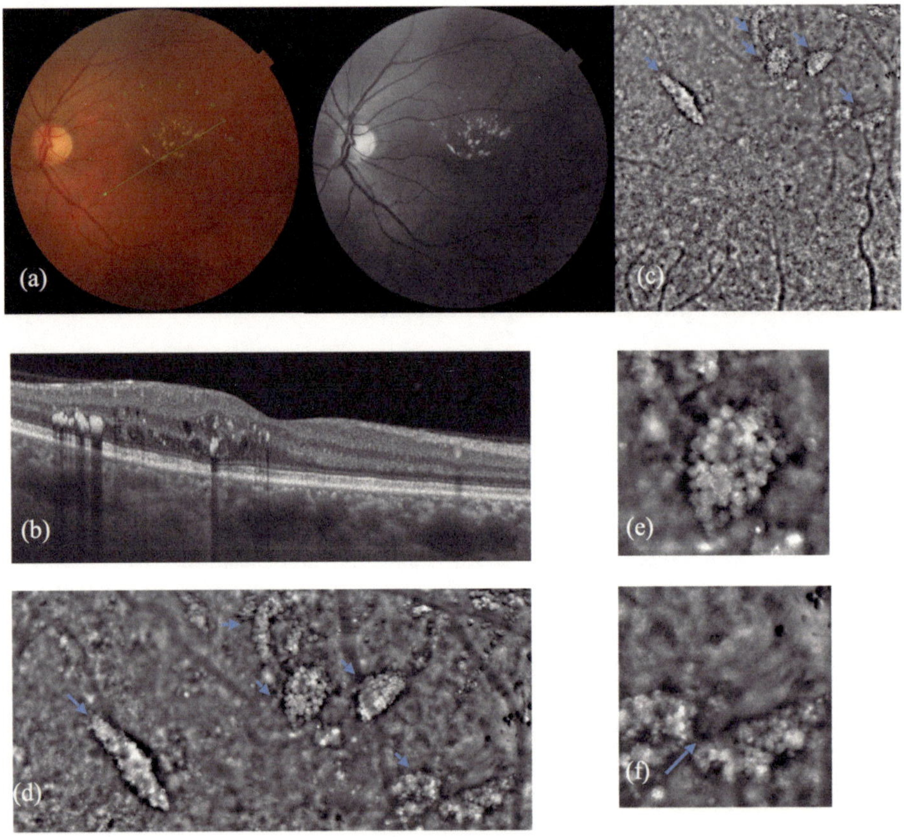

Figure 1.
(a) Color fundus photo and red free photo of a patient with hard exudates and retinal edema. (b) Optical coherence tomography corresponding to the green line in (a) shows hard exudates in the middle retinal layers. (c) Adaptive optics imaging cone mosaic; small arrows indicate the hard exudates. (d) Magnification of the upper part in (c), in which besides the hard exudates (small arrows), edema blurring the retinal image can be noticed. (e) Magnification of (d), detail of a hard exudate showing foci of hyper- and hypo-reflectivity. (f) Magnification of (d), detail of two hard exudates and retinal edema; the cystic spaces have a sharp demarcation line indicated by the big arrow. (Reproduced from [46]. Copyright by the ©Romanian Society of Ophthalmology.)

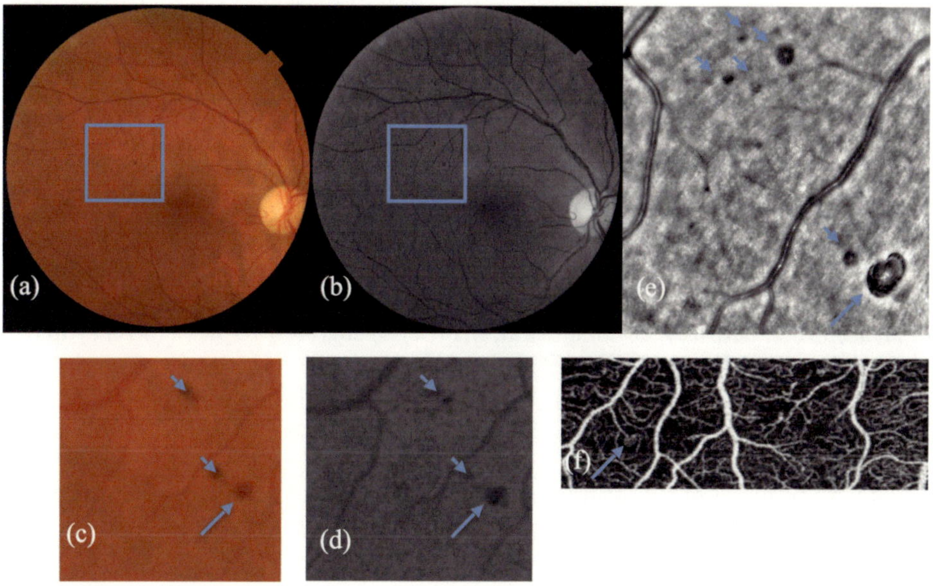

Figure 2.
(a) and (b) Color fundus photo and red free photo of a patient with microaneurysms and hemorrhages. (c) and (d) Larger magnification of the area delimited in the previous photos, (a) and (b). The big arrow indicates a microaneurysm and the arrowheads show hemorrhages. (e) Adaptive optics image corresponding to (c) and (d). The black lesion with inner hyper-reflectivity marked by a big arrow is a microaneurysm. The black lesions marked by small arrows are retinal hemorrhages. (f) OCT angiography revealed only one lesion from the ones above which is the microaneurysm. (Reproduced from [46]. Copyright by the ©Romanian Society of Ophthalmology.)

2.1 Imaging the cone mosaic in diabetic retinopathy

Biological systems are characterized by symmetrical spatial arrangements as in hexagonal systems. These structures can have equal angles and sides. Even when they are not clearly delimited [52], Voronoi diagrams can generate the limits between elements, taking the starting points as generators. It is known that the regular hexagon is the maximum-sided polygon that could be used to cover a plane without overlaps. The immediate advantage of this organization is the maximization of number of neighbors of each element and the consequent optimization of cell signaling, resolution, and isotropy (photoreceptors, retinal neurons).

2.1.1 Cone parameters

2.1.1.1 Photoreceptor density

The density of photoreceptors is usually assessed by dividing the number of detected cones by the analyzed area. This method implies a normal distribution within the analyzed area and will underestimate the density if this area overlaps over regions for which no data are available. These limitations motivate the need for Voronoi local density analysis [53]. The density of photoreceptors can be expressed in metric (cones/mm^2) or angular (cones/degree) units. The value of the antero-posterior axis can influence the values expressed in metric units. At a certain eccentricity, the distance from the fovea may be different depending on the antero-posterior axis. For example, an eccentricity of 2° corresponds to a distance between 0.53 and 0.64 mm from the fovea, given an axis of 22–26 mm. As the axis gets longer, the retinal area increases and the cones density gets lower when expressed in metric units [54].

2.1.1.2 Cone spacing

This indicator is useful to be used in conjunction with photoreceptor density. It considers only the closest photoreceptor for each cone detected in the region of interest, regardless of the measured distance [17]. This can lead to high values for isolated cells. On the other hand, it has been shown that the distance between photoreceptors is less sensitive to subsampling (compared to cones) and to the correlation with a certain pathology. Thus, photoreceptor spacing overestimates the overall health of the photoreceptor mosaic (e.g., a mosaic with sporadic photoreceptor losses may have normal distances between photoreceptors, but in the presence of an abnormal density). In conclusion, in order to correctly depict a mosaic, all biomarkers should be considered [55].

2.1.1.3 Voronoi diagrams

Given a finite set of two or more points in an Euclidean plane, we associate all locations of that plane with the nearest element of the set. The result is a tessellation of the plane in a series of regions associated with the elements of the set of points. This tiling is called the Voronoi diagram generated by the set of points, while the regions that make up the Voronoi diagram are called Voronoi polygons [56]. Li and collaborators showed that less than 30% of Voronoi polygons are non-hexagonal in the vicinity of the fovea and that their percentage increases to 50–60% at higher eccentricities [57]. Cones at higher eccentricities are unevenly distributed and protect the visual system from perceiving a distorted signal [58].

AO ophthalmoscopy is an accessible tool for clinicians to visualize the human retina *in vivo* [59, 60]. Cones parameters have been analyzed in healthy, adult population [15, 61, 62] and correlated to several factors (age, gender, refractive error, antero-posterior axis, race, ethnicity). These studies showed a variability of photoreceptor densities in normal population [15, 63], which makes it difficult to detect small variabilities of this parameter in comparative studies. The inclusion of all photoreceptor parameters (distance from the nearest photoreceptor and Voronoi diagrams—with the analysis of their spatial arrangement) in study protocols promises to provide more conclusive results [17]. Nevertheless, the first measurements of cone density come from the postmortem histological analysis of the human retina [64]. It has been shown that in the center of the fovea, there is a density of 199,000 cells/mm^2, which decreases to about 20,000 cells/mm^2 to 1 mm from the center of the fovea.

2.1.2 Cone parameters in diabetic retinopathy

AO ophthalmoscopy has been used to assess the parafoveal cone parameters in diabetic patients (type I or type II diabetes) and controls in various studies (**Figure 3**) [16, 17, 48, 66, 67].

Lombardo et al. [17] studied the differences between cone parameters at 1.5 degrees eccentricity in patients diagnosed with DM I without DR or with nonproliferative DR and in healthy subjects. Their results showed that cone density was higher in the control group as compared with the study group, on both vertical and horizontal meridians. Another study [47, 68] showed that cone density was 10% lower in type I diabetic subjects with no DR than in controls. Moreover, cone densities were also investigated in type II diabetic patients with or without DR and in healthy subjects, at 0 and 2 degrees eccentricity [16]. The results showed a positive correlation of the extent of cone loss on AO imaging with DR severity in

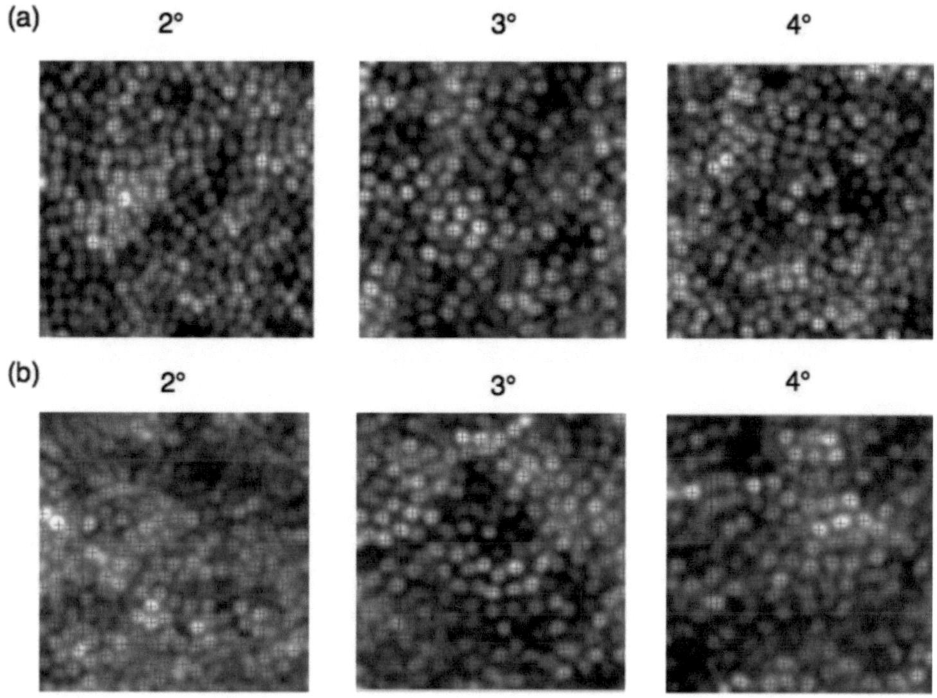

Figure 3.
Examples of regions of interest (red square) at 2, 3, and 4 degrees nasally analyzed in a control subject (a) and in a diabetic patient (b). (Reproduced from [65]. Copyright by the ©Romanian Society of Ophthalmology.)

type II diabetic patients. On the other hand, Tan and collaborators [69] found no cone densities differences at 7 degrees eccentricity between patients with DM I and healthy subjects, probably due to the short duration of diabetes in the study group.

In addition to this, cone spacing was found to significantly increase in diabetic patients, when compared with healthy controls [70]. Results show lessening of hexagonal mosaics of cones (Voronoi 6 tiles) with increased severity of DR.

The horizontal meridian was proved to have a higher average cone density than the vertical one in both controls and type I diabetic patients with no DR [47, 68]. However, the asymmetry was higher in the control group. Another study reported this pattern in normal subjects [15]. This asymmetry, also called "horizontal–vertical anisotropy," could be related to the way we are using our vision. When reading, the horizontal meridian is more in demand than the vertical one. Psychophysical studies have shown a higher contrast sensitivity and spatial resolution of the horizontal meridian as compared with the vertical one at a given eccentricity [71]. Further studies including more subjects are needed to describe the cone parameters in diabetic and age-matched volunteers.

2.2 Imaging the retinal microvasculature in diabetic retinopathy

Retinal microcirculation is a network of arterioles, capillaries, and venules with diameters that do not exceed 150 μm, whose main function is to assure and regulate an optimal tissue perfusion [72]. Microcirculation alterations, also called microangiopathy, lead to organ damage and clinical events in patients with DM.

A microvascular network is assessed from a structural and functional point of view, taking into consideration both its topology and geometric abnormalities [73].

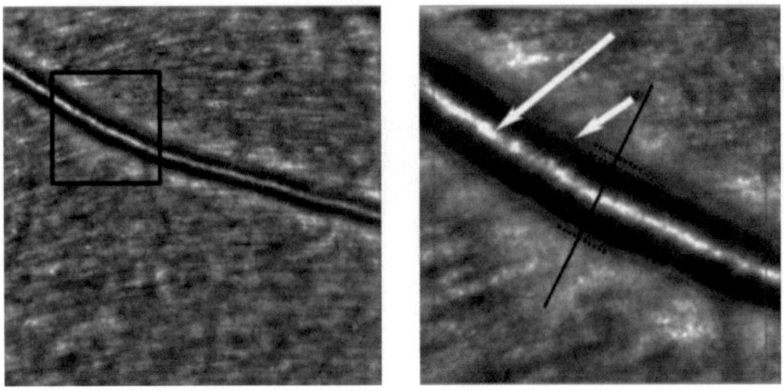

Figure 4.
Image of the retinal artery of a patient with diabetes mellitus, with visualization of the walls (short arrow) and lumen (long arrow), employing AO detect artery software.

The retinal vascular branching model is similar to a fractal, having a complex pattern of distribution, where each part has similar features to the main structure. DR is associated with a decreased fractal dimension, which is probably correlated with the shortcoming of the retinal circulation [74]. The network geometry is appreciated using the length and the diameters of the vessels, by calculating different derived parameters.

Vascular-addressing diseases encounter different patterns of vascular remodeling. The inward eutrophic remodeling, seen in stages 1 and 2 of essential hypertension, is characterized by a reduced lumen diameter, with consecutive rearrangement of the surrounding smooth muscle cells, but without a marked growth response [75]. The media-to-lumen ratio is increased due to reduced lumen diameter and external diameter of the wall and due to increased media thickness, with minimum changes in the total amount of wall tissue. All these result in decreased vasodilation potential of the vessel and altered arteriolar distensibility [76, 77]. In contrast, the hypertrophic remodeling, found in diabetes mellitus and in long-standing, severe and secondary hypertension, exhibits a significant growth response with vascular smooth muscle cell hypertrophy or hyperplasia [78, 79]. This leads to the increase of both media-to-lumen ratio and the media cross-sectional area of the vessel [80].

The bedside morphological assessment of human retinal microcirculation is not facile, the gold standard being the media-to-lumen ratio evaluated by wire or pressure micromyography on bioptic samples [81]. Recently, noninvasive techniques for the evaluation of retinal arterioles prove rather good agreement with micromyographic measurements, in particular scanning laser Doppler flowmetry and adaptive optics [81, 82]. Preliminary data suggest that AO has a substantial advantage over Doppler flowmetry, having a better correlation with the gold standard, but invasive procedure [81].

Adaptive optics ophthalmoscopy uses a cutting-edge technique, visualizing the retinal arterioles lumen as a bright band, while the walls correspond to the darker neighboring regions (**Figure 4**). The wall thickness of the blood vessels depends on the vessels' size, with large lumens requiring thicker walls. The AO-related vascular parameters of interest are:

- wall thickness (WT);
- lumen diameter (LD);
- vessel diameter (VD—the algebraic sum between the thickness of the arterioles' walls and the lumen diameter);

- wall-to-lumen ratio (WLR—the ratio between the wall thickness and the lumen diameter);
- the cross-sectional area of the vascular wall (WCSA—the calculation is based on the lumen diameter and vessel diameter values).

Zaleska-Żmijewska et al. [48] found statistically significant differences between the control group and the prediabetic group with respect to LD and to WLR. Furthermore, the same scientific team demonstrated that WLR, WCSA, and the average WT exhibit significant differences between the control group and type II diabetic patients [70]. An AOSLO study confirms that retinal arterial WT is significantly greater in patients with type 2 diabetes than in controls [83].

When it comes to DM type I, the average capillary LD proved to be significantly narrower in eyes with nonproliferative diabetic retinopathy and type I DM, when compared with healthy subjects (6.27 ± 1.63 μm versus 7.31 ± 1.59 μm, $p = 0.002$) [50]. When investigating the retinal microcirculation changes in type I and II diabetic patients without retinopathy, among all studied parameters, only WLR was significantly different between the control group and each group of diabetic patients taken individually, while no statistically significant differences were found between the two diabetic groups [47, 68].

New data characterize retinal arterioles according to DR classification, showing that LD, WT, and WLR significantly correlate with the stage of DR [84]. AO was even used to establish the effects of a multinutrient complex on retinal microvasculature in diabetic patients. After 3 months of food supplements administration, WLR, WT, and WCSA had significantly decreased, when compared with initial observations [85].

AO proved its potential to detect retinal microvascular changes in prediabetic subjects and diabetic patients, as well as to reveal differences between the diabetic groups. Providing useful information about the topological and geometrical features of the retinal microvasculature from early onset of diabetic disease, AO has a promising role in the future, providing valuable prognostic, diagnostic, and therapy-related information in diabetic retinopathy.

Conflict of interest

The authors declare no conflict of interest.

Author details

Florian Baltă[1,2,3], Irina Elena Cristescu[3]* and Ioana Teodora Tofolean[1,2]

1 "Carol Davila" University of Medicine and Pharmacy, Bucharest, Romania

2 Emergency Eye Hospital, Bucharest, Romania

3 "Retina" Clinic, Bucharest, Romania

*Address all correspondence to: cristescu.irina@gmail.com

References

[1] Hardy J. Adaptive optics—A progress review. Proceedings of SPIE on Active and Adaptive Optical Systems. 1991; **1542**:2-17

[2] Park JH, Kong L, Zhou Y, Cui M. Large-field-of-view imaging by multi-pupil adaptive optics. Nature Methods. 2017;**14**(6):581-583

[3] Takayama K, Ooto S, Hangai M, Arakawa N, Oshima S, Shibata N, et al. High-resolution imaging of the retinal nerve fiber layer in normal eyes using adaptive optics scanning laser ophthalmoscopy. PLoS One. 2012; **7**(3):e33158

[4] Takayama K, Ooto S, Hangai M, Ueda-Arakawa N, Yoshida S, Akagi T, et al. High-resolution imaging of retinal nerve fiber bundles in glaucoma using adaptive optics scanning laser ophthalmoscopy. American Journal of Ophthalmology. 2013;**155**(5):870-881

[5] Choi SS, Zawadzki RJ, Keltner JL, Werner JS. Changes in cellular structures revealed by ultra-high resolution retinal imaging in optic neuropathies. Investigative Ophthalmology & Visual Science. 2008;**49**(5):2103-2119

[6] Ramaswamy G, Lombardo M, Devaney N. Registration of adaptive optics corrected retinal nerve fiber layer (RNFL) images. Biomedical Optics Express. 2014;**5**(6):1941-1951

[7] Hunter JJ, Masella B, Dubra A, Sharma R, Yin L, Merigan WH, et al. Images of photoreceptors in living primate eyes using adaptive optics two-photon ophthalmoscopy. Biomedical Optics Express. 2010;**2**(1): 139-148

[8] Liu T, Jung H, Liu J, Droettboom M, Tam J. Noninvasive near infrared autofluorescence imaging of retinal pigment epithelial cells in the human retina using adaptive optics. Biomedical Optics Express. 2017;**8**(10):4348-4360

[9] Doble N, Choi SS, Codona JL, Christou J, Enoch JM, Williams DR. In vivo imaging of the human rod photoreceptor mosaic. Optics Letters. 2011;**36**(1):31-33

[10] Zhang B, Li N, Kang J, He Y, Chen XM. Adaptive optics scanning laser ophthalmoscopy in fundus imaging, a review and update. International Journal of Ophthalmology. 2017;**10**(11):1751-1758

[11] Scoles D, Sulai YN, Dubra A. In vivo dark-field imaging of the retinal pigment epithelium cell mosaic. Biomedical Optics Express. 2013;**4**(9): 1710-1723

[12] Zwillinger S, Paques M, Safran B, Baudouin C. In vivo characterization of lamina cribrosa pore morphology in primary open-angle glaucoma. Journal Français d'Ophtalmologie. 2016;**39**(3): 265-271

[13] Dong ZM, Wollstein G, Wang B, Schuman JS. Adaptive optics optical coherence tomography in glaucoma. Progress in Retinal and Eye Research. 2017;**57**:76-88

[14] Liang J, Williams DR, Miller DT. Supernormal vision and high-resolution retinal imaging through adaptive optics. Journal of the Optical Society of America. A, Optics, Image Science, and Vision. 1997;**14**(11):2884-2892

[15] Legras R, Gaudric A, Woog K. Distribution of cone density, spacing and arrangement in adult healthy retinas with adaptive optics flood illumination. PLoS One. 2018;**13**(1): e0191141

[16] Soliman MK, Sadiq MA, Agarwal A, Sarwar S, Hassan M, Hanout M, et al.

High-resolution imaging of parafoveal cones in different stages of diabetic retinopathy using adaptive optics fundus camera. PLoS One. 2016;**11**(4): e0152788

[17] Lombardo M, Parravano M, Serrao S, Ziccardi L, Giannini D, Lombardo G. Investigation of adaptive optics imaging biomarkers for detecting pathological changes of the cone mosaic in patients with type 1 diabetes mellitus. PLoS One. 2016;**11**(3):e0151380

[18] Koch E, Rosenbaum D, Brolly A, Sahel JA, Chaumet-Riffaud P, Girerd X, et al. Morphometric analysis of small arteries in the human retina using adaptive optics imaging: Relationship with blood pressure and focal vascular changes. Journal of Hypertension. 2014;**32**(4):890-898

[19] Lermé N, Rossant F, Bloch I, Paques M, Koch E, editors. Coupled Parallel Snakes for Segmenting Healthy and Pathological Retinal Arteries in Adaptive Optics Images. Cham: Springer International Publishing; 2014

[20] Tumahai P, Moureaux C, Meillat M, Debellemaniere G, Flores M, Delbosc B, et al. High-resolution imaging of photoreceptors in healthy human eyes using an adaptive optics retinal camera. Eye (London, England). 2018;**32**(11): 1723-1730

[21] Bedggood P, Metha A. Optical imaging of human cone photoreceptors directly following the capture of light. PLoS One. 2013;**8**(11):e79251

[22] Roorda A, Romero-Borja F, Donnelly Iii WJ, Queener H, Hebert TJ, Campbell MCW. Adaptive optics scanning laser ophthalmoscopy. Optics Express. 2002;**10**(9):405-412

[23] Godara P, Dubis AM, Roorda A, Duncan JL, Carroll J. Adaptive optics retinal imaging: Emerging clinical applications. Optometry and Vision Science. 2010;**87**(12):930-941

[24] Zhang Y, Rha J, Jonnal R, Miller D. Adaptive optics parallel spectral domain optical coherence tomography for imaging the living retina. Optics Express. 2005;**13**(12):4792-4811

[25] Kolb JP, Pfeiffer T, Eibl M, Hakert H, Huber R. High-resolution retinal swept source optical coherence tomography with an ultra-wideband Fourier-domain mode-locked laser at MHz A-scan rates. Biomedical Optics Express. 2018;**9**(1): 120-130

[26] Jonnal RS, Kocaoglu OP, Zawadzki RJ, Liu Z, Miller DT, Werner JS. A review of adaptive optics optical coherence tomography: Technical advances, scientific applications, and the future. Investigative Ophthalmology and Visual Science. 2016;**57**(9):OCT51-OCT68

[27] Pircher M, Zawadzki RJ. Review of adaptive optics OCT (AO-OCT): Principles and applications for retinal imaging [invited]. Biomedical Optics Express. 2017;**8**(5):2536-2562

[28] Nentwich MM, Ulbig MW. Diabetic retinopathy—ocular complications of diabetes mellitus. World Journal of Diabetes. 2015;**6**(3):489-499

[29] Wong TY, Sun J, Kawasaki R, Ruamviboonsuk P, Gupta N, Lansingh VC, et al. Guidelines on diabetic eye care: The international council of ophthalmology recommendations for screening, follow-up, referral, and treatment based on resource settings. Ophthalmology. 2018;**125**(10):1608-1622

[30] Fletcher EL, Phipps JA, Wilkinson-Berka JL. Dysfunction of retinal neurons and glia during diabetes. Clinical & Experimental Optometry. 2005;**88**(3):132-145

[31] Ding J, Wong TY. Current epidemiology of diabetic retinopathy and diabetic macular edema. Current Diabetes Reports. 2012;**12**(4):346-354

[32] Yau JW, Rogers SL, Kawasaki R, Lamoureux EL, Kowalski JW, Bek T, et al. Global prevalence and major risk factors of diabetic retinopathy. Diabetes Care. 2012;**35**(3):556-564

[33] Stem MS, Gardner TW. Neurodegeneration in the pathogenesis of diabetic retinopathy: Molecular mechanisms and therapeutic implications. Current Medicinal Chemistry. 2013;**20**(26):3241-3250

[34] Nian S, Lo ACY, Mi Y, Ren K, Yang D. Neurovascular unit in diabetic retinopathy: Pathophysiological roles and potential therapeutical targets. Eye and Vision. 2021;**8**(1):15

[35] Abràmoff MD, Lavin PT, Birch M, Shah N, Folk JC. Pivotal trial of an autonomous AI-based diagnostic system for detection of diabetic retinopathy in primary care offices. npj Digital Medicine. 2018;**1**(1):39

[36] Sohn EH, van Dijk HW, Jiao C, Kok PH, Jeong W, Demirkaya N, et al. Retinal neurodegeneration may precede microvascular changes characteristic of diabetic retinopathy in diabetes mellitus. Proceedings of the National Academy of Sciences of the United States of America. 2016;**113**(19): E2655-E2664

[37] Tyrberg M, Lindblad U, Melander A, Lövestam-Adrian M, Ponjavic V, Andréasson S. Electrophysiological studies in newly onset type 2 diabetes without visible vascular retinopathy. Documenta Ophthalmologica. 2011;**123**(3):193-198

[38] Kern TS, Berkowitz BA. Photoreceptors in diabetic retinopathy. Journal of Diabetes Investigation. 2015;**6**(4):371-380

[39] Calderon GD, Juarez OH, Hernandez GE, Punzo SM, De la Cruz ZD. Oxidative stress and diabetic retinopathy: Development and treatment. Eye (London, England). 2017;**31**(8):1122-1130

[40] Kodl CT, Seaquist ER. Cognitive dysfunction and diabetes mellitus. Endocrine Reviews. 2008;**29**(4):494-511

[41] Friedenwald J, Day R. The vascular lesions of diabetic retinopathy. Bulletin of the Johns Hopkins Hospital. 1950; **86**(4):253-254

[42] Duh EJ, Sun JK, Stitt AW. Diabetic retinopathy: Current understanding, mechanisms, and treatment strategies. JCI Insight. 2017;**2**(14):e93751

[43] Paques M, Meimon S, Rossant F, Rosenbaum D, Mrejen S, Sennlaub F, et al. Adaptive optics ophthalmoscopy: Application to age-related macular degeneration and vascular diseases. Progress in Retinal and Eye Research. 2018;**66**:1-16

[44] Lombardo M, Parravano M, Lombardo G, Varano M, Boccassini B, Stirpe M, et al. Adaptive optics imaging of parafoveal cones in type 1 diabetes. Retina. 2014;**34**(3):546-557

[45] Bek T. Fine structure in diabetic retinopathy lesions as observed by adaptive optics imaging. A qualitative study. Acta Ophthalmologica. 2014; **92**(8):753-758

[46] Cristescu I-E, Ochinciuc R, Balta F, Zagrean L. High-resolution imaging of diabetic retinopathy lesions using an adaptive optics retinal camera. Romanian Journal of Ophthalmology. 2019;**63**(1):29-34

[47] Cristescu IE. Diabetic retinopathy evaluation through high resolution imaging techniques. Bucharest: "Carol Davila" University of Medicine and Pharmacy; 2019

[48] Zaleska-Żmijewska A, Piatkiewicz P, Smigielska B, Sokolowska-Oracz A, Wawrzyniak ZM, Romaniuk D, et al. Retinal photoreceptors and microvascular changes in prediabetes measured with adaptive optics (rtx1): A case-control study. Journal Diabetes Research. 2017;**2017**:4174292

[49] Rosenbaum D, Mattina A, Koch E, Rossant F, Gallo A, Kachenoura N, et al. Effects of age, blood pressure and antihypertensive treatments on retinal arterioles remodeling assessed by adaptive optics. Journal of Hypertension. 2016;**34**(6):1115-1122

[50] Lombardo M, Parravano M, Serrao S, Ducoli P, Stirpe M, Lombardo G. Analysis of retinal capillaries in patients with type 1 diabetes and nonproliferative diabetic retinopathy using adaptive optics imaging. Retina. 2013;**33**(8):1630-1639

[51] Loganadane P, Delbosc B, Saleh M. Short-term progression of diabetic hard exudates monitored with high-resolution camera. Ophthalmic Research. 2019;**61**(1):3-9

[52] da Fontoura CL, Rocha F, Araújo de Lima SM. Characterizing polygonality in biological structures. Physical Review E. 2006;**73**(1):011913

[53] Costa Lda F, Bonci DM, Saito CA, Rocha FA, Silveira LC, Ventura DF. Voronoi analysis uncovers relationship between mosaics of normally placed and displaced amacrine cells in the thraira retina. Neuroinformatics. 2007;**5**(1): 59-78

[54] Obata R, Yanagi Y. Quantitative analysis of cone photoreceptor distribution and its relationship with axial length, age, and early age-related macular degeneration. PLoS One. 2014;**9**(3):e91873

[55] Garrioch R, Langlo C, Dubis AM, Cooper RF, Dubra A, Carroll J. Repeatability of in vivo parafoveal cone density and spacing measurements. Optometry and Vision Science. 2012; **89**(5):632-643

[56] Okabe A, Boots B, Sugihara K, Spatial Tessellations: Concepts and Applications of Voronoi Diagrams. J. Wiley and Sons, Chichester, New York, Brisbane, Toronto and Singapore: Wiley Series in Probability and Mathematical Statistics; 1992

[57] Li KY, Roorda A. Automated identification of cone photoreceptors in adaptive optics retinal images. Journal of the Optical Society of America. A, Optics, Image Science, and Vision. 2007;**24**(5):1358-1363

[58] Williams DR, Collier R. Consequences of spatial sampling by a human photoreceptor mosaic. Science. 1983;**221**(4608):385-387

[59] Burns SA, Elsner AE, Sapoznik KA, Warner RL, Gast TJ. Adaptive optics imaging of the human retina. Progress in Retinal and Eye Research. 2019; **68**:1-30

[60] Paques M, Meimon S, Grieve K, Rossant F. Adaptive Optics for In-Vivo Exploration of Human Retinal Structures. Munich, Germany: SPIE Optical Metrology; 2017.

[61] Park SP, Chung JK, Greenstein V, Tsang SH, Chang S. A study of factors affecting the human cone photoreceptor density measured by adaptive optics scanning laser ophthalmoscope. Experimental Eye Research. 2013; **108**:1-9

[62] Chui TY, Song H, Burns SA. Individual variations in human cone photoreceptor packing density: Variations with refractive error. Investigative Ophthalmology & Visual Science. 2008;**49**(10):4679-4687

[63] Lombardo M, Serrao S, Devaney N, Parravano M, Lombardo G. Adaptive

optics technology for high-resolution retinal imaging. Sensors (Basel). 2012;**13**(1):334-366

[64] Curcio CA, Sloan KR, Kalina RE, Hendrickson AE. Human photoreceptor topography. Journal of Comparative Neurology. 1990;**292**(4):497-523

[65] Cristescu IE et al. Cone photoreceptor density in type I diabetic patients measured with an adaptive optics retinal camera. Romanian Journal of Ophthalmology. 2019;**63**(2):153-160

[66] Sawides L, de Castro A, Burns SA. The organization of the cone photoreceptor mosaic measured in the living human retina. Vision Research. 2017;**132**:34-44

[67] Lammer J, Prager SG, Cheney MC, Ahmed A, Radwan SH, Burns SA, et al. Cone photoreceptor irregularity on adaptive optics scanning laser ophthalmoscopy correlates with severity of diabetic retinopathy and macular edema. Investigative Ophthalmology and Visual Science. 2016;**57**(15): 6624-6632

[68] Cristescu IE, Zagrean L, Balta F, Branisteanu DC. Retinal microcirculation investigation in type I and II diabetic patients without retinopathy using an adaptive optics retinal camera. Acta Endocrinologica (Bucharest). 2019;**15**(4):417-422

[69] Tan W, Wright T, Rajendran D, Garcia-Sanchez Y, Finkelberg L, Kisilak M, et al. Cone–photoreceptor density in adolescents with type 1 diabetes. Investigative Ophthalmology and Visual Science. 2015;**56**(11): 6339-6343

[70] Zaleska-Żmijewska A, Wawrzyniak ZM, Dąbrowska A, Szaflik JP. Adaptive optics (rtx1) high-resolution imaging of photoreceptors and retinal arteries in patients with diabetic retinopathy. Journal Diabetes Research. 2019;**2019**:9548324

[71] Fuller S, Rodriguez RZ, Carrasco M. Apparent contrast differs across the vertical meridian: Visual and attentional factors. Journal of Vision. 2008;**8**(1): 1-16

[72] Smits MM, Tonneijck L, Muskiet MH, Hoekstra T, Kramer MH, Diamant M, et al. GLP-1-based therapies have no microvascular effects in type 2 diabetes mellitus: An acute and 12-week randomized, double-blind, Placebo-Controlled Trial. Arteriosclerosis, Thrombosis, and Vascular Biology. 2016;**36**(10):2125-2132

[73] Yu PK, Balaratnasingam C, Cringle SJ, McAllister IL, Provis J, Yu DY. Microstructure and network organization of the microvasculature in the human macula. Investigative Ophthalmology & Visual Science. 2010;**51**(12):6735-6743

[74] Huang F, Dashtbozorg B, Zhang J, Bekkers E, Abbasi-Sureshjani S, Berendschot TT, et al. Reliability of using retinal vascular fractal dimension as a biomarker in the diabetic retinopathy detection. Journal of Ophthalmology. 2016;**2016**:6259047

[75] Rizzoni D, Agabiti RE. Small artery remodeling in hypertension and diabetes. Current Hypertension Reports. 2006;**8**(1):90-95

[76] Laurent S, Boutouyrie P. The structural factor of hypertension: Large and small artery alterations. Circulation Research. 2015;**116**(6):1007-1021

[77] Gliemann L, Buess R, Nyberg M, Hoppeler H, Odriozola A, Thaning P, et al. Capillary growth, ultrastructure remodelling and exercise training in skeletal muscle of essential hypertensive patients. Acta Physiologica (Oxford, England). 2015;**214**(2):210-220

[78] Schiffrin EL. Remodeling of resistance arteries in essential hypertension and effects of

antihypertensive treatment. American Journal of Hypertension. 2004;**17** (12 Pt 1):1192-1200

[79] Izzard AS, Rizzoni D, Agabiti-Rosei E, Heagerty AM. Small artery structure and hypertension: Adaptive changes and target organ damage. Journal of Hypertension. 2005;**23**(2):247-250

[80] Rizzoni D, Porteri E, Guelfi D, Muiesan ML, Valentini U, Cimino A, et al. Structural alterations in subcutaneous small arteries of normotensive and hypertensive patients with non-insulin-dependent diabetes mellitus. Circulation. 2001;**103**(9): 1238-1244

[81] De Ciuceis C, Caletti S, Coschignano MA, Rossini C, Duse S, Docchio F, et al. [OP.8C.03] comparison between three non-invasive techniques of evaluation microvascular morphology vs. the gold-standard locally invasive micromyography. Preliminary data. Journal of Hypertension. 2017;**35**:e90

[82] Virdis A, Savoia C, Grassi G, Lembo G, Vecchione C, Seravalle G, et al. Evaluation of microvascular structure in humans: A 'state-of-the-art' document of the working group on macrovascular and microvascular alterations of the Italian society of arterial hypertension. Journal of Hypertension. 2014;**32**(11):2120-2129, discussion 9

[83] Arichika S, Uji A, Murakami T, Suzuma K, Gotoh N, Yoshimura N. Correlation of retinal arterial wall thickness with atherosclerosis predictors in type 2 diabetes without clinical retinopathy. The British Journal of Ophthalmology. 2017;**101**(1):69-74

[84] Ueno Y, Iwase T, Goto K, Tomita R, Ra E, Yamamoto K, et al. Association of changes of retinal vessels diameter with ocular blood flow in eyes with diabetic retinopathy. Scientific Reports. 2021;**11**(1):4653

[85] Baltã F, Cristescu IE, Mirescu AE, Baltã G, Tofolean IT. Effect of a multinutrient complex on retinal microcirculation in diabetic patients investigated using an adaptive optics retinal camera. Acta Endocrinologica (Bucharest). 2020;**16**(4):389-395

Chapter 8

Anatomic and Topographic Vitreous and Vitreoretinal Interface Features during Chromovitrectomy of A, B, C Stages of Proliferative Diabetic Vitreoretinopathy (P. Kroll's Classification of Proliferative Diabetic Vitreoretinopathy, 2007): Fyodorov's Eye Microsurgery Complex

Natalia Kislitsyna and Sergei Novikov

Abstract

Methods and results of the developed vitreous body imaging technique in proliferative diabetic vitreoretinopathy diagnostics using new contrast dye during operation. The P. Kroll"s classification of proliferative diabetic retinopathy was modified after receiving new data about vitreoretinal interface structures during investigation using chromovitrectomy.

Keywords: vitreous, anatomy, diabetes, retinopathy, diagnostics chromovitrectomy

1. Introduction

Vitreous body is a clear, light-transparent eye part. The visualization of vitreous structures and their changes after and during pathological processes caused by diabetes did not provide yet. The purpose of this study was to study the possibility of developed vitreous body developed technique in proliferative diabetic vitreoretinopathy diagnostics.

Since 2010 chromovitrectomy with the original dye "Vitreocontrast" is developing for all intravitreal pathologies in the Fyodorov's Eye Microsurgery Complex. This method, called "vitreocontrastography", allows contrast and visualize all Worst J. described vitreous structures [1–9].

2. Materials and methods

The aim of this work was to study the anatomic and topographic specifics of the vitreous body (VB) and vitreoretinal interface (VRI) changes at different proliferative diabetic vitreoretinopathy (PDVR) stages.

The inclusion criteria of patients into the study corresponded to the traditional PDVR classification (A, B, C stages by P. Kroll et al., 2007 [10]), according to it, patients were divided into three groups.

The first group of patients included 52 patients (52 eyes) with diagnosed PDVR, stage A. 10 patients had diabetes mellitus II type, 6 out of them had insulin-dependent, 4 – insulin-related. Best-corrected visual acuity (BCVA) varied from 0.01 to 0.3; IOP varied within 12 mm–22 mm of mercury; the length of the eye-ball was 23 mm. and less. According to B-scanning, all patients had PVD with local fixations causing local tractional elevation 0.7–0.9 high; 30 patients had hemophthalmia.

In the second group 47 patients (47 eyes) with PDVR, stage B were followed up. Diabetes mellitus I type was diagnosed in 16 patients; diabetes mellites was diagnosed in 31 patients, 14 of them had insulin diabetes. In this group, the BCVA varied from fingers at face to 0,1 non-corrigible; IOP varied within 12 mm–22 mm of mercury; the length of the eyeball was 23 mm and less. According to B-scanning, all patients had PVD with local fixations causing tractional retinal detachment 1,2–1,7 high, 34 patients had hemophthalmia.

In the third group 32 (32 eyes) with PDVR, stage C was followed up. Fourteen patients were diagnosed with diabetes mellitus type I; 18 patients had diabetes mellitus type II, 14 out of them had had insulin-related diabetes. BCVA left pr. certae – 0.03 non-corrigible; IOP varied 14 mm–20 mm of mercury. B-scanning found PVD in all patients, the tractional retinal detachment was up to 2,2–2,7 mm. Hemophthalmia was in 18 cases.

All the patients had 25 G vitrectomy with the Constellation Vision System (Alcon, USA) under the operational microscope Topcon OFFISSOMS 800 (Japan). The visocontrastophy method was used to contrast the structures.

The distinctive feature of the vitrectomy performed within this study was contrasting VB structures for the intra vitam imaging of cisterns and canals, the assessment of their integrity, and anatomic and topographic specifics at each stage of the disease.

For this purpose, 3 ports at 4.00, 14.30, and 9.30 o'clock positions were installed pars plana 4 mm from the limbus. 0.1–0.2 ml of vitreocontrast suspension was injected sequentially through each of the installed ports into the vitreous body with a 30 G needle in order to contrast retrociliary and equatorial cisterns.

After contrasting the VB structures and video recording of their specific anatomical and topographic arrangement, an irrigation cannula was installed, an infusion solution was supplied into the vitreous cavity, and a median vitrectomy was performed. In the course of the vitrectomy, sequential isolated removal of VB cisterns was possible. At the next stage, by repeated contrasting, VB cortical layers were sequentially visualized followed by their removal until the surface of the retinal ILM was exposed. Then, retinal ILM was contrasted and its peeling in the macular zone was performed. Peeling was done by shaping ILM petals, followed by their partial removal with a vitreotome needle in a shave mode, and leaving the ILM in the foveolar zone in order to prevent the development of neuroepithelial atrophy in the long-term postoperative period.

The results of the studies proved the fact that under contrasting VB structures, in the first group, retrociliary and equatorial cisterns were preserved. The contrasted structures fully corresponded to their normal architectonics. The wall of the discovered structures was preserved, the boundaries were clear, and the contrasting composition did not go beyond the cisterns in 36 (97%) cases (**Figure 1**).

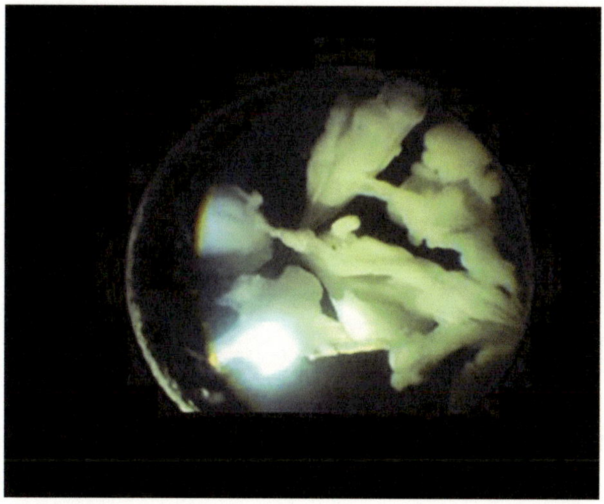

Figure 1.
Normal architectonics of retrociliary and equatorial cisterns in PDVR, stage a (the first group of patients).

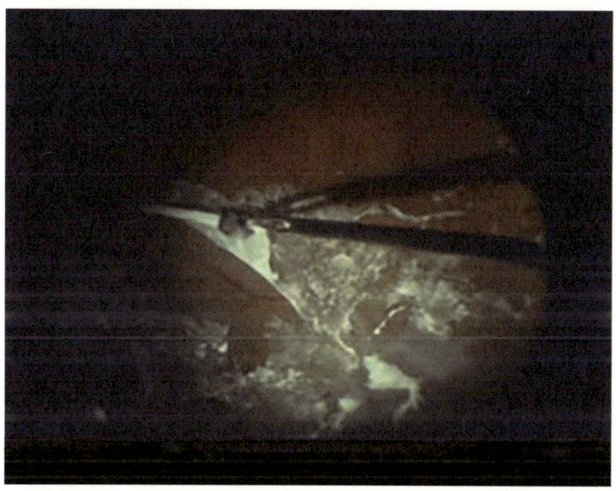

Figure 2.
The cortical layer on the retinal surface after vitrectomy for PDVR, stage a (the first group of patients).

During central vitrectomy, VB was completely removed without cortex contrasting. After complete VB removal in all the cases, the retina was attached, no cortical layers or residual fibers were visualized on its surface. After repeated staining of the retinal surface with the suspension, a thin layer of fibers was visualized (**Figure 2**).

In 94% of cases it had a similar configuration and took the central zone of the eye fundus limited by vascular arcades. In other cases, this thin layer took the entire extent of the retina up to the extreme periphery. We managed to remove the contrasted layer from the retinal surface by endovitreal forceps in 24 patients. In 28 patients, it had a very loose and fibrous structure and was quite tightly fixed to the ILM along its entire length and to remove it partially from the retinal surface was possible only by Tano scraper (**Figure 3**).

To remove it in a single layer in the macular region was not possible. In all the cases it was removed only in a single block with ILM. The foveolar zone was left intact to prevent the development of retinal neuroepithelia atrophy (**Figure 4**).

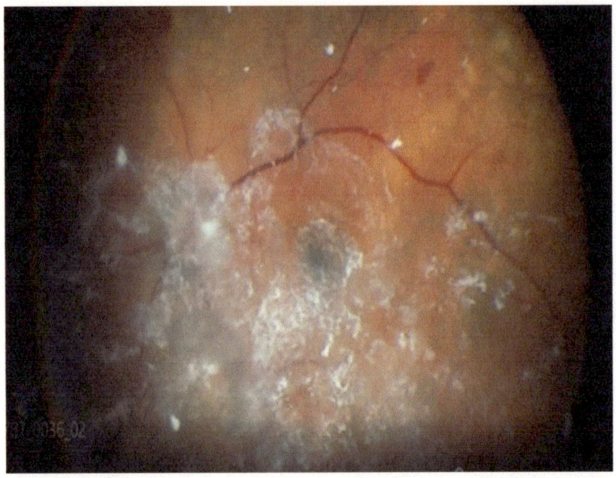

Figure 3.
Thin vitreous layer in the central zone limited by vascular arcades after putting the suspension on the retinal surface under PDVR, stage a (the first group of patients).

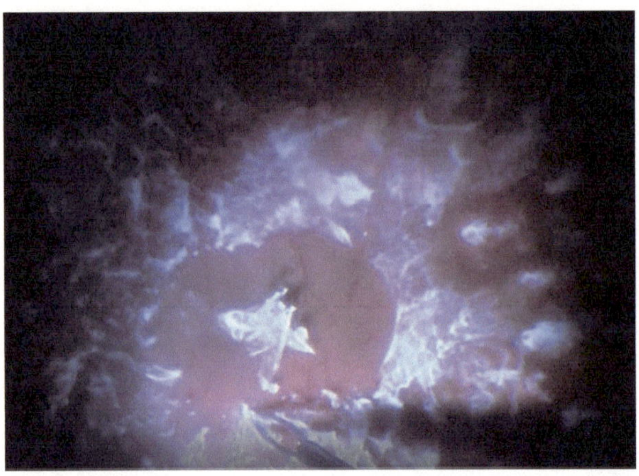

Figure 4.
The removal of the cortical layer soldered with ILM keeping the foveolar fixation in PDVR patients, stage a (the first group of patients).

It is necessary to note that the application of the developed technique of VB imaging (in comparison with the reference classification) made it possible to identify the new stage of PDVR defined by us A-1.

The classification features of this stage are:

- Full visualization of the vitreous and the VB layer attached to it at the background of ophthalmoscopically unchanged ILM;
- Full contrasting of the main VB structures (bursa-like cavities) cisterns with clear boundaries 1,5–1,7ᴍᴍ and 0,2–0,3 ᴍᴍ wide, the surface is preserved (the contrasting agent does not go beyond the boundaries
- Lack of the fixation of posterior cortical layers to the retinal surface;
- Tight adhesion of VB layers to ILM;

- Vitreous layers in the central zone of VB layers in the central area of VRI vascular arcades.

It should be noted that the last classification sign (as a suggested PDVR stage A – 1) is presented by new scientific facts. In 70% of the cases this layer can be quite easily separated from the retina by the forceps (average level of adhesion), in 30% the VB layer is characterized by a high level of adhesion with the possibility of their partial removal (**Figure 5**).

According to basic classification [10], stage A is characterized by proliferative changes of VB and retina especially around the optic disk and posterior cortical layers. The application of the developed VB imaging technique made it possible to design the following classification signs of the A-2 stage:

- The presence of well visualized bursa-like cavities in VB 1.5–1.7 mm long and 0.3–0.5 mm wide with equal clear boundaries, the walls of the cavities are preserved;
- Cortical layers have areas of fixation to the VB. They are removed only by intraoperative PVD induction (in 40% of the cases) or cannot be completely removed, staying fixed in the places of firm contact with the retina;
- On the retinal surface in the VRI zone a multilayered (in 94% of cases 2–3 layers) cortical layered with vitreoschisis areas;
- VB layer adjacent to the retina can be completely removed in 30%, partially in 50% of cases. In other cases, it is characterized by the firm degree of adhesion to the retina;
- In the macular zone, in 80% of cases this layer has such firm adhesion to the ILM that can be removed only in a single block with ILM;
- In the periphery, true PVD is visualized.

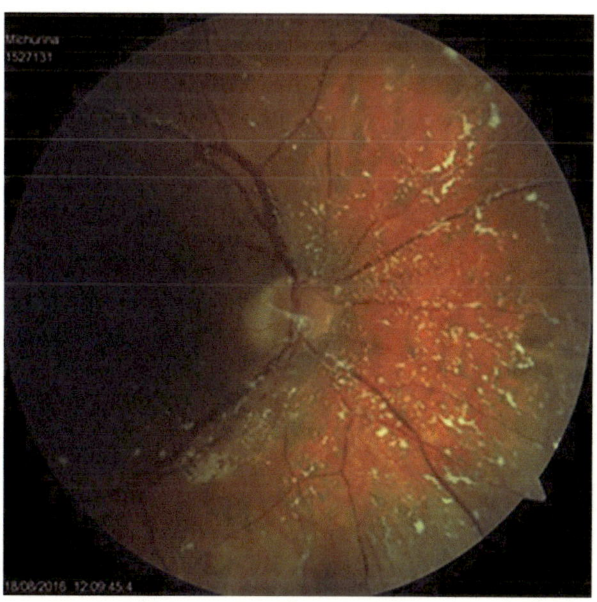

Figure 5.
Cortical VB layer that cannot be mechanically removed intraoperatively.

Thus, at stage A-2 the tractional element develops in the areas of VB splitting (but not its complete posterior detachment) that eventually causes a tractional retinal detachment. At this stage, local tractional detachment localizes in the periphery in 85% of cases.

The results of the anatomic and morphological assessment of the 2-nd group patients showed that during vitreocontrastograpy retrociliary and equatorial cisterns had fully preserved architectonics, unchanged wall, and clear boundaries. In most cases (95%) there is no exit of the contrast agent, and only in 5% of the cases, the structure was disrupted (**Figure 6**).

After central vitrectomy and removal of contrasted VB structures, the cortical layers were sequentially stained. At the same time, in 96% of cases, the VB layer extending to the region of vascular arcades and removed as a single layer was visualized. After repeated contrasting, another VB layer was visualized in 63% of the patients. It was also attached to the retina up to the zone of the vascular arcades. In 41% of the patients, the area of this layer was limited by the macular zone. Thus, VB cortical layers is a multilayered structure consisting of several formed layers, each of which has a certain topography and fixation (**Figures 7–9**).

The discovered VB layers do not get to the peripheral retina being firmly fixed in the zone limited by vascular arcades. Besides, in this group patients' true PVD was discovered in 94% and only in the periphery. After the removal of cortical layers in the central zone and the retinal surface visualization as well as after repeated staining with the suspension, in all the cases a thin vitreous layer firmly fixed to the ILM surface was visualized on the retinal surface (**Figure 10**).

This layer's mechanical removal was complicated and possible only partially because of its insufficient thickness and its loose and unformed structure. Besides, in the macular zone, this layer removal separately from ILM was not possible (**Figures 11, 12**).

According to basic classification [10] stage B is characterized by the shrinkage of the posterior vitreous cortical layer that leads to its tractional detachment in the areas of VB fixation to the retina. Proliferative and tractional changes in the temporal lobe (along the upper and/or lower vascular arcades) without the engagement of the macular zone are related to stage Bt proliferative changes of VB and retina especially around the optic disc and posterior vitreous cortical layers.

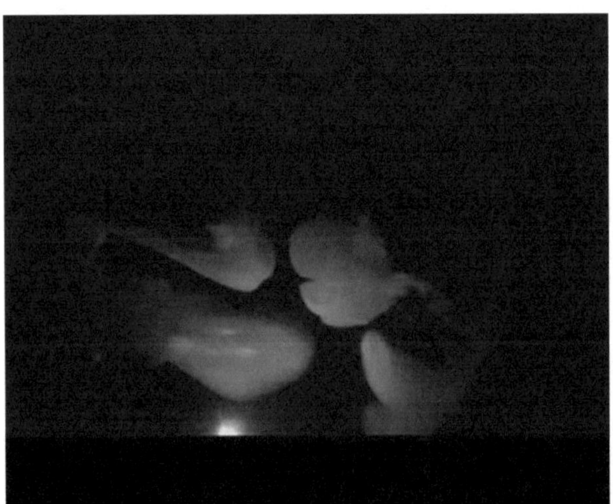

Figure 6.
Fully preserved architectonics, unchanged wall, and the clear boundaries of cisterns under PDVR, stage B (2-nd group of patients).

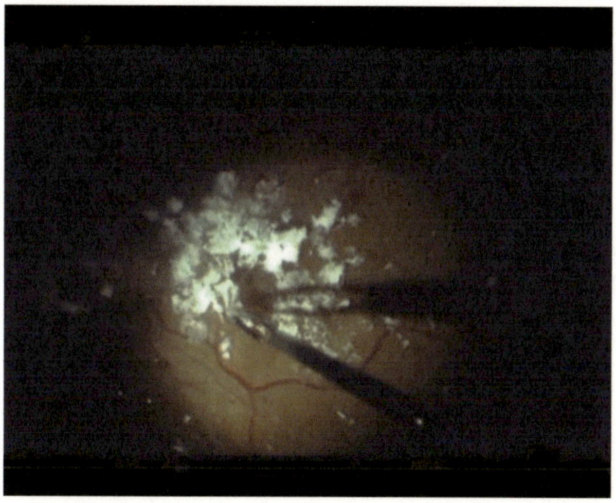

Figure 7.
Splitting of cortical layers (vitreoschisis) extending to vascular arcades in PDVR, stage B (2-nd group of patients).

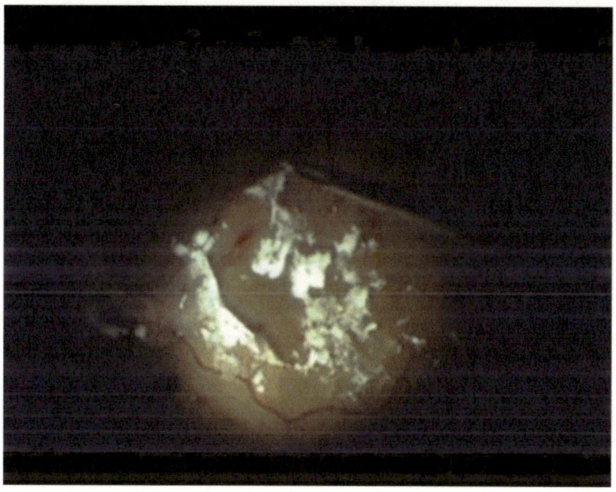

Figure 8.
Splitting of cortical layers (vitreoschisis) extending to vascular arcades in PDVR, stage B (2-nd group of patients).

The application of the developed VB imaging technique made it possible to design the following classification signs of stage B:

- The presence of bursa like cavities 1.5–1.7 mm high and 0.3–0.5 mm wide with equal clear boundaries well visualized in VB, the walls of the cavities are preserved;

- Cortical layers in the central zone have a lamellar structure including up to 5–7 vitreous layers forming numerous vitreoschisis zones that cause tractional retinal detachment 1.1 to 2.2 high in different segments while using vitreous layers in vitreoschisis zones as a substrate. Along with the vitreous layers, neovascularization proliferates and cellular proliferation occurs forming a typical picture of eye fundus changes;

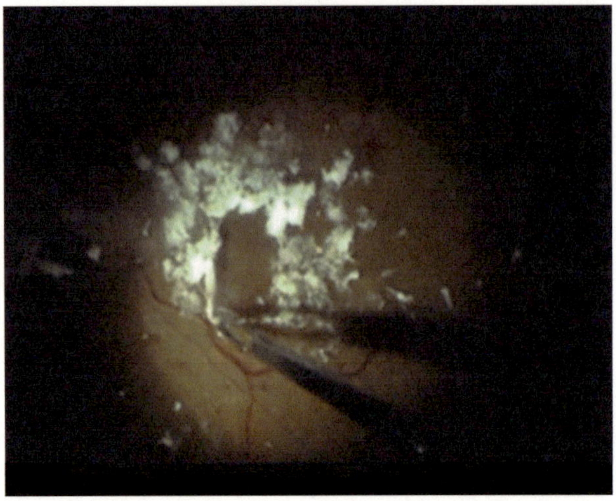

Figure 9.
Splitting of cortical layers (vitreoschisis) extending to vascular arcades in PDVR, stage B (2-nd group of patients).

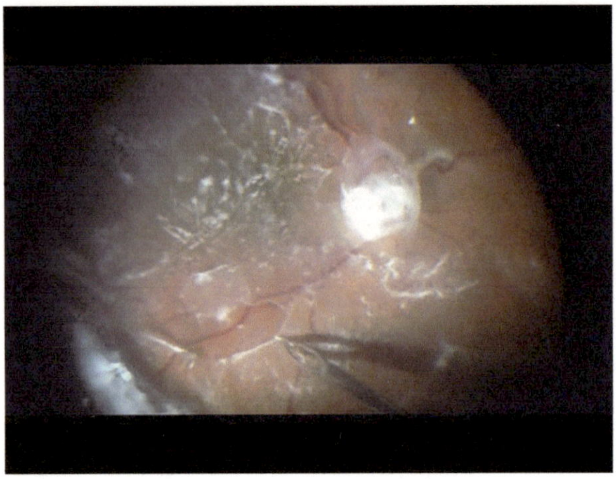

Figure 10.
Preretinal VB layer extending to vascular arcades after repeated contrasting under PDVR, stage B (2-nd group of patients).

- VB layer adjacent to the retina may be partially mechanically removed. In 80% of cases it stays in the places of firm fixation to the retina;

- In the macular zone, in 80% of cases, this layer can be removed in a single block with ILM.

In general, it is necessary to say that during the preoperative period and during the surgical intervention, PDVR hemorrhagic manifestations do not complicate the performance of sequential (lamellar) vitreocontrastography. Besides, the VRI condition makes it possible to study the exact topography of each vitreous layer formed in the course of the pathological process (collagen crosslinking), vitreoschisis zones with the possibility of their exact measurement, configuration sizes, the localization of the fixation points to the underlying vitreous layers. Vessels, and retinal surface.

The results of the anatomic morphologic assessment of the 3-d group showed that during vitreocontrastography all the retrociliary and equatorial cisterns

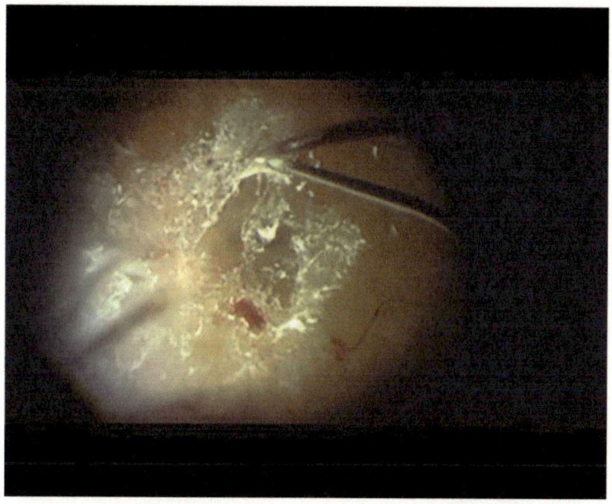

Figure 11.
Removal of the layer soldered with ILM under PDVR, stage B (2-nd group of patients).

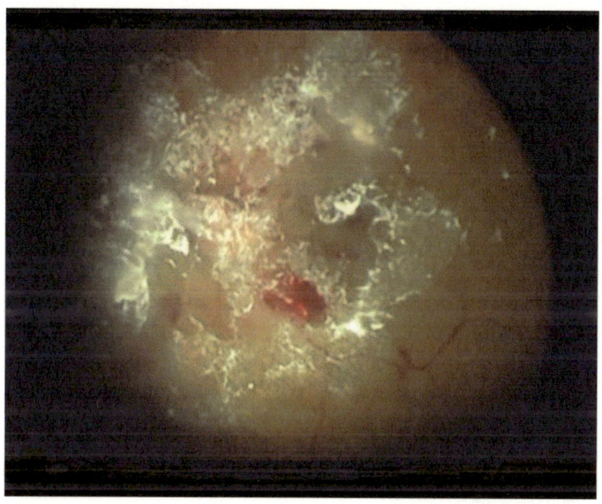

Figure 12.
Removal of the layer soldered with ILM under PDVR, stage B (2-nd group of patients).

had fully preserved architectonics, unchanged wall, and clear boundaries (**Figure 13**).

After central vitrectomy, in the zone limited by vascular arcades, a fibrovascular membrane with multiple zones of the fixation to the retina and causing tractional retinal detachment was visualized. In 11% of the cases, this structure had a multi-layered structure. However, in other (89%) cases we failed to perform layer-by-layer contrasting and to identify the zones of layers attachment (**Figures 14, 15**).

According to the basic classification [10] stage B is characterized by a tractional retinal detachment that extends to the macular zone. And stages from C1 to C4 are identified by the number of detached macular quadrants.

Developed VB imaging technique made it possible to develop the following classification signs of stage C:

- The presence of well-visualized bursa like cavities 1.5–1.7 mm high and 0.3–0.5 mm wide with equal clear boundaries in VB, the walls of the cavities are preserved;

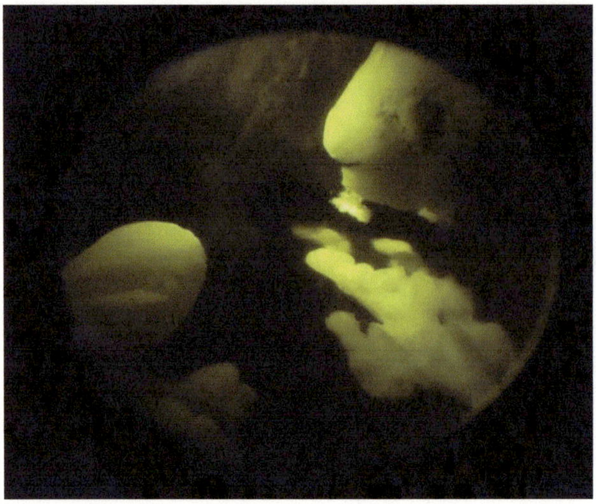

Figure 13.
Preserved anatomy and topography of retrociliary and equatorial cisterns in PDVR, stage C (3-d group of patients).

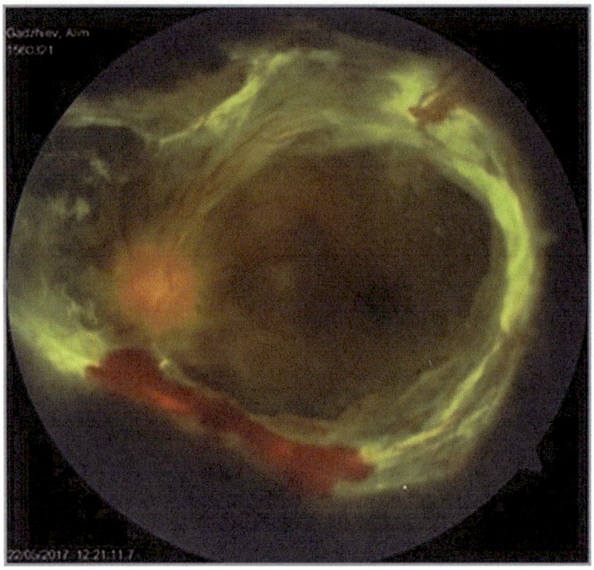

Figure 14.
Multi-layered fibrovascular membrane that has numerous zones of fixation to the retina and causes tractional retinal detachment in the region limited by vascular arcades under PDVR, stage C (3-d group of patients).

- In 18% of cases, VB partial destruction is visualized. It is manifested in the elongation of bursa like structures (cisterns) up to 2.0–2.5 mm, their disrupted walls, and the exit of the contrast beyond the cavity boundaries;

- VB cortical layers have fibrosis, and in 80% of cases, are not differentiated. Besides, in the central zone, under the possibility of its visualization, stratified cortical layers are identified (thicker than at the previous stage, no more than 2–3 layers);

- In the central zone, VB has a firm attachment to the retinal ILM.

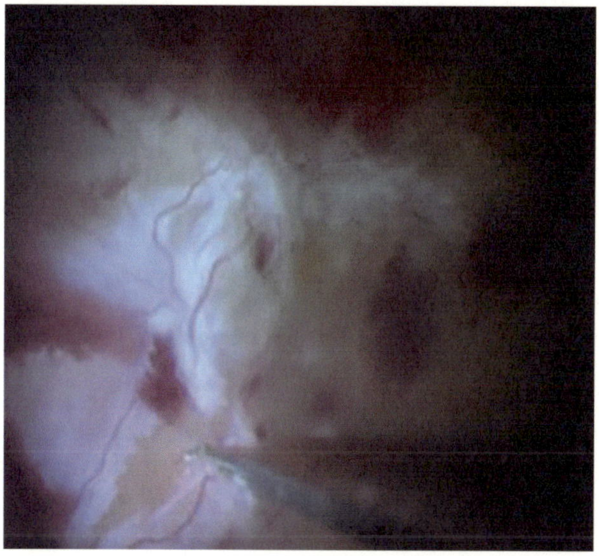

Figure 15.
Multi-layered fibrovascular membrane that has numerous zones of fixation to the retina and causes tractional retinal detachment in the region limited by vascular arcades under PDVR, stage C (3-d group of patients).

When discussing the presented results, it is necessary to single out four main positions. The first one deals with the PDR basic classification choice. In this regard, we should note that some classifications proposed before do not take into account the role of the vitreous in the development of changes under diabetes. They mostly address retinal vascular changes and are usually based on ophthalmoscopic data that predominantly reviews the relevance of these classifications for the laser treatment tactics [citation according to 402]. The classification offered by P. Kroll et al. [10] is not that much based on PDR classification characteristics but rather on those of PDVR that determined its choice for the aims of this work. It should be mentioned again that our analysis of classification signs under different PDVR stages provided for the application of the developed VB imaging technique based on the original method of vitreocontastograthy.

The second position defines the main aspects of PDVR pathogenesis from the perspective of anatomic topographic changes of the vitreous structure. In this regard, the first thing that draws attention is quite clear delineation into anatomically preserved pre-equatorial vitreous section and pathologically changed cortical layers, and the VRI zone. In all the cases irrespective of the stage of the disease retrociliary and equatorial cisterns preserved their changed cortical layers, and there was no exit of the contrasting agent deeper than the stained structures. Another interesting fact is that under the unchanged anatomy of the vitreous structures, the suspension localizes only in the cisterns and does not reach cortical layers on the retinal surface. This circumstance may explain the fact that preserved cisterns prevent the circulation of inflammatory and VGF factors and their occurrence in the anterior segment of the eye-ball.

It is also important to note that, in the ILM zone, the thinnest VB layer lining this area, reaching vascular arcades, and having tight adherence to ILM was found for the first time. This layer was discovered after multiple contrasts of cortical layers that again confirm their stratified structure and the ability to split. Such anatomic localization of the vitreous layer and pathological changes in the area of vascular arcades may be explained by PDRV development pathogenic specifics. Such anatomic localization of the vitreous layer and pathologic changes in the area of vascular arcades can be explained by the pathogenic changes of PDVR development. The trigger mechanism in PDVR is known to be vascular permeability disorder, more often in the zone of vascular arcades, which leads to the release of inflammation factors, VGF, PGF. This probably provokes the tight fixation of VB preretinal layer to the ILM directly in the zone limited by vascular arcades. This is the discovered VB layer that plays a leading role in the development of following changes under the disease progression. Propagating to the macular zone and being tightly fixed to the ILM, these VB changes condition macular edema development, especially, due to the tangential tractions. They are the risk factor for the development of further proliferative changes.

Besides, due to the abnormal PVD in the zone limited by vascular arcades further changes of cortical layers take place by sort of crosslinking (adhesion) of vitreous fibers, and as a result, they turn into numerous multilayered vitreoschisis zones tightly fixed to the retina. These structure layers are the risk factors of neovascularization and further proliferation with the formation of fibrous membranes with the course of time. These anatomic specifics explain tractional retinal detachment development during the progression of VB proliferative changes that also have a specific topography.

The third position is connected to the results of our comparative analytical assessment of PDVR clinical diagnostic efficiency using the developed technique of VB imaging and the traditional classification (**Tables 1–3**). The data presented in the tables prove to the principally higher level of anatomic and morphologic diagnosis at different PDVR stages using the new VB imaging technique (based on the original method of vitreocontrastography) that, in our opinion, is related to the following general weaknesses of the traditional classification:

VB imaging technique	Traditional classification	Main weaknesses of the traditional classification
Definition of the *new stage–A-1:* 1. Anterior cortical layers are preserved. 2. VB structures are preserved (cisterns). 3. The retina is fully attached without the visible ophthalmological changes of the vitreous and retina. 4. VB layer with certain topography (taking the central area of the eye fundus). *Stage A-2:* 1. Anterior cortical layers and VB structures are preserved 2. In the central zone 2–3 layered VB cortical layer is 3. preserved. The layers are formed by vitreoschisis zones 4. On the retinal surface VB layer firmly fixed to the ILM in the macular zone is contrasted.	Characterized by proliferative changes of VB and retina especially around the optic disc and VB posterior cortical layers.	1. Based on the ophthalmoscopy data. 2. Optically transparent media are required. 3. Cannot be performed under hemophthalmia and vitreous opacification (or in such a case should be based on B-scanning data). 4. Based only on the assessment of the vitreous and retinal changes visible with the use of ophthalmoscopy (judging by pathogenesis, epiretinal membranes become visible only at the fibrosis stage) 5. Anterior and central structures are not assessed.

Table 1.
Results of the comparative analytical assessment of the main classification signs of PDVR, stage a found using the developed VB imaging technique and traditional classification (Kroll et al. [10]).

VB imaging technique	Traditional classification	Main weaknesses of the traditional classification
1. Anterior vitreous cortical layers are preserved. 2. In the central zone, there are cortical layers with numerous vitreoschisis zones causing tractional retinal detachment 1.7–2.2 mm high. 3. Normal PVD is at the retinal periphery. In the central zone, there is abnormal PVD with numerous vitreoschisis 4. zones.	Shrinkage of VB posterior cortical layers in the places of VB fixation to the retina results in retinal tractional detachment.	1. The assessment is possible only under transparent media by ophthalmoscopy or (under hemophthalmia) should be based on b-scanning data that is not indicated in the classification. 2. Takes into account retinal detachment localization and height but the analysis of VB changes with the account of the localization of vitreoschisis zones is not possible. 3. Only irreversible changes (tractional retinal detachment) is possible. 4. Only (fibrosis) changes of the vitreous (epiretinal membranes) visible by ophthalmoscopy can be seen 5. There is no analysis of the layer-by-layer changes of the posterior cortex and VRI as the main areas of the pathological process.

Table 2.
Results of the comparative analytical assessment of the main classification signs of PDVR, stage C, found using the developed imaging technique and according to the.

VB imaging technique	Traditional classification	Main weaknesses of the traditional classification
1. Anterior cortical layers and VB structures are intact. 2. Partial destruction of VB structures manifested in the disrupted integrity and changed sizes of some its sizes. 3. Vitreroschisis areas in the central zone are not visualized due to fibrous changes in VB cortical layers. 4. After the removal of fibrous membranes in the central zone, VB layer tightly fixed to the ILM of the retina is visualized.	Tractional retinal detachment covers the macular zone. According to the number of detached macular from C1 to C4 stages are identified.	1. Evaluate the final result of pathological changes (tractional retinal detachment area by segments), VB changes are not included into the analysis. 2. Practically does not provide data about the pathological process pathogenesis related to the retinal detachment configuration and topography.

Table 3.
Results of the comparative analytical assessment of classification signs of PDVR, stage C found using the developed imaging technique and according to the traditional classification (Kroll et al. [10]).

- Classification signs are based on ophthalmoscopy data (assessment of VB and retina changes seen only by ophtolmoscopy);
- There are sufficient limitations related to the transparency of optical media (in particular, under hemophthalmia and vitreous opacification, B-scanning data is required;
- There is no assessment of anterior and central vitreous structures;

- Lack of the visualization of layer by layer posterior vitreous cortex and VR interface in general, the structures of which are recognized as the main areas of the pathological process development under PDVR [11, 12];

- Classification signs are based on the assessment of irreversible changes (localization and the height of tractional retinal detachment) without taking into account VB changes related to vitreoschisis zones.

The fourth position defines the cumulation of PDVR classification anatomic morphological signs (CAMS) developed using the original VB imaging technique with the position of vitreoretinal surgery improvement (**Table 4**).

The data presented in **Table 4** makes it possible to formulate the following main areas of surgical intervention improvement under PDVR that is supported by the application of the developed VB imaging technique on the basis of the original vitreocontrasting method:

1. Maximum full visualization of all the pathological changes including the area of VB layer (CAMS - 1,2,3,8);

2. Maximum possible (without accompanying iatrogenic retinal damages) removal of the VB layer on the retinal surface as a prognostic factor of the pathological process severity increase (CAMS-6,7);

3. In the cases of the partial removal of the layer firmly adhered to the retina, it is viable to correct these retinal zones by selective, pathogenetically based endolazocoagulation or by endovitreal tamponade (either the gas-air one or the silicon one). Anti VGF therapy to prevent hemorrhagic complications (CAMS – 6,7) is also indicated;

4. In the cases of visible tractional component and the VB layer firm fixation to the ILM in the macular zone, retinal ILM peeling is advisable to remove the traction component (CAMS – 4,5).

Thus, the application of the developed VB imaging technique (based on the vitreocontrastography) in patients with PDVR provides a principally new approach

##	Classification anatomic morphological sign	A-1	A-2	B	C
1.	Visualization of VB structures (cisterns, cavities)	+++	+++	+++	+++
2.	Visualization of VB cortical layers with the possibility of their complete removal only in the periphery	+++	+++	+++	+++
3.	Partial VB destruction (structural integrity is disrupted)	—	—	+	++
4.	The presence of stratified cortical layers with vitreoschisis zones	+	+	++	+++
5.	Tractional retinal detachment manifestation	—	+	++	+++
6.	The adhesion degree of the VB layer adjacent to the retina	+	++	+++	+++
7.	The adhesion degree of the VB layer in the macular zone	+	++	++	+++
8.	Visualization of true PVD in the retinal periphery	+	+	++	+++

Sign: "-" – no sign, "+" – the sign is insignificant; "++" – the sign is moderate; "+++" – the sign is distinctly manifested.

Table 4.
Classification of PDVR anatomic and morphological signs developed on the basis of the original VB visualization technique.

to clinical diagnostic research based on the development of anatomic and morphological signs (imaging of VB structures and cortical layers (including on the retina), the VB adhesion level, etc). and characterized by principal advantages comparing to PDVR traditional classifications. In general, on the basis of the given recommendations, this makes it possible to increase the level of vitreoretinal surgery efficiency.

The above given positions are illustrated by the following clinical case.

The clinical case:

Patient F-va, 52 years old, medical record #1469012, diagnosis – PDVR, hemophthalmia, condition after transpupillary retinal laser coagulation. Hemophthalmia. Visual acuity – 0.03. IOP 16 mm. of mercury. Anterior posterior axis – 22.8 mm. The main stages of diagnosis and treatment are presented in **Figures 16–23**.

The first stage was the step-by-step consistent contrasting of vitreous structures (**Figure 16**). Thus, the presence of nontransparent optic media does not influence the quality of the imaging technique of complex VB structures and gives the opportunity to build the three-dimensional image of the topographic anatomy of VB structures.

After the vitrectomy, eye fundus imaging with the assessment of its pathological changes was performed. Without vitreocontrastography, vitreous cortical layers are not visualized on the eye fundus, no major pathological changes are seen, and the

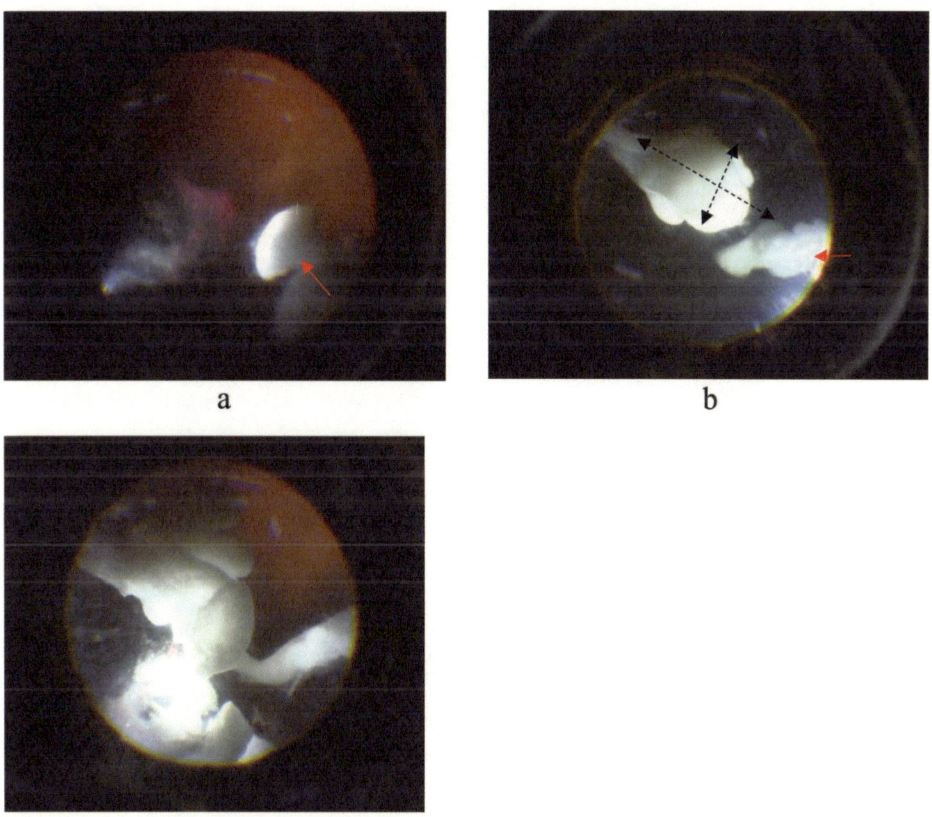

Figure 16.
a – Contrasting of vitreous cisterns at the backdrop of hemophthalmia does not influence the quality of vitreocontrastographia. The contrasted vitreous cavity with clearly outlined boundaries, preserved walls (red arrow), patient F-va, medical record # 1469012. b – Contrasting of VB structures. Contrasted vitreous cavities (cistern according to J. Worst) with clear boundaries are visualized, no exit of a contrasting agent, possibility to perform a vitreocontrastometry (changes of sizes) (black arrow), patient F-va, medical record #1469012. c – Contrasting of vitreous structures. Partial destruction of VB (blue arrow). changes of the cavity (cistern) clear boundaries, no exit of a contrasting agent, patient F-va, medical record #1469012.

eye fundus looks quite good to complete the surgery. However, the further application of VRI contrasting made it possible to visualize a cortical VB layer on the retinal surface. Besides, vitreocontrastography made it possible to assess the topographic anatomy (boundaries, area, relation to other anatomic structures) of the visualized layer (**Figures 17–19**). Since there is no cito and phototoxicity of the contrasting suspension, these manipulations are not limited by time. At the next stage, the attempt of the discovered VB layer mechanical removal with the concurrent assessment of its adhesion to underlying tissues is made (**Figure 20**). The role of this very layer in the pathological process, and in the support and development of its complications, is expressed in the development of hemorrhagic complications during the attempt to remove the cortical layer in the places of its tight fixation to the retinal ILM and (or) to the vessels (**Figure 21**).

The highest level of the contrasted layer adhesion is observed in the macular and paramacular zone (**Figure 22**).

At this stage of the process, the cortical layer can be removed from the retinal ILM surface in the macular and paramacular zone both as a separate layer and in a single block with retinal ILM. After the VB layer removing from the ILM surface in the macular and paramacular zones, retinal ILM is contrasted. If on the ILM surface there is the residual VB layer, its thickness is assessed, and the need in ILM peeling is reviewed. In this case, in order to maximally eliminate the tractional component

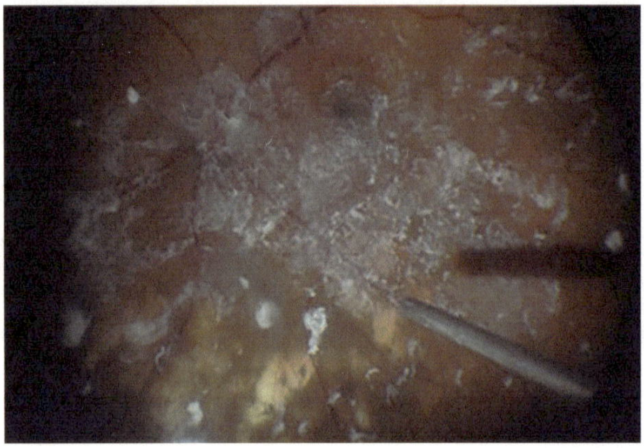

Figure 17.
Putting the contrasting agent on the retinal surface (patient F-va, medical record #1469012).

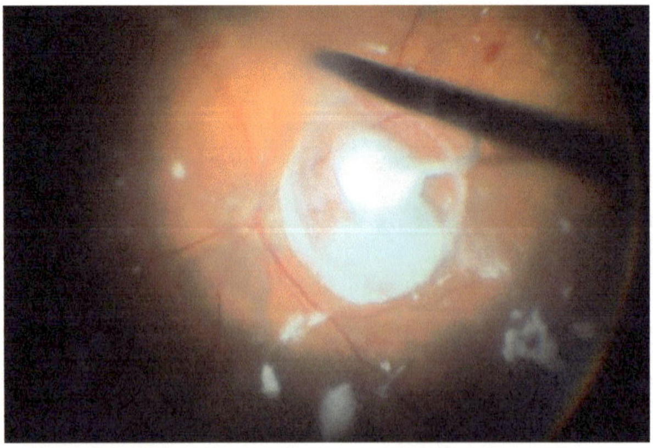

Figure 18.
Removal of the contrasting suspension excess by aspirational canula (patient F-va, medical record #1469012).

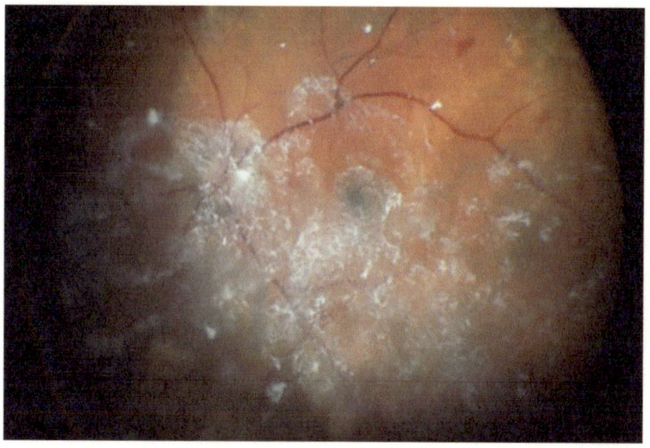

Figure 19.
Visualization of VB cortical layer on the retinal surface (patient F-va, medical record #1469012).

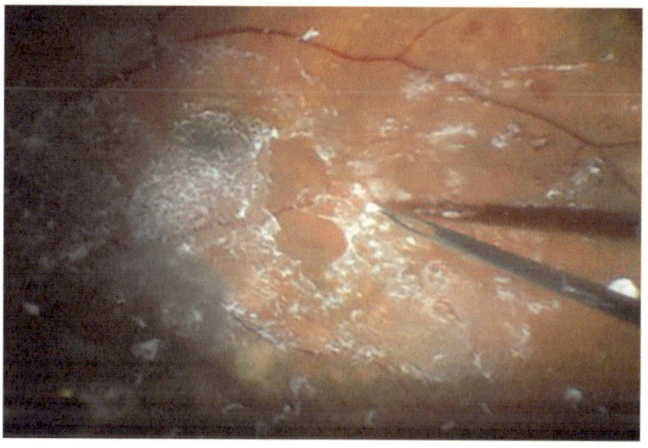

Figure 20.
Removal of the contrasted VB layer from the retinal surface by endivitreal forceps (patient F-va, medical record #1469012).

and to prevent the development of neuroepithelial atrophy in the long-term follow-up period, the ILM was removed in the paramacular zone without affecting the macular zone. The VB contrasted layer was removed from the retinal surface as much as it was possible leaving the areas of tight fixation to ILM, vessels, and optic disc to prevent hem Due to the adhesion of the contrasting suspension particles to the VB fibers, this layer becomes more formed, denser and well visualized, which makes this delicate process easy to manage and control. Retinal endolaser coagulation was carried out selectively, in the areas of this VB layer dense fixation to the retinal ILM, to the vessels, in the zones where this layer mechanical removal is impossible, and in the neovascularization zones. The tamponade of the vitreous cavity with the air completed the surgery.

Neither in the early nor in the late postop period, the patient had complications. Two years after the surgery, visual acuity – 0.7; IOP 16 мм of mercury, the photo of the eye fundus is presented in **Figure 23**.

The clinical case:

Patients P 49 years old.

Female: Diabetes mellitus type 2, noninsulin-dependent. Glycemia level 8–9 mmol/l.

Diagnosis: Proliferative diabetic retinopathy. Tractional retinal detachment 2,2–2,5 mm.

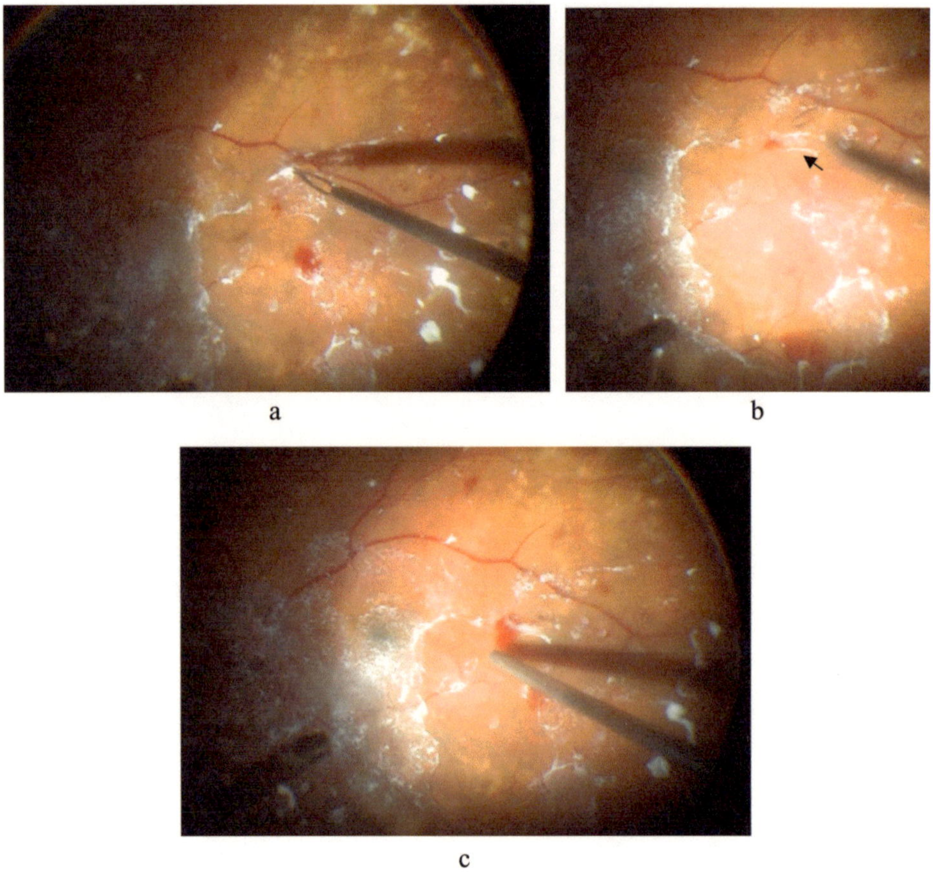

Figure 21.
a, b. the photo of the VB layer fixation place to the retinal ILM (black arrow), patient F-va, medical record #1469012. c, the development of hemorrhagic manifestations under the attempt to remove the VB cortical layer in the places of the tight fixation to the ILM (patient F-va, medical record #1469012).

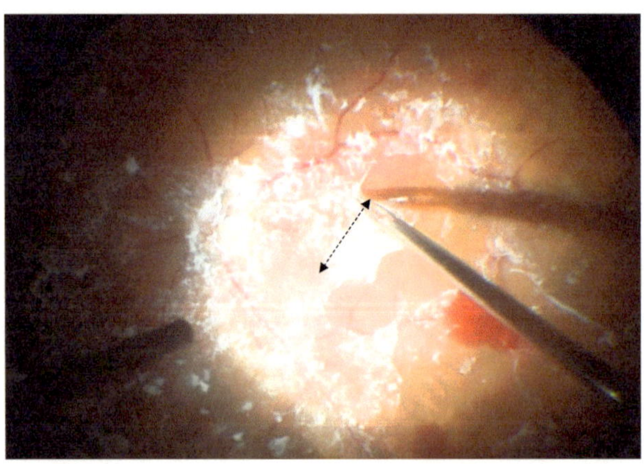

Figure 22.
During the removal of the contrasted VB layer from the retinal surface, its tight fixation to the retinal ILM is seen in the macular zone (indicated by the black arrow). In the indicated zone VB layer mechanical separation is complicated (patient F-va, medical record #1469012).

Visual acuity 0,06, IOP 19 mm. of mercury. APA 22,1 mm.

B scan: Strong destruction of the vitreous body, PVD causing tractional retinal detachment 2,2–2,5 mm high.

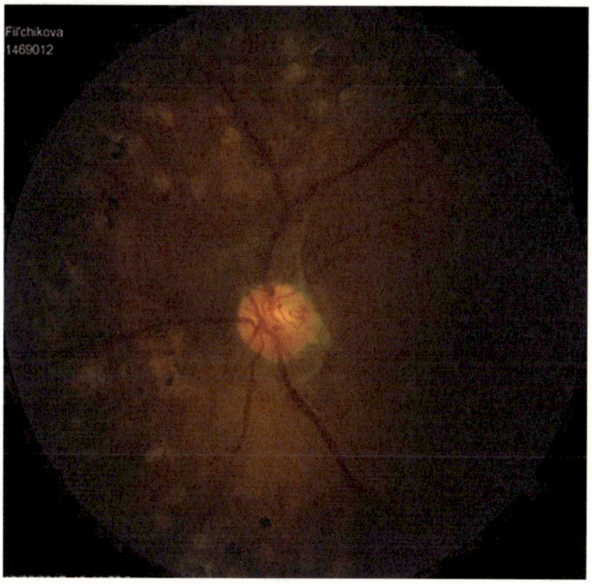

Figure 23.
Photo of the eye fundus 2 years after the surgery (patients F).

According to the ophthalmological picture, this stage corresponds to stage 2 by Kroll classification.

Vitreocontrastography.

Visualization of vitreous structures.

The first stage of the vitreocontrastography is step-by-step staining of vitreous structures. This investigation can be carried out in any of relevant quadrants.

In this example, cavities (cisterns by J. Worst) filled with the dye are visualized. Stained cavities have clear borders, unchanged size, suspension vitreocontrast did not go beyond the cavities.

It is possible to do vitreocontastomentry with the identification of the sizes of stained cisterns (**Figure 1**).

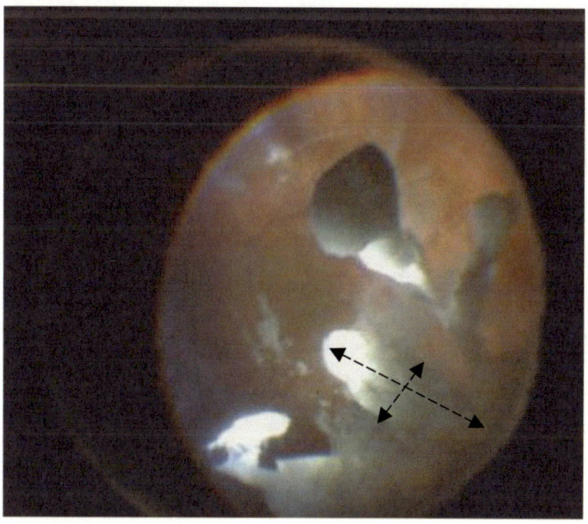

Figure 24.
Vitreocontrastography. The preserved cisterns of the vitreous body with clear-cut borders are visualized. The measurement of stained structures is possible.

Haemhorragic and neurotrophic complications (**Figure 24**).

The next step is the central vitrectomy with the removal of all stained endovitreal structures. After that, the possibility to investigate the cortical layers of the vitreous body by vitreocontrastography is given.

The staining composition is applied to the cortical layer of the vitreous body (**Figure 25**).

The use of vitreocontrastography in the course of the vitreoretinal surgery makes it possible to execute the step-by-step lamellar removal of vitreous cortical layers with the precise visualization of their topography (**Figure 26a–d**).

The interoperative image of the eye fundus after the removal of one vitreous cortical layer (**Figure 27**).

Vitreous body visualization using vitreocontrastography method. Applying of suspension Vitreocontrast (**Figure 28**) makes it possible to visualize the next cortical layer of the vitreous body (**Figure 28**). After staining it is possible to remove the isolated vitreous cortical layer both by vitreotome needle (**Figure 28**) and endovitreal forceps (**Figure 28a, b**) (**Figures 29** and **30**).

To evaluate the topographic anatomy of the second layer of the vitreous body and to identify the places of its fixation to underlying tissues for its separation and removal we used the endovitreal forceps (**Figure 31a** and **b**).

After the intraoperative dissection and the delicate removal of the second layer of the vitreous body, the underlying layers of the vitreous body remain transparent and practically are not visualized. Intraoperatively, it is possible to evaluate only irrepressibly changed areas of the vitreous body (**Figure 31**).

During the vitreocontrastography, the dye was applied for the second time for further intraoperative diagnostics (**Figures 32** and **33**).

After this stage of vitreous staining, another cortical layer of the vitreous body is visualized (**Figure 34a–d**).

In the course of the third vitreous layer removal, its tense fixation to the retinal ILM in the macular area was discovered. The removal of the discovered layer separately is impossible (**Figure 35**). Under the accurate dissection of this layer in

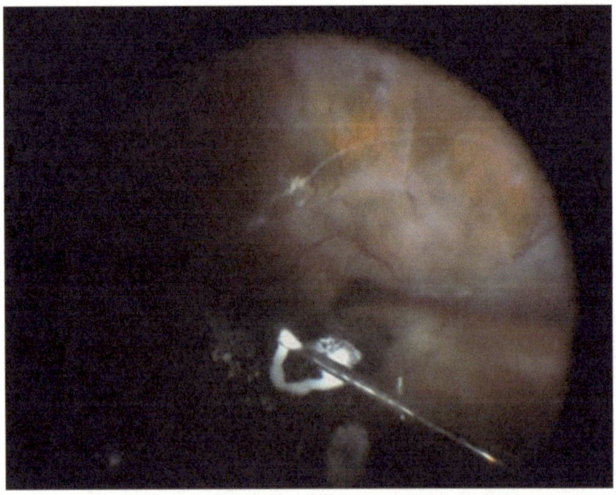

Figure 25.
Visualization of the topographic anatomy of cortical layers. Staining of the first layer of the vitreous body.

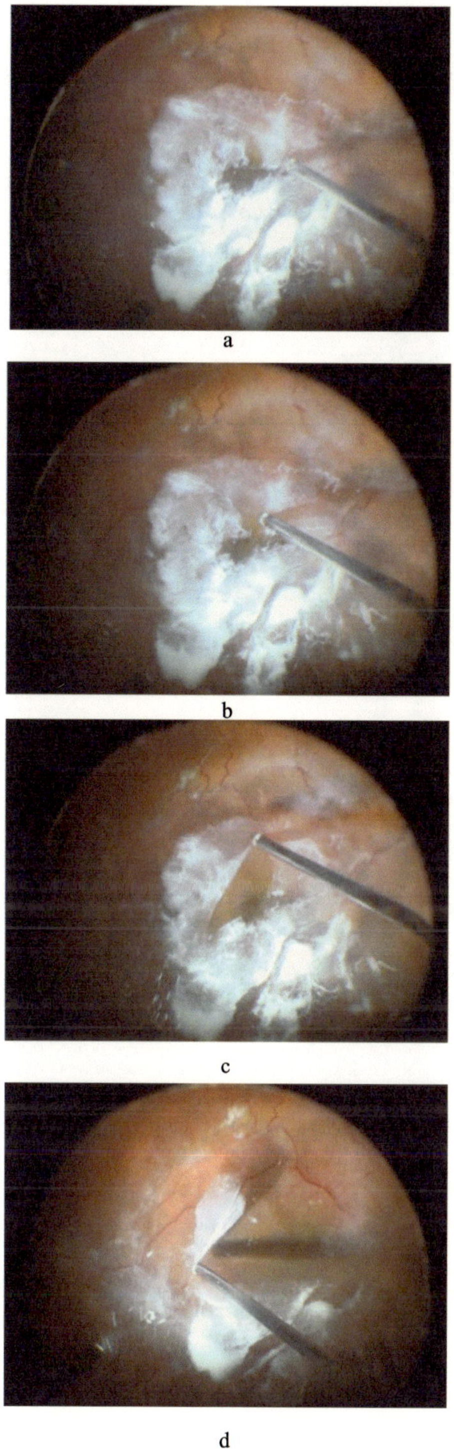

Figure 26.
Removal of the stained layer of the vitreous body. When the vitreotome needle has used the particles of the dye do not change the degree of adhesion making it possible to remove the vitreous body consistently strictly within the limits of one layer. The lack of the shaking effect facilitates surgical procedures.

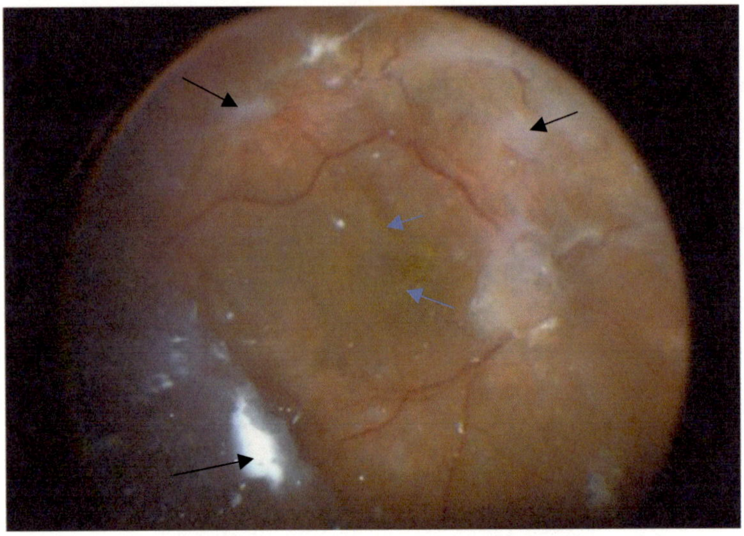

Figure 27.
One layer of the vitreous body is removed. Visually accessible changes of the vitreous body are visualized in the form of the proliferative tissue niduses that cause tractional retinal detachment (black arrows). In the macular zone puckers can be seen (blue arrow). the visualization of other pathological changes is hampered.

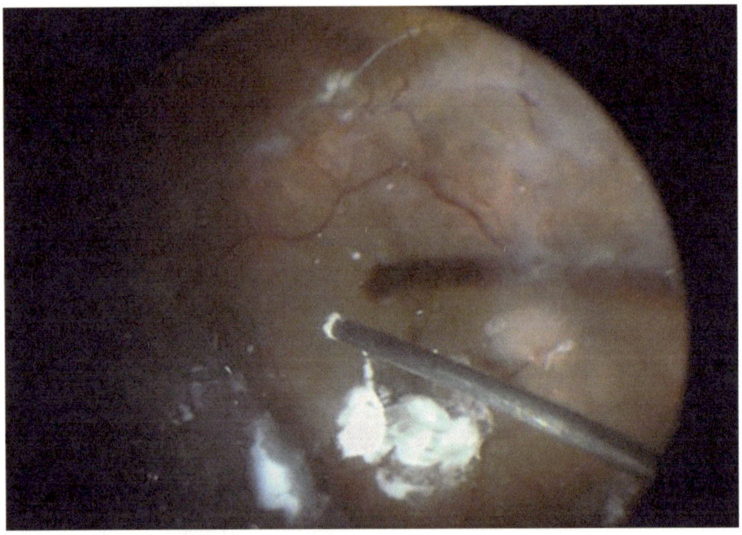

Figure 28.
Applying suspension vitreocontrast on the retinal surface.

the macular zone, it showed a very high level of adhesion, and its removal without ILM is impossible in this zone.

In the macular zone, the removal of this layer is possible only as a single block with retinal ILM (**Figure 35**).

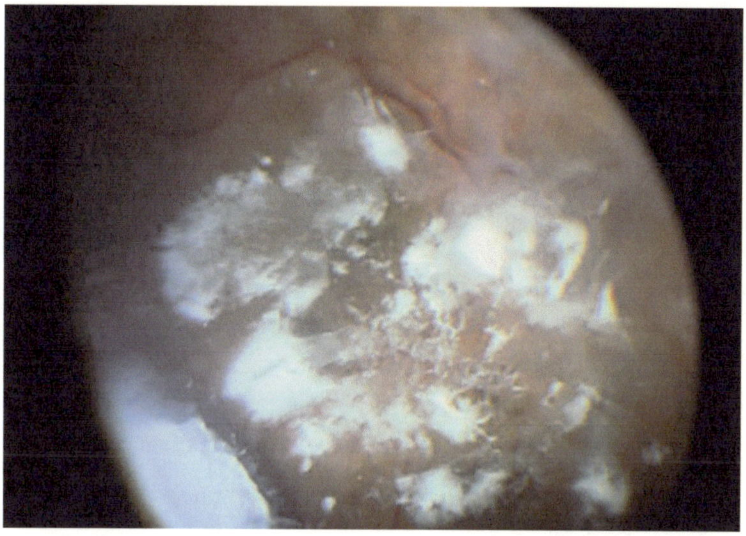

Figure 29.
Visualization of the second layer of the vitreous body.

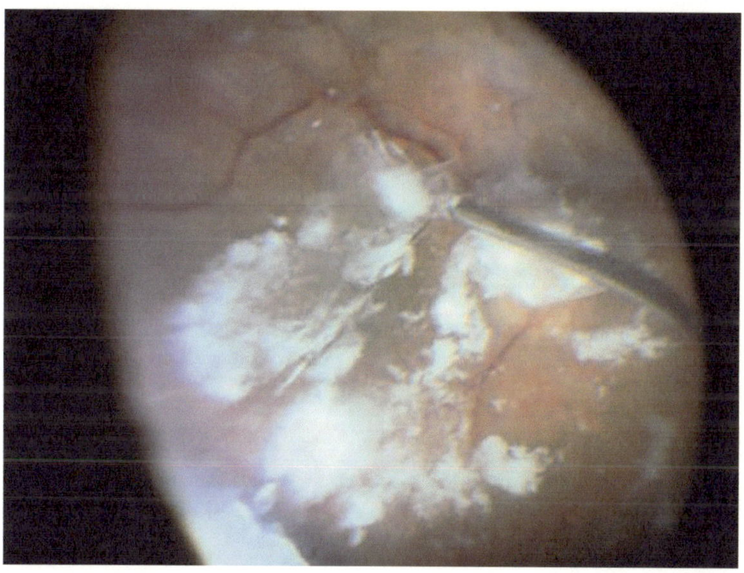

Figure 30.
Isolated step-by-step removal of the second stained layer of the vitreous body by the vitreotome needle.

To prevent the development of neuroepithelium atrophy in the long-term follow-up period ILM segment is not removed in the macular zone (**Figure 36**).

The changes of ILM physical properties in the course of staining make any manipulations with retinal ILM easily performed, manageable, and well visualized.

Thus, during vitreocontastography and practical lamellar intraoperative dissection of the structures and layers of the vitreous body, it is possible to

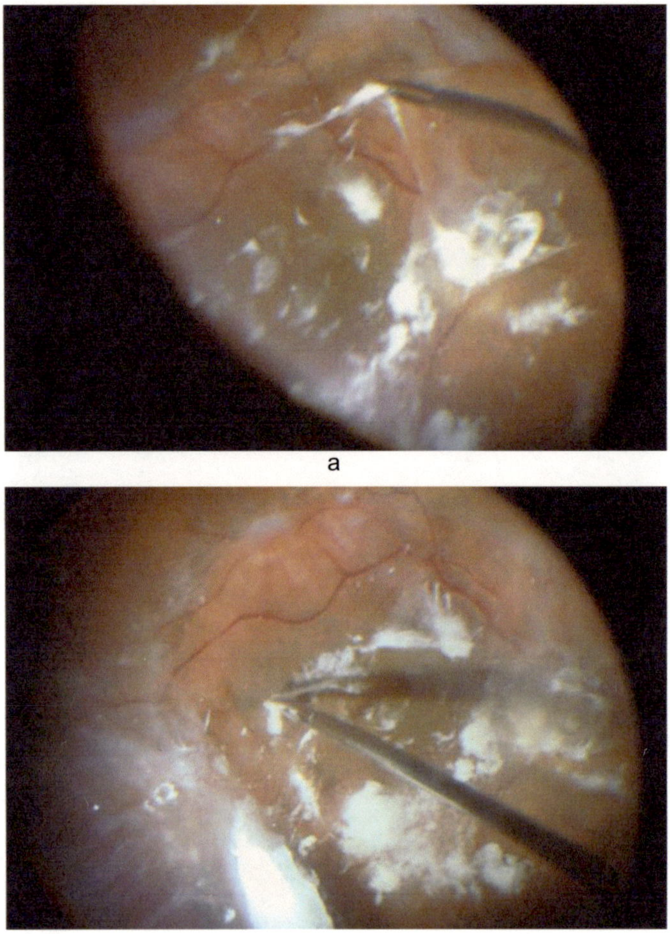

Figure 31.
A—Isolated lamellar intraoperative dissection of the second cortical layer of the vitreous body. b—Identifying the places of the second vitreous layer fixation to the underlying tissues (designated by the black arrow).

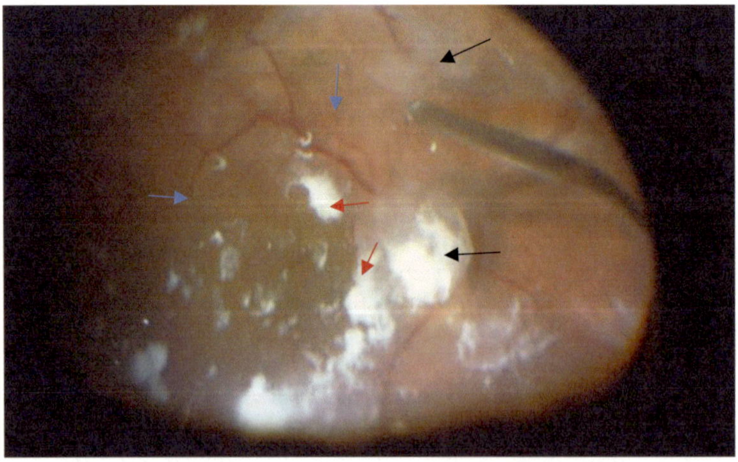

Figure 32.
The image of the eye fundus after the removal of the second layer of the vitreous body. The underlying cortical layers are transparent (blue arrows), only the changed areas of the vitreous body are visualized (black arrows), some insignificant amount of the staining suspension on the surface (red arrows).

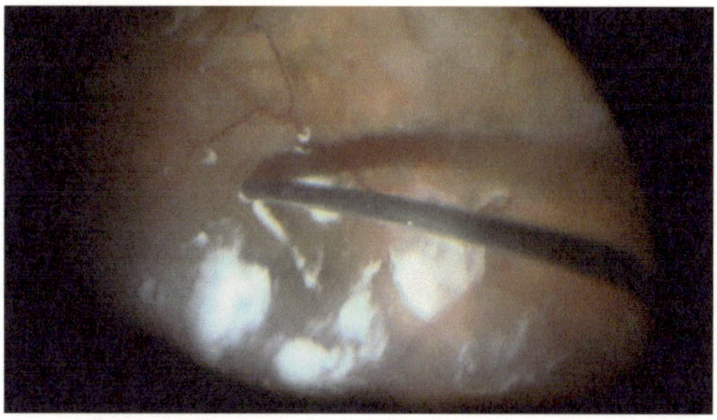

Figure 33.
The second application of the dye to identify the topographic anatomy of underlying tissues.

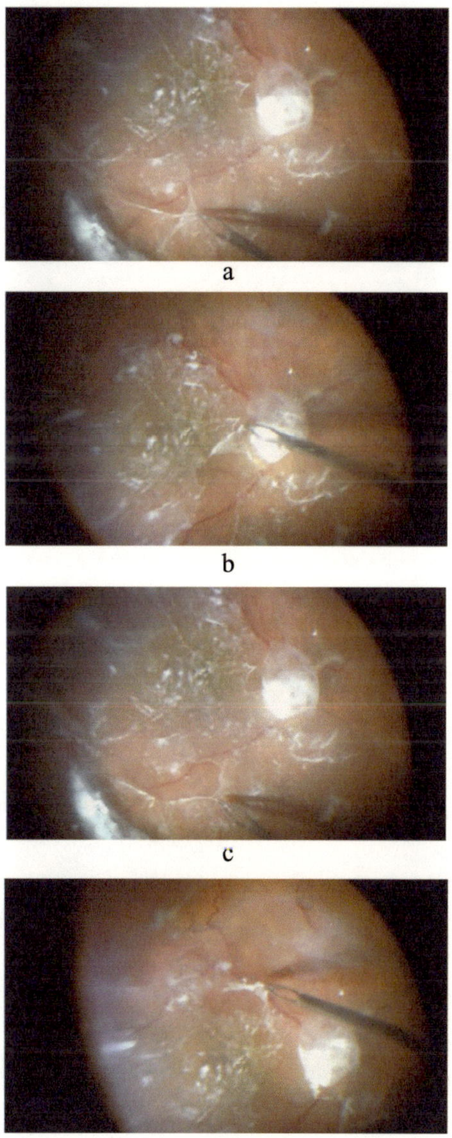

Figure 34.
Cortical layers visualizing.

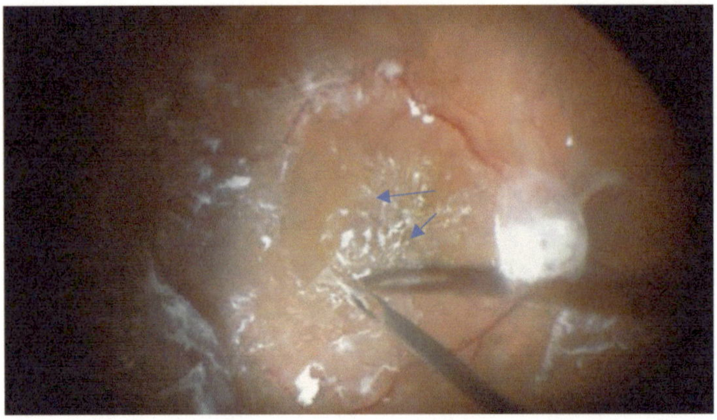

Figure 35.
The lamellar removal of the stained layer from the retinal surface is impossible in the macular zone due to the high level of adhesion between the cortical layers and ILM (blue arrows).

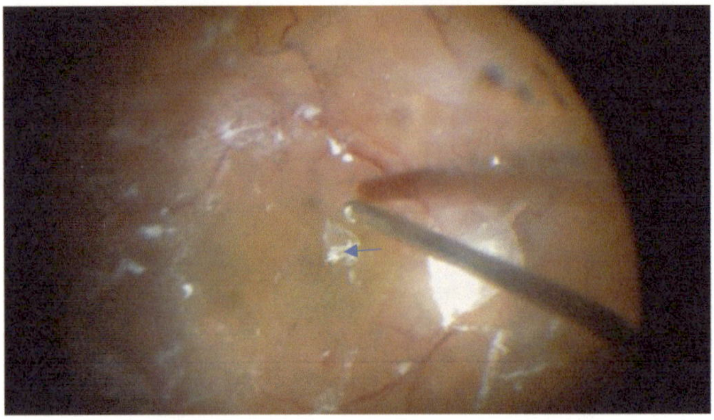

Figure 36.
In the course of the removal of the vitreous layer as a single block with ILM we refrain from performing this manipulation (blue arrow).

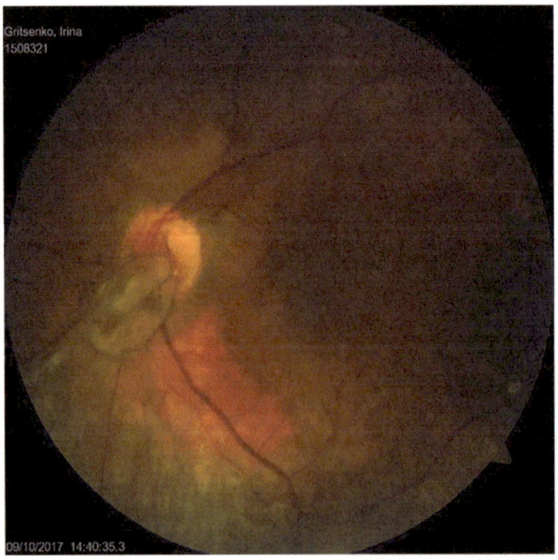

Figure 37.
Foto of the eye fundus 2 years after surgery.

visualize numerous areas of vetreoschisis that are the substrate for the process of proliferation and the growth of neovessels (**Figure 37**).

3. Conclusion

Developed method of vitreocontrastography during vitrectomy allowed to find and describe new structures and interactions in VRI. It is shown that vitreococn-trastography method is very simple, safe, and effective for the ultrathin and transparent eye structures visualization. Due to vitreocontrastography new classification of PDVR was proposed.

Author details

Natalia Kislitsyna[1]* and Sergei Novikov[2]

1 The S. Fyodorov Eye Microsurgery Federal State Institution, Moscow, Russian Federation

2 "SEP" Ltd, Scientifical Medical Research Center for Eye Microsurgery, Moscow, Russian Federation

*Address all correspondence to: natalikislitsin@yandex.ru

References

[1] Kislitsyna NM, Novikov SV, Belikova SV. [The use of a new vital dye for the visualization of vitreous structures (experimental study)] Primeneni kontrastnogo veshchestva dlya vizualizatsii struktur steklovidnogo tela (eksperimental'noe issledovanie) // Obshchestvo oftal'mologov Rossii FGU MNTK «Mikrokhirurgiya glaza» im. akad. S.N. Fedorova. 2010;**11**:55. (in Russ)

[2] Kislitsyna NM et al. [Clinical and morphological study of the influence of "Vitreocontrast" suspension on rabbit eye tissues] Kliniko-morfologicheskoe issledovanie vliyaniya suspenzii «Vitreokontrast» na tkani glaza krolikov// Oftal'mokhirurgiya. 2011;**4**: 59-64

[3] Kislitsyna NM, Kolesnik SV, Novikov SV et al. [Anatomical and topographic features of the posterior vitreous detachment in various vitreoretinal diseases] Anatomo-topograficheskie osobennosti zadney otsloyki steklovidnogo tela pri razlichnoy vitreoretinal'noy patologii// Sovremennye tekhnologii v oftal'mologii// Современные технологии в офтальмологии .2017;**1**:123-126

[4] Kislitsyna NM, Novikov SV, Kolesnik SV, Veselkova MP, Dibirova S. "Anatomic-Topographic Features of the Anterior Cortical Layers of the Vitreous Body". EC Ophthalmology. 2019;**10**(12): 1-10

[5] Kislitsyna NM, Kolesnik SV, Novikov SV, Kolesnik AI, Veselkova MP. Modern Possibilities for the Vireoretinal Interface Contrasting (Experimental Study). Ophthalmology in Russia. 2018; **15**(2S):231-238. (In Russ). DOI: 10.18008/1816-5095-2018-2S-231-238

[6] Kislitsyna NM, Novikov SV, Kolesnik SV, Kolesnik AI, Veselkova MP. Anatomic and Topographic Vitreous and Vitreoretinal Interface Features in Proliferative Diabetic Vitreoretinopathy. Ophthalmology in Russia. 2020;**17**(2):249-257. (In Russ). DOI: 10.18008/1816-5095-2020-2-249-257

[7] Worst JGF. Comparative anatomy of the vitreous body in rhesus monkeys and man. Doc. Ophthalmol. 1992;**71**(1): 169-178

[8] Worst JGF. A SEM-correlation of the anatomy of the vitreous body: making visible the invisible. Doc. Ophthalmol. 1986;**64**(1):117-127

[9] Kroll P. The role of the posterior hyaloids membrane in the diseases of diabetic vitreoretinopathy Focus on Diabetic Retinopathy. 1995;**2**(1):63-64

[10] Kroll P. Pathogenesis and Classification of Proliferative Diabetic Vitreoretinopathy Ophthalmologica. 2007;**221**:78-94

[11] Sebag J. Abnormalities of human vitreous structure in diabetes. Graefes Arch Clin. Exp. Ophthalmol. 1993;**231** (5):257-260

[12] Sebag J. Anomalous posterior vitreous detachment: A unifying concept in vitreo-retinal disease Graefe's archive for clinical and experimental ophthalmology. 2004;**242**(8):690-698

Section 3

Management of Diabetic Retinopathy

Chapter 9

Current Management of Diabetic Macular Edema

Ogugua Ndubuisi Okonkwo, Toyin Akanbi and Chineze Thelma Agweye

Abstract

Diabetic macular edema is a complication of diabetes mellitus (DM) which contributes significantly to the burden of visual impairment amongst persons living with diabetes. Chronic hyperglycemia triggers a cascade of pathologic changes resulting in breakdown of the retinal blood barrier. Understanding the pathophysiological and biochemical changes occurring in diabetes has led to developing novel therapeutics and effective management strategies for treating DME. The clinical utility of optical coherence tomography (OCT) imaging of the retina provides a detailed assessment of the retina microstructure, valid for individualization of patient treatment and monitoring response to treatment. Similarly, OCT angiography (dye-less angiography), another innovation in imaging of DME, provides an understanding of retinal vasculature in DME. From the earlier years of using retinal laser photocoagulation as the gold standard for treating DME, to the current use of intravitreal injection of drugs, several clinical trials provided evidence on safety and efficacy for the shift to intravitreal steroids and anti-vascular endothelial growth factor use. The short durability of available drugs leading to frequent intravitreal injections and frequent clinic visits for monitoring constitute an enormous burden. Therefore, extended durability drugs are being designed, and remote monitoring of DME may be a solution to the current challenges.

Keywords: Diabetes Mellitus, Hypertension, Diabetic Macular Edema, Diabetic Macular Ischemia, Intravitreal Anti Vascular Endothelial Growth Factor, Intravitreal Steroids, Retinal Laser Photocoagulation, Optical Coherence Tomography, Clinical Trials

1. Introduction

The rising number of persons living with diabetes worldwide has significant implications for global blindness. Diabetes is a condition of public health importance and paramount health concern in our time, with about 463 million adults worldwide living with diabetes as of 2019 [1]. The prevalence of diabetes for all age groups worldwide is 2.8% in 2000 and will increase to 4.4% in 2030 [2]. Projections suggest that the total number of individuals with diabetes will more than double from 171 million in 2000 to 366 million by 2030 [2]. Diabetic retinopathy (DR) is a microangiopathy and a significant finding amongst people living with diabetes. About 140 million patients are estimated to have diabetic retinopathy, and 10% of this number, i.e., about 14 million, have impaired vision. Diabetic macular edema (DME) is the commonest cause of visual impairment amongst persons living with diabetes [3].

The prevalence of DME is influenced by the type of diabetes and the use or non-use of insulin treatment [4]. The ten-year incidence of DME is highest amongst older onset patients on insulin, in which a rate as high as 25% has been reported. In research examining the prevalence and risk factors for DME in the United States, non-Hispanic blacks had a higher odd of developing DME than non-Hispanic whites [5]. There was a more significant burden of DME among non-Hispanic blacks, individuals with high hemoglobin A1c, and those with a longer duration of diabetes. It would appear that race plays a vital role in developing DME.

Development of DR and DME is associated with well-researched risk factors, including long duration of diabetes, suboptimal glycemic control as evidenced by elevated HbA1c, hypertension, obesity, elevated serum lipid levels, anemia, pregnancy, associated kidney disease, and smoking [6–10]. DME patients are at increased risk of cerebrovascular accidents (stroke) and cardiovascular disease (CVD) when compared to other DM patients without DR [11]. Also, DME has been shown to negatively impact the quality of life (QoL) of the patient [12]. The most feared complication of all the complications associated with diabetes is a loss of vision [13].

The management of a patient living with diabetes requires the input of a multidisciplinary team [14, 15]. It includes such psychosocial support as can be provided by the family, peers, and even the workplace. This kind of support will help improve patient compliance to treatment and result in an overall healthier patient. There are physician and patient challenges in the care of DR and DME. Physician challenges include managing wide variations in patient responses to treatment, the complex comorbidity profile of the high-risk population, and the suboptimal outcomes associated with delayed initiation of treatment with intravitreal anti-VEGF therapy. Obvious patient challenges include compliance to treatment and clinic attendance for monitoring, the cost of treatment and medical insurance, the burden associated with long-term follow-up and management, problems with access to health care and treatment (especially amongst the low and medium-income), and the time spent on treatment, visits, and follow-up, particularly for the working-age population. Nonetheless, to prevent visual impairment and blindness from DR and DME amongst patients living with diabetes, timely intervention is required. It is possible through the early detection of treatable retinopathy.

2. Screening for DR and DME

DR and DME occur in DM patients, and risk factors are as outlined previously. Therefore, this disease lends itself to early detection through screening of at-risk persons. DR is a progressive disease. The early stages of DR, which can be asymptomatic, can progress to more advanced sight-threatening forms of the disease. The role of ophthalmic screening for early detection of vision-threatening disease in at-risk patients living with diabetes is an essential and practical strategy for preventing vision loss from DR and DME. Though systematic screening is preferred and has proven to reduce rates of blindness from DR effectively, few nations have this in place. In most countries, only some form of opportunistic screening is available or no screening at all [16].

There are different real-world examples of the benefit gained through DR screening. The English national health service (NHS) diabetic retinopathy screening program is a successful model of a screening program that has evolved from opportunistic to effective systematic screening [16]. The UK's systematic screening has effectively reduced the prevalence of DR-related blindness in the UK. The UK national screening program was established in 2004 to provide standardized, quality-assured DR screening across England. All patients living with diabetes above the age of 12 years are invited at least annually for an ophthalmic screen. Those patients at higher risk could have more frequent visits, while those at least level of risk could be considered for more extended visits. Screening is done by qualified screeners who carry out two-field retinal photography, using an updated list of persons living with DM. Images are then digitally transferred to a centralized location for retinal grading by qualified individuals (graders). A comprehensive quality-assurance system is set up, including regular auditing of grading carried out by individuals grading within the English screening program. The UK's screening program has a coverage of 83% and screened close to 3 million persons in 2018/2019. The entire program has reported successes, such that after seven years of the program, a review of the causes of blindness in the UK showed that DR was no longer the most common cause of blindness amongst the working-age [17]. This UK experience of DR screening provides compelling evidence that systematic diabetic retinopathy screening, coupled with timely treatment of sight-threatening disease, can reduce vision impairment and blindness.

For a DR screening program to be effective, it should be composed of the following seven component pathways, 1. identifying the population eligible for screening; 2. invitation and information; 3. testing; 4. referral of screen positives and reporting of screen-negative results; 5. appropriate diagnosis; 6. intervention, treatment, and follow-up; 7. reporting of outcomes [16].

The entire framework of the screening program should be based on the following, resources and infrastructure, a pathway for screening, quality of screening, and equity in access to high-quality screening. In addition, standardization of the process, quality assurance, and auditing of the screening program should be implemented to ensure effectiveness and a high level of sensitivity for timely detection of sight-threatening disease and appropriate referral. Although there are well-designed guidelines for DR screening, considerable gaps exist in deciding the best screening methods and how often to screen, infrastructure and resources for screening, and the fact that several patients living with diabetes fail to keep screening appointments. In addition, in several low- and mid-income countries, healthcare coverage is not countrywide. There is a scarcity of updated information on persons living with diabetes who are the targets of such DR screening programs [16].

In consideration of the economic aspect of DR screening, issues relating to the overall cost-effectiveness of ophthalmic care, the cost-effectiveness of systematic versus opportunistic screening, how screening should be organized and delivered, how often screening should be performed, have all been raised. It has been shown that systematic screening for DR is cost-effective in terms of sight years preserved than no screening [18]. In addition, teleophthalmology screening offers remote screening by trained paramedics in out-of-hospital facilities, including rural and hard-to-reach communities [19, 20]. Other remote screening initiatives include healthcare kiosks and smartphone tele screening, which provide teleophthalmology solutions for a broader range of patients, including in underserved locations and rural communities. In countries with inadequate primary care systems, without a routine systematic screening program, a holistic approach to screening for diabetes is recommended to prevent end-organ damage. This holistic approach should include at least retinal screening, foot examinations, blood pressure monitoring, urine albumin testing, HbA1c, and lipid testing [19]. A significant side benefit of DR screening is that it can also identify other ophthalmic conditions, including cataracts, glaucoma, and other retinal and retinovascular diseases.

In recent times, the entry of artificial intelligence (AI) algorithms further provides immediate grading and feedback on fundus photographs acquired by trained personnel in an out-of-hospital location (including primary care clinics and pharmacies) [21–23]. These AI-backed systems feature automated retinal image analysis (ARIA) [24, 25]. The image to be graded or analyzed can be acquired using digital fundus cameras, and now even handheld mobile devices, including smartphones, can be used. Internet access is required to upload the image for grading to the AI software. The software then compares the uploaded image with cloud-based images. It can provide information on if there is a presence of sight-threatening DR or not with a high level of sensitivity and specificity. This AI software-based screening is the future of DR screening. Utilizing ARIA, detection of DR can be done without the need for human image graders. ARIA, in turn, standardizes the process, is more efficient, and covers a larger area within a shorter period. The EMERALD Study is a recent multicenter study conducted in 13 centers within the UK [26]. This study examined the sensitivity, specificity, and acceptability of an alternative pathway using spectral-domain OCT to detect DME and 7-field Early Treatment Diabetic Retinopathy Study [ETDRS] and ultra-widefield fundus images for PDR. These images were interpreted by trained nonmedical staff (ophthalmic graders) to detect reactivation of previously treated disease. The authors compare this alternative pathway with the current standard of care (face-to-face examination by ophthalmologists). They concluded that this new alternated pathway has acceptable sensitivity and offers a significant release of resources.

At this time, home screening using optical coherence tomography (OCT) device has been explored, "Home OCT device" [27]. Success and experience gained from using the Foresee Home Device in monitoring eyes with AMD have evolved into the idea that patients at risk of DME can be monitored remotely from their homes using the Home OCT device, reducing the number of hospital visits [28]. Home OCT can be combined with home monitoring of visual acuity and other aspects of visual function. This innovative idea also provides information on DME's entire clinical evolution and history, which is missed between clinic visits for several patients. The patient uses the Home OCT device to scan the macula for early disease detection constantly. Therefore, home teleophthalmology and home monitoring combined can detect early disease, lead to intervention early in the disease process, and prevent vision loss from DR and DME. This home screening and monitoring of DME is another current reality in the COVID 19 era and provides a way out for a future lockdown, as happened during the COVID 19 pandemic.

To conclude, DR screening of at-risk patients living with diabetes is essential for the early detection of sight-threatening disease to enable timely, effective treatment. With increasing numbers of patients diagnosed with diabetes, DR-related visual disabilities will likely increase in the coming years. An interdisciplinary organized public health approach will provide the best approach to achieving screening for many patients. Collaboration amongst all different partners is required to reduce the incidence of vision loss resulting from DME and DR. This multidisciplinary approach will ensure that relevant information about diabetes and the eye screened is shared with the screened patient and across the system responsible for diabetes care. This will facilitate integrated care for the patient. Other incidental findings diagnosed during eye screening, such as cataracts or glaucoma, should be referred to the appropriate eye care team.

3. Pathophysiology of DME

3.1 Pathophysiology

The pathophysiology of DME is multifactorial and has not been clearly and completely defined since it involves various complex pathological processes [29–31]. In health, the retinal circulation is unique in that retinal capillaries are non-fenestrated, and their endothelial cells have tight junctions which do not allow fluid leakage. A lymphatic system does not exist in the retina, but leakage can occur in the presence of retinal pathology, causing edema and swelling [32]. Chronic capillary non-perfusion and retinal ischemia are said to be the primary contributors to DME [33]. Signaling molecules such as insulin-like growth factor-1 (IGF-1), platelet-derived growth factor (PGF), angiopoietin, and most importantly, vascular endothelial growth factor (VEGF) all play a role in the subsequent development of diabetic microangiopathy [33].

The trigger for the vascular damage has been convincingly linked to the chronic hyperglycemia present in DM. Vessel damage occurs via the glucose metabolic pathways, which include the Diacylglycerol (DAG)–protein kinase C (PKC) pathway, Advanced glycation end-products (AGE), Polyol (sorbitol) pathway, Hexosamine pathway, and the plasma kallikrein-kinin system (KKS) [34–36]. The blood-retinal barrier (BRB) is an essential structure that regulates normal visual function [31, 37]. It is a physiologic barrier that tightly regulates the balance of electrolytes, protein, solute, and water movement in and out of the retina. It is composed of both an outer and an inner portion [31, 37]. The inner BRB comprises tight junctions between retinal capillary endothelial cells, basement membrane surrounding it, and pericytes outside [31, 37]. The outer BRB tight junctions exist between retinal pigment epithelial cells located between them the fenestrated choriocapillaris and the outer retina [31, 37].

In DME, disruption of the BRB is common, leading to increased vasopermeability associated with vascular leakage, neovascularization, and inflammation [38]. In chronic hyperglycemia, cellular and structural alteration in the BRB is characterized by the breakdown of cell–cell junctions between endothelial cells, pericyte loss, basement membrane thickening, increased deposition of extracellular matrix components, and Muller cell metabolism disturbance heralding the beginning of the microangiopathy [30, 37, 39]. Over time, continued retinal microvasculature damage results in the release of reactive oxygen species and inflammatory mediators and capillary nonperfusion, giving rise to retinal hypoxia and ischemia that drives upregulation of angiogenic factors, such as vascular endothelial growth factor (VEGF) and breakdown of the BRB [29, 39]. The breakdown of the inner BRB then results in the accumulation of plasma proteins such as albumin, which exerts a high oncotic pressure in the neural interstitium, inducing interstitial edema, neural tissue impairment, and ultimately vision loss if there is a delay in treatment or no treatment at all [29, 31, 40].

Patients with DME have elevated vitreous levels of VEGF, Intracellular Adhesion Molecule-1 (ICAM-1), interleukin-6 (IL-6), and monocyte chemoattractant protein-1 compared to nondiabetic patients [41]. VEGF-A mediates angiogenesis by promoting endothelial cell migration, proliferation, and survival [41]. VEGF-A also possesses inflammatory properties through its capacity to mediate microvascular permeability and increase the adhesion of leukocytes. It has been noted to stimulate expression of ICAM-1 and vascular cell adhesion molecule –1 (VCAM-1), thus incorporating the inflammatory cascade, initiating early diabetic retinal leukocyte adhesion, and aiding the development of diabetic vasculopathy [39, 41]. VEGF-A inhibitors have been shown to reduce vascular permeability [30, 31]. Anti-VEGF agents such as Ranibizumab, Aflibercept, and Bevacizumab administered according to various treatment protocols are currently the gold standard for treating center-involving DME [31, 37, 42]. The introduction of intravitreal anti-VEGF therapy has led to notably improved outcomes for some patients with DR/DME [39]. Nevertheless, there are several practical limitations to the treatment with anti-VEGF. They include; cost, need for frequent intravitreal injections, undertreatment, and incomplete response in some patients [39, 43].

3.2 Alternative pathways

Furthermore, clinical trials have demonstrated that only 33–45% of DME patients on intravitreal anti-VEGF agents showed three lines or more of visual improvement. Other DME patients showed an intermediate response (5–9 letters of improvement) or inadequate response (<5 letters of improvement or worse). Eyes with suboptimal early vision response showed poorer long-term visual outcomes than eyes with pronounced early response [37, 44, 45]. In the clinical setting, available data have shown that anti-VEGF therapy does not live up to the high goals set by clinical trials, leaving patients with suboptimal vision [46]. These limitations have resulted in exploring alternate pathways involved in aberrant angiogenesis, including the Tie-2 pathway and the effect of genetics [39].

The angiopoietin-tyrosine-protein kinase (Ang-Tie) system plays an essential and complementary role alongside VEGF-mediated vessel formation and vascular stability [42]. The angiopoietins, Ang-1 and Ang-2, are a family of growth factors that interact with one another to play a vital role in vessel homeostasis, angiogenesis, and vascular permeability via interacting with the Tie-2 transmembrane receptor tyrosine kinase [37, 39, 42]. Ang-1 plays a protective role in pathological angiogenesis, supports quiescent vessel maturation, and prevents intravesical inflammation [39, 42]. In contrast, Ang-2 promotes vascular instability through its competition with Ang-1 and inhibition of Tie-2, contributing to DME [47]. Ang-2 is upregulated in response to hyperglycemia and plays a vital role in altering the BRB in DME [37]. Increased Ang-2 leads to decreased phosphorylation of Tie-2, which results in increased retinal vascular permeability [37]. Together Ang-2 and VEGF-A have been reported to produce accelerated neovascularization in the developing retina and ischemic retina [39].

3.3 Systemic control

The UKPDS and FIELD studies concluded that good control of modifiable risk factors of diabetic retinopathy delayed its development and progression [48–51]. Howbeit, findings of the ADVANCE trial came to a contrary conclusion [52]. Moreover, it has been observed in clinical practice that despite prolonged periods of poor control of glycemic and systemic blood pressure in some patients, DR was not observed, contrary to expectations. On the other hand, some other patients would develop DR within a relatively shorter period of diabetes, despite better control [53, 54]. These observations suggest that mechanisms other than hyperglycemia, elevated blood pressure, and hyperlipidemia contributes to the development and progression of DME and diabetic retinopathy in some patients [55]. In addition, disparities in the risk of developing diabetic retinopathy have been noted among patients of different ethnic groups even after correcting for environmental factors, alluding to the fact that genetic factors may play a role in the pathogenesis of diabetic retinopathy [56–59]. This ethnic bias and variable predisposition bring to the fore the consideration of a concept of genetic predisposition to DME and DR in individuals of diverse ethnicity and genetic constitution.

3.4 Genetics of DME and DR

Gene mapping has been employed to identify novel genetic variants underlying DME and DR. However, only weak associations have resulted [55, 60]. The Genome-wide association studies (GWAS) had identified loci of interest MRPL19 and NRXN3 as novel loci with suggestive association with DME and PDR, respectively, which are sight-threatening complications of DR [61]. Although DR-associated genes have yet to be replicated and confirmed, these early findings represent the initial groundwork and maybe a preview of DR genetics' complexity [55, 60, 62].

3.5 Macular ischemia

Retinal ischemia has been recognized as a primary risk factor for developing proliferative diabetic retinopathy (PDR); it sometimes occurs with DME. A paucity of studies describing diabetic macula ischemia (DMI) exists, mainly due to difficulty in its detection using fluorescein angiography and limited treatment options [63]. Clinically, DMI is defined by an enlargement of the foveal avascular zone (FAZ) and paramacular areas of capillary nonperfusion [64]. Two anatomical changes can be characteristically seen in the retina of patients with DMI. First, due to marked cellular and extracellular damage, there is extensive loss of neuro-retinal tissue. Secondly, there is notable occlusion of the vessels supplying the retina [63]. DMI results in the upregulation of growth factors such as VEGF, which contribute to DME development [65], making it difficult to observe and anatomically characterize DMI in isolation. The anatomical and physiological basis of this disease is still very poorly studied [63]. Recently optical coherence tomography angiography (OCTA) offers a better image of macular microvasculature and is superior to conventional FA in assessing DMI. Anatomically the microcirculation supply to the retina is divided mainly into superficial capillary plexus (SCP) and deep capillary plexus (DCP) [66]. Choroidal circulation seems to be the most critical blood supply to the central macula, including the photoreceptor inner segment (IS) band, which appears to be the most critical consumer of oxygen [67]. It is thought that the DCP is responsible for up to 15% of the blood supply to the photoreceptors, especially during dark adaptation [65, 66].

3.6 Classification of DME

3.6.1 The classification of diabetic retinopathy (DR) and DME

The classification of diabetic retinopathy (DR) and DME have evolved over the years. About five decades ago, experts in ophthalmology gathered in Airlie House for a symposium to review the state of knowledge of DR; an outcome from that meeting was developing a standardized classification of DR [68–70]. Afterward, this classification was modified for use by the Diabetic Retinopathy Study (DRS) [69, 70]. The modified Airlie House classification of diabetic retinopathy used in the DRS was further developed for the Early Treatment Diabetic Retinopathy Study (ETDRS). This randomized, prospective study evaluated the efficacy of laser treatment for macular edema [68]. It became the gold standard for many years. The ETDRS introduced the term clinically significant macular edema (CSME). CSME was defined using slit-lamp biomicroscopy, when it met any of the three criteria viz. "(1) thickening of the retina at or within 500 μm of the center of the macula; or (2) hard exudate at or within 500 μm of the center of the macula associated with thickening of the adjacent retina; or (3) a zone of retinal thickening one disc area or larger, any part of which is within one disc diameter of the center of the macula" [71]. After that, fluorescein angiography was used to guide laser treatment [72]. The ETDRS found that macular laser photocoagulation effectively reduced moderate visual loss by at least 50% in laser-treated eyes with CSME compared to untreated eyes [68, 70]. In 2003, an international classification called the Diabetic macular edema disease Severity Scale with greater simplicity was proposed [29, 73]. The DME disease severity scale put forward that DME is 'apparently present' when some apparent retinal thickening or hard exudates exist in the posterior pole; DME is proposed to be 'absent' otherwise [29, 70]. When DME is present, it is classified into mild, moderate, or severe if the retinal thickening or hard exudate is distant from the center of the macula, approaching the center of the macula but not involving the center and involving the center of the macula, respectively [29, 70]. Ten years after ETDRS, Optical Coherence Tomography (OCT) became the new imaging modality that enabled ophthalmologists to utilize the qualitative and quantitative measurement of central subfield macular thickness (CSMT) and visual acuity to diagnose and determine the response of DME to treatment [29, 72]. OCT is invaluable due to its reliability and reproducibility; its importance in evaluating and monitoring DME cannot be over-emphasized [41, 74].

A classification based only on slit-lamp biomicroscopic evidence of retinal thickening is grossly insufficient to precisely describe DME and determine the appropriate therapeutic modalities for the various morphologies [72, 75].

3.6.2 DME classification based on OCT

DME classification based on OCT is described using various morphology (1) diffuse edema type (sponge-like diffuse retinal thickening), (2) cystoid macular edema (CME) type (thickening of the fovea with intraretinal cystoid change), (3) serous retinal detachment (SRD) type (thickening of the fovea with subretinal fluid) and (4) vitreomacular interface abnormalities as seen in incomplete or complete posterior vitreous detachment and epiretinal membrane (ERM) formation or vitreomacular traction or both [74–76].

Other parameters deployed by the OCT in DME diagnosis include retinal thickness, volume (quantitative data), and inner and outer layers of the retina [72, 74].

3.7 Clinical presentation (symptoms and signs)

Patients with DME may be asymptomatic if the macula center is not involved. However, some eyes having center involving DME (CI-DME) have been seen to have no visual disturbance, presumably because of the recent involvement of the center [32]. Depending on the degree of fovea involvement and the chronicity of the edema, patients may present with an array of visual symptoms [32]. These include gradual progressive diminution and distortion of central vision over some time (usually moderate, unlike the severe loss after vitreous hemorrhage or retinal detachment involving the macula in proliferative diabetic retinopathy), metamorphopsia, and loss of color vision. They may also experience poor night vision and 'washing-out of vision in bright sunlight with poor dark–light adaptation [32, 77, 78].

On dilated biomicroscopic examination, retinal thickening may be observed in commonly identified patterns. Focal edema often occurs in association with a cluster of microaneurysms, sometimes surrounded by an incomplete ring of hard exudates. Diffuse DME may be very difficult to identify clinically if the retina is uniformly thickened due to the lack of reference landmarks. Clues include the height of the retinal blood vessels over the pigment epithelium, cystoids spaces, or even loss of the foveal depression. Other features that are sometimes seen with macular edema include variable loss of retinal transparency, a significant number of microaneurysms, intraretinal hemorrhages, and dispersed areas of hard exudates [32].

3.8 Evaluation of DME

3.8.1 The control of systemic metabolic abnormalities

The control of systemic metabolic abnormalities observed in diabetes mellitus has a significant effect on the development and progression of diabetic microvascular complications, including DME [79]. The United Kingdom Prospective Diabetes Study (UKPDS) and the Diabetes Control and Complications Trial (DCCT) did demonstrate that optimal metabolic control could reduce the incidence and progression of DR [50, 80]. To achieve good management of a patient with DME, a multidisciplinary approach involving different medical subspecialists such as ophthalmology, endocrinology, nephrology, neurology, cardiology, orthopedics is key [29]. Systemic workup involving blood investigations helps monitor the systemic status of these patients. These investigations including fasting blood glucose (FBG), glycosylated hemoglobin levels (HbA1C), serum electrolyte, urea, creatinine, and fasting lipid profile. Other investigations that may be required would be based on systemic complaints, examination findings, and other suspected comorbidities [29]. The recommended values for HbA1c, blood pressure, and LDL cholesterol are $< 6.5–7\%$, $<130/<85$ mmHg, and < 100 mg/dl, respectively [81]. However, many patients fail to achieve or maintain these levels of metabolic control. In patients who significantly reduce HbA1c, there is an associated increased risk of severe hypoglycemia [33, 50, 80]. Managing physicians must recognize correctable risk factors of DR and DME, such as hyperglycemia, hypertension, and/or hyperlipidemia, to ensure appropriate monitoring and referral for eye care.

3.8.2 Ophthalmic evaluation

I. Over the last two decades, a wide range of imaging modalities, including fundus photography, fluorescein angiography (FA), optical coherence tomography (OCT), and OCT-Angiography (OCT-A), have been utilized not only for the diagnosis and classification of disease but also to monitor disease progression and treatment [82]. **Figures 1–5** illustrate the significance of these imaging technologies in DR and DME. DME is diagnosed clinically with the slit-lamp biomicroscopy or indirect ophthalmoscopy with features such as visible microaneurysms, hard exudates, cysts, and retinal thickening. However, stereoscopic fundus photography and fluorescein angiography have greater sensitivity in detecting DME than ophthalmoscopy because of superior optics of the former, the enhanced contrast of fluorescein angiography, ability to make confirmation of vascular leakage, and the ability of the observer to evaluate magnified images without the interference of patients moving or blinking [83].

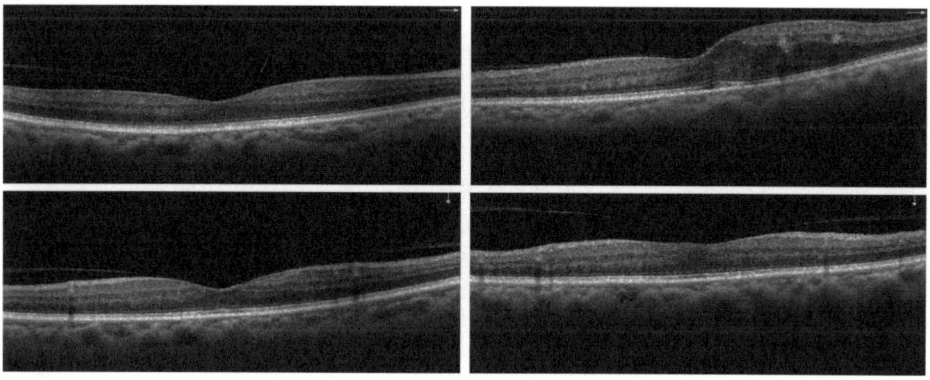

Figure 1.
OCT image of both eyes of a patient who suffers from DME in the left eye. The right eye shows typical retinal microstructure, while the left eye shows thickening in the foveomacula area from intraretinal cystic spaces due to diabetic macular edema. Notice that the posterior vitreous membrane is "partly" attached to the retina in both eyes.

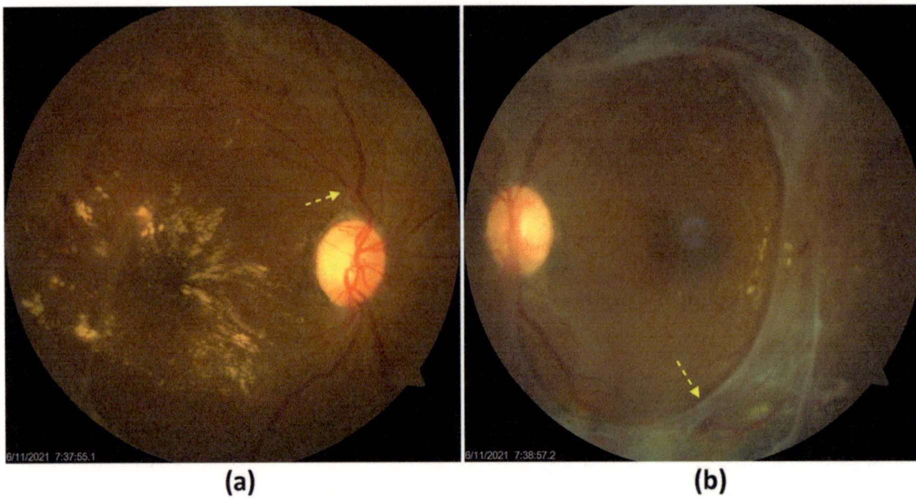

Figure 2.
(a) Right eye fundus photograph, with the star shaped appearance of hard exudation, the nasal portion of which involves the fovea. There are dot hemorrhages and microaneurysms involving the temporal macula and superiorly within the superotemporal arcade. Notice the arteriovenous nipping (broken yellow arrows) suggestive of co-existing hypertensive retinopathy. There are opacities within the vitreous. (b) Left eye fundus photograph, a ring of fibrovascular tissue extends from the retina into the pre retinal space and vitreous cavity. Hard exudates, hemorrhages, and microaneurysms are present within the temporal macula beneath the fibrovascular tissue. Contraction of fibrovascular proliferative tissue creates a tractional effect on the inferotemporal arcade (broken yellow arrows).

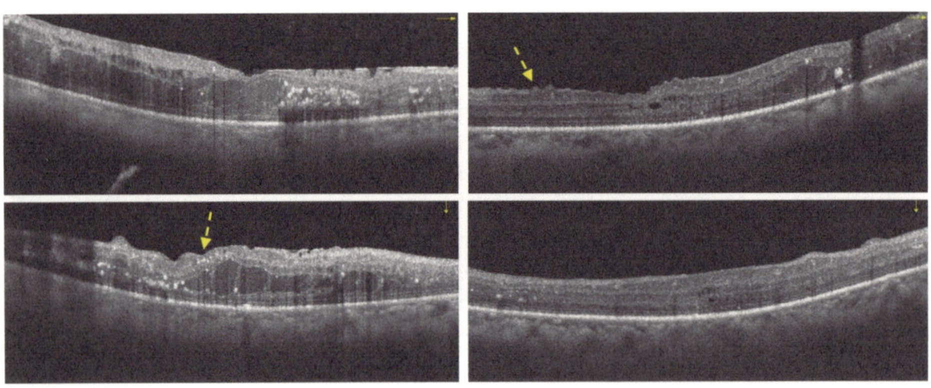

Figure 3.
OCT images of both eyes as in ***Figure 2a*** *and* ***b****. There is intraretinal cluster of hard exudates and intraretinal cystoid spaces, worse in the right eye (correlating with the fundus photographs). Epiretinal membrane is present in both eyes (broken yellow arrows).*

Stereoscopic fundus photographs provide an opportunity to evaluate and document long-term changes in the retina [32, 82]. The ETDRS study used the 7 standard fields (7SF) 30° photographs of the retina (three horizontally across the macula and four around the optic nerve). This combination gave nearly 75° of visualization [29]. Mydriatic or nonmydriatic fundus imaging with $\geq 30^0$ mono- or stereo photography is used with or without OCT [84]. Ultra-wide-field imaging is currently used for the screening and detection of DR, as is ultra-wide-field angiography [83].

Fundus fluorescein angiography (FFA) visualizes the retinal vasculature. It identifies lesions of diabetic retinopathy, patchy areas of hypo fluorescence representing ischemia as demonstrated by capillary dropout, areas of impaired BRB function, and microaneurysms manifest as areas of hyper fluorescence demonstrated by leakage of dye and visualize expansion of the foveal avascular zone (FAZ) [59, 82].

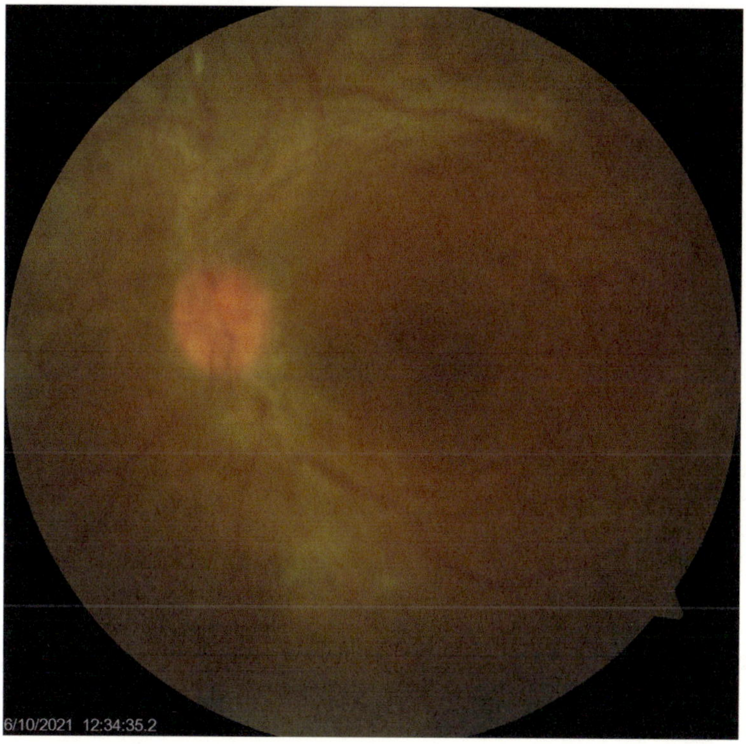

Figure 4.
Left eye fundus photograph showing extensive fibrovascular tissue proliferation across the macula and optic disc. There is a faint view of retinal hemorrhages in the temporal macula.

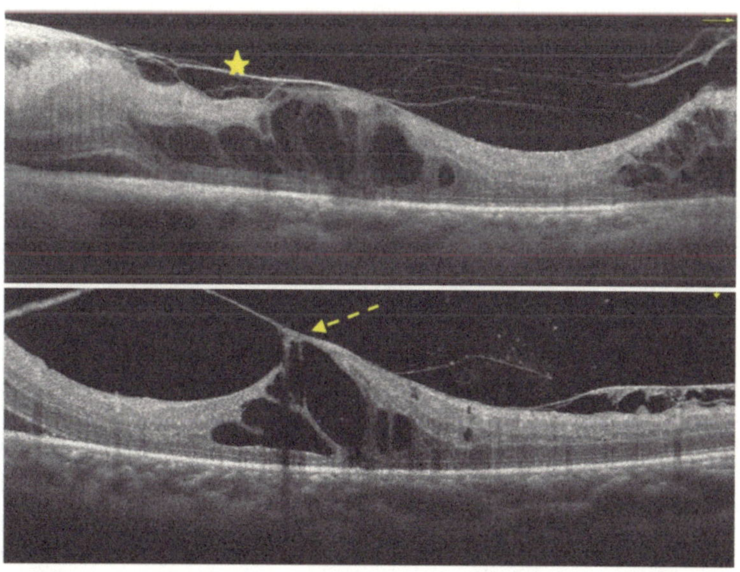

Figure 5.
The OCT image of the left eye fundus photograph in ***Figure 4****. Tangential (yellow star) and vertical (yellow dotted arrow) tractional elements in the preretinal space extend into the vitreous. This thick taut hyaloid creates foveomacular traction-induced macular edema (evident as the large cystoid spaces within the macula).*

Previously FFA helped predict prognosis and response to treatment in DME [59]. A case of diffuse DME was defined by fluorescein leakage involving most of the macula. This form of DME is more challenging to treat than focal DME involving leakage from identified lesions [85]. FFA also revealed the degree of capillary non-perfusion and macular ischemia, shown by an enlarged foveal avascular zone [59]. With the development of ultra-widefield imaging, FFA can now be performed with visualization of up to 200° of the retina. Extensive ischemia in the retinal periphery has been associated with recalcitrant disease, and the ultra-widefield FFA may help identify DME that is likely to be treatment-resistant [59]. It reveals areas of peripheral ischemia and non-perfusion, which can be promptly treated with pan-retinal laser photocoagulation. The significant advantage of FFA is that it was the only imaging modality commonly used in DR that provides information on vascular flow and vessel permeability over time by visualizing leakage and pooling [82]. The disadvantage of FFA is that it is an invasive procedure that involves the administration of intravenous dye. It should be performed carefully, especially in patients with severe DR and associated systemic vascular complications such as severe renal disease and clinical or subclinical cardiovascular disease [29, 82, 86, 87]. The most common adverse reactions are nausea and vomiting, but more severe side effects include localized reactions, urticaria, seizures, and, very rarely, anaphylaxis [29, 82]. Before performing FFA, the ophthalmologist must carefully consider whether the information provided is necessary to make therapeutic decisions and whether the same or equivalent information can be provided by OCT which is non-invasive [83].

II. Since its first introduction, OCT has become the most frequently used diagnostic tool in ophthalmology for the past two decades and has revolutionized clinical imaging for diagnosis and disease management in most retinal diseases, including DME [78, 82]. The diagnostic utility of the OCT can be seen in the case illustrated by **Figures 6** and **7**. The fast, non-invasive, high-resolution imaging available with OCT of the posterior segment allows for close study of the retinal anatomy and assessing retinal thickness profile and morphology in DME [82, 83]. A significant advantage of OCT is that it can be easily repeated several times, within the same day, with a high degree of reproducibility. Therefore, it can be used to monitor the effect of therapy, e.g., intravitreal anti-VEGF given the same day or shortly after, to detect or objectively quantify response to therapy [82, 83]. This value of the OCT to monitor treatment is illustrated with **Figures 8** and **9**.

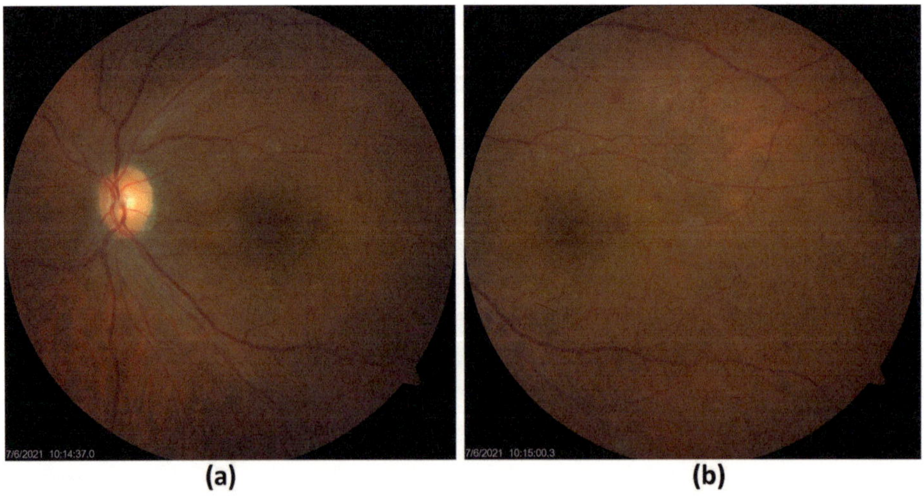

Figure 6.
(a and b) The left eye fundus photograph shows dot hemorrhages, microaneurysms, and few hard exudates, over the macula (a) and extending to the temporal retina (b). This is a clinical diagnosis of non-proliferative diabetic retinopathy and DME.

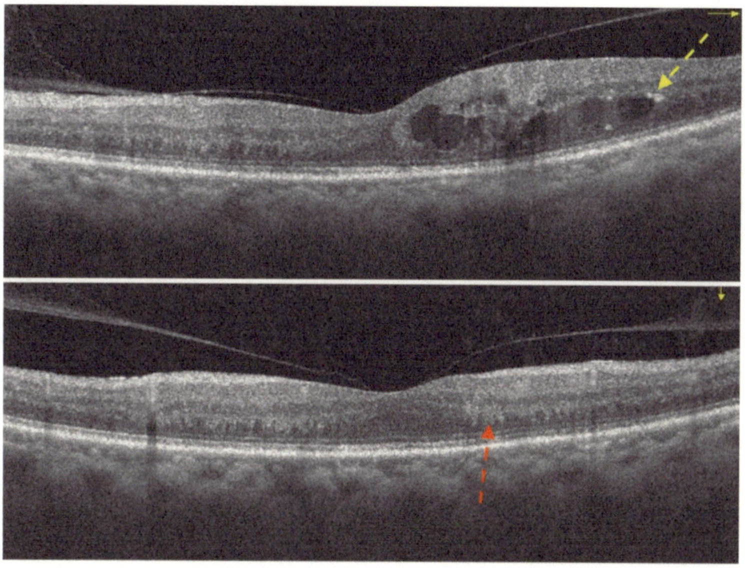

Figure 7.
*OCT of fundus image in **Figure 6** showing intraretinal cystoid spaces and a few hard exudates clustering around the cystoid (broken yellow arrows). Hyper reflective digitations are extending into the outer nuclear layer (broken red line).*

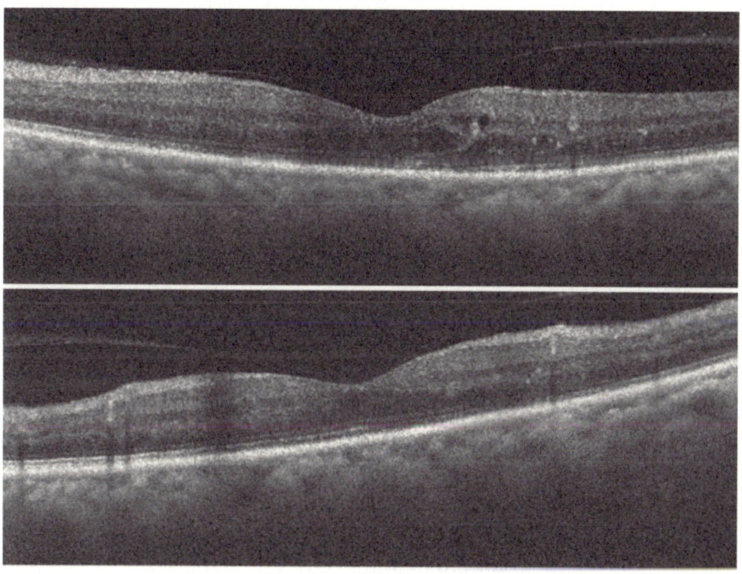

Figure 8.
*This is the OCT image of the same eye as in **Figure 7** after intravitreal injection of Bevacizumab. Notice the reduction in intraretinal cystoid space size. The foveomacular retina is no longer thickened, as in **Figure 7**.*

There are three types of OCT: time-domain (TD), spectral-domain (SD), and swept-source (SS) [82]. Spectral-domain OCT is the most commonly used, allowing three-dimensional raster scans of up to a few hundred B-scans, also creating high-resolution images. It supersedes time-domain (TD)-OCT, the first generation that allowed imaging of 6 radial cuts only [78, 83]. The most recent third-generation OCT technology uses a swept-source (SS) light source that allows high-speed imaging and provides three-dimensional raster images of high microstructural resolution, also referred to as optical histology [78]. OCT is highly sensitive and more accurate in

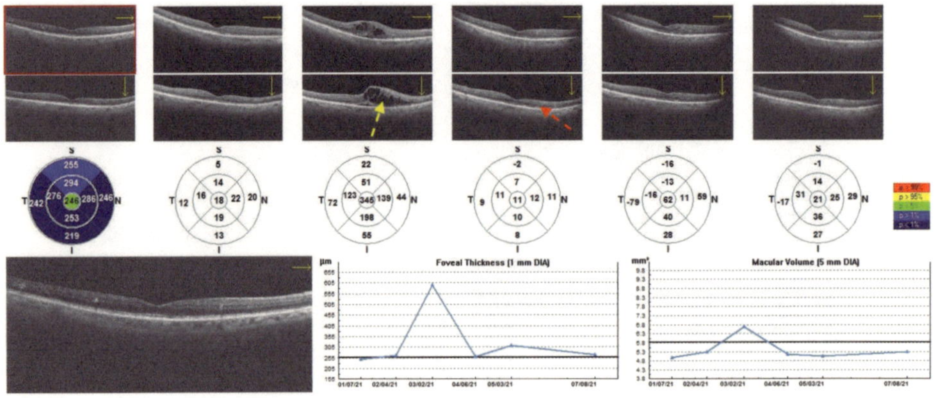

Figure 9.
This serial OCT shows longitudinal follow-up of a case of recurrent macular edema, which resolves after initial treatment with intravitreal Ranibizumab. However, recurrence of edema (broken yellow arrow) occurs after an attempt at extending the injection interval from monthly to two monthly, then three monthly (treat and extend protocol). The resolution of edema (broken red arrow) occurs again after repeating intravitreal injection of Ranibizumab. The macula remains dry at subsequent visits.

diagnosing DME when compared to fundus stereo photography and biomicroscopy [78], see **Figures 1, 3** and **5**. It is currently the gold standard for the diagnosis and monitoring of DME.

It is used to determine whether DME is center-sparing or center -involving, an essential criterion in determining treatment [78]. A limitation noted is that image segmentation could be a problem in eyes with marked DME and dome-shaped macula [88].

OCT not only identifies the presence or absence of disease activity such as the intra-retinal fluid (IRF) and the sub-retinal fluid (SRF) as seen in DME, it localizes them in the retina. It allows for quantification to assess the disease's response to anti-VEGF therapy [89], as demonstrated in **Figure 9**. It has been demonstrated that OCT using microstructural changes seen in IRF and SRF at baseline can prognosticate response to intravitreal treatments [90].

III. Certain features of retinal morphology seen on the SD-OCT, such as central subfoveal thickness (CST), vitreoretinal interface abnormalities, and the epiretinal membrane (ERM), can be used as surrogate markers and act as predictive factors for visual acuity (VA) outcomes in the treatment of DME [91–93]. CST was initially used as a predictor of visual outcome after treatment due to the ease of identifying and obtaining this parameter, but this had limitations [92]. Consequently, other aspects of OCT have been investigated to determine their usefulness as possible biomarkers and correlations for VA and treatment outcomes. These include an external limiting membrane (ELM) and ellipsoid zone (EZ) disruption, and disorganization of retinal inner layers (DRIL) [91, 92]. Sun et al. described an OCT feature termed disorganization of the inner retinal layers (DRIL) [94]. It was observed that an improvement in DRIL following treatment for DME was predictive of better VA outcomes. There was an association with VA after the resolution of centre-involving DME [95, 96]. An association between DRIL, the disruption of the outer retina, and increasing DR severity have been observed [91].

IV. The role of OCT-A is evolving as a tool in the evaluation of DME. OCT-A is an imaging technique that uses motion contrast and faster scan speeds, including spectral-domain (SD) and swept-source (SS), to obtain three-dimensional cubes, which then undergo automated segmentation into layers [82], as seen in **Figure 10**. In DME, as with FFA, OCTA can visualize the increase in the size of the fovea avascular zone (FAZ) and perifoveal intercapillary area [97], seen in **Figure 11**. It can also

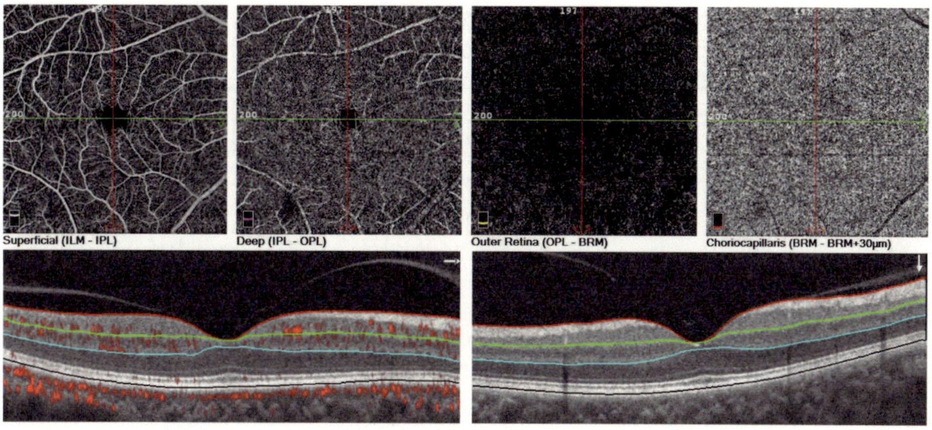

Figure 10.
A normal OCT-Angiography (OCT-A) scan of the right eye, showing the four segmented layers, including superficial and deep plexi, outer retina and the choriocapillaris layers. Also shown are the cross sectional OCT scans, highlighting the borders and planes of tissue segmentation.

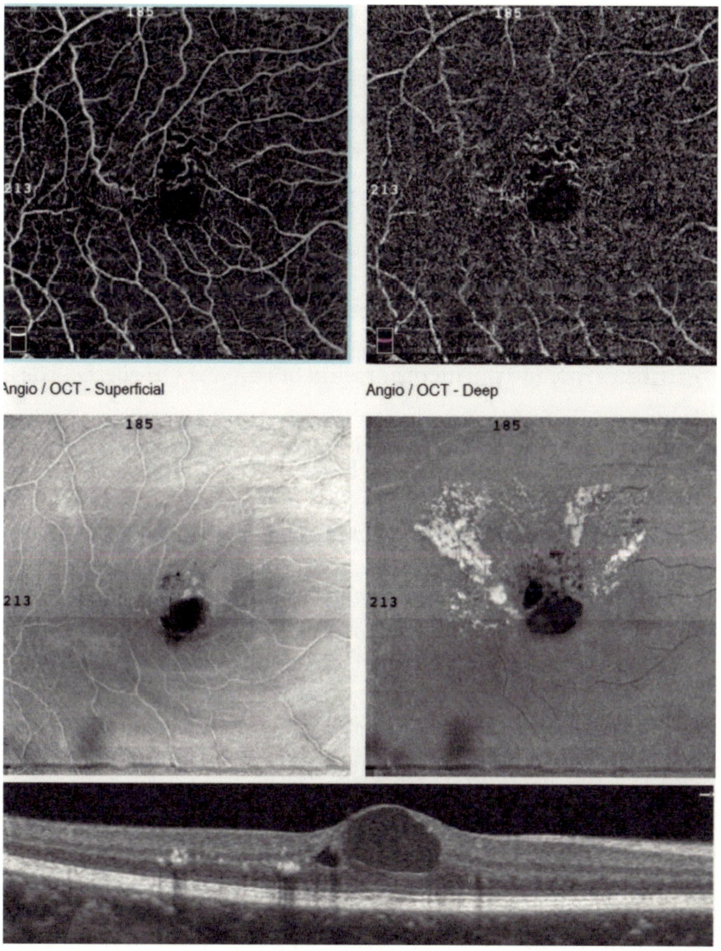

Figure 11.
OCT-A, showing a well perfused macular and what looks like shunt vessels within the foveal avascular zone. The en face OCT images show radiating hard exudates centered on the fovea. The cross sectional OCT shows large intra retinal cystic space in the fovea, and there is aggregation of hard exudates observed within the retina (outer nuclear layer) microstructure.

study the retinal vascular plexuses in layers, determine microvascular parameters, and correlate them with functional and morphological data [98].

The advantages of OCT-A are: It provides "3-D" imaging information of the macula and visualizes peripapillary capillaries [99]. It is dye-free, thereby suitable for patients with adverse reactions to the dyes and poor intravenous access or renal failure [100]. It is reproducible with a faster acquisition time [99, 101]. An advantage of OCT-A over conventional FA is that the absence of dye leakage using OCT-A enables visualization of the distinct margins and sizes of neovascularization since there is no leaking of dye to obscure the neovascularization complex's margins seen in the later frames of the FFA [33]. The disadvantages of OCT-A include its inability to visualize leakage of dye in the retina, a common feature of inflammatory vascular pathology, and a sign of blood-retinal barrier breakdown [100]. Limitation to detecting peripheral retinal ischemia as it can scan mostly the posterior pole [100]. Studies suggest that in the future management of DME, OCT-A could be used to prognosticate the evolution of visual acuity with the help of biomarkers such as low vascular density (VD) and enlargement of the foveal avascular zone (FAZ) [102–104]. OCT-A could also be used to aid in the monitoring of the response of DME to anti-VEGF treatment such as Ranibizumab since poor responders show significant damage to the DCP, but not SCP [105, 106].

Initially, the major limitation of OCTA was the small field of view, with the greatest resolution achieved at smaller scanning sizes such as the commonly used 3 × 3 mm scan [33, 82]. Wider field OCTA scans are already available such as the 9 × 9 mm and 12 × 12 mm. Experimental wide-field OCTA using faster scanning OCTA is being researched and could be available in the future [102, 103, 107].

Other drawbacks noted are that OCTA is subject to projection artifacts. Vasculature from outer layers is projected onto the deep plexuses and choriocapillaris, affecting the accurate interpretation of vascular pathology in the deeper layers. It is also prone to movement artifact; patient movement presents as horizontal white lines, and artifact blinking appears as black lines across the image [83]. Solutions to artifacts include the incorporation of software to correct the motion artifacts [108].

Visual acuity is still viewed as the gold standard in clinical settings for assessing vision using the Snellen or ETDRS charts, but it does not entirely reflect functional vision [109, 110]. Functional vision depicts the impact of sight on the quality of life as expressed by the patient [109]. Various visual function disturbances such as waviness, relative scotoma, and reduction in contrast sensitivity are known to precede loss of visual acuity in patients with DME. However, they are not assessed and quantified during a routine eye examination. For assessing these abnormalities, microperimetry is used to identify vision-threatening retinopathy before visual acuity is affected. Microperimetry is a diagnostic tool used to assess retinal sensitivity while the fundus is directly examined; it enables exact topographic correlation between macular pathology and corresponding functional abnormality [109, 110]. It is rapid, safe, and non-invasive [110]. Microperimetry is of value in prognosticating the functional outcome as foveal thickness returns to normal following the treatment of DME [109]. Microperimetry has been used to demonstrate low retinal sensitivity present in the areas of capillary drop out in eyes with ischemic DME [111].

Multifocal electroretinogram is an electrophysiologic test. It is used to objectively identify functional changes of the retina in the early phases of DR and DME [112] and is also helpful for objectively monitoring eyes on intravitreal antiVEGF treatment such as Ranibizumab for DME [113].

4. Treatment of DME

4.1 Systemic control

The control of all systemic risk factors is vital in the treatment of DME. Optimizing control of diabetes, hypertension, and serum lipids should be emphasized. Optimization of care involves visits to the internist. The intervention aims to reduce glycated hemoglobin, elevated blood pressure, and elevated serum lipids to produce measurable effects in macular thickness in as little as six weeks [114].

The Diabetes Control and Complications Trial (DCCT) reported that tight blood glucose control in patients with type 1 diabetes reduced the cumulative incidence of macular edema at 9-year follow-up by 29% and reduced the application of focal laser treatment for DME by half [115, 116].

The United Kingdom Prospective Diabetes Study (UKPDS), a randomized clinical trial of patients with type 2 diabetes, reported that tighter blood glucose control reduced the requirement for laser treatment at ten years by 29%, compared with looser control; 78% of the laser treatments were for DME [50]. This study also demonstrated that a mean systolic blood pressure reduction of 10 mm Hg and a diastolic blood pressure reduction of 5 mm Hg over a median follow-up of 8.4 years led to a 35% reduction in retinal laser treatments 78% were for DME [51].

The Action to Control Cardiovascular Risk in Diabetes (ACCORD) eye study compared the progression of DR in a Simvastatin plus placebo group, Simvastatin plus fenofibrate group. The rate of progression of DR was lower in the fenofibrate group than in the placebo group [117].

High plasma cholesterol may be associated with more severe hard exudates at the macula [118, 119]. It has been reported that oral Atorvastatin reduced lipid migration to the subfoveal region and decreased the severity of hard exudates in type 2 DM patients with dyslipidemia who had CSME [120]. Nephropathy and anemia can contribute significantly to the risk of DR and DME. Weight loss and cessation of smoking are also crucial in preventing DR and DME.

4.2 Observation

The DRCR Network, Protocol V study, addressed the management of well-controlled DM with center involving DME (CI - DME) and good vision. Randomization of study participants was to observation, focal laser, and intravitreal Aflibercept [121]. The results suggest that patients with CI-DME and good vision (20/25 or better) can be managed initially with observation and close follow-up. These eyes should receive treatment if they suffer a decrease in vision.

For many years, focal and or grid macular laser photocoagulation (MLP) was the gold standard for DME treatment; newer laser techniques are now available. These minimize the side effects of a traditional laser. Intravitreal anti-Vascular endothelial growth factor (anti-VEGF) injections are now the mainstay of CI-DME. Although intravitreal anti-VEGFs have become popular, intravitreal steroids are often indicated in the treatment of DME. Vitrectomy is also used to treat DME. Combination therapy is another strategy employed for treating DME.

4.3 Intravitreal anti-vascular endothelial growth factors (anti VEGF).

Anti VEGFs inhibit upregulated VEGF, which has been implicated in the pathogenesis of DME. The efficacy of anti-VEGF injections in DME has been demonstrated by several studies [122–125]. Anti-VEGF therapy, however, requires frequent intravitreal injections that are difficult to transpose to clinical practice. Thus, fewer injections are administered in clinical practice than in clinical trials; this contributes to decreased efficacy as the results of clinical trials have been difficult to replicate in real life [126].

4.3.1 Pegaptanib

The first anti-VEGF drug used to treat DME was Pegaptanib (Macugen®, Bausch and Lomb, Rochester, NY, USA), which selectively blocks the 165-isoform of VEGF [127]. A phase II trial by the Macugen Diabetic Retinopathy Study Group reported that at 36 weeks, Pegaptanib led to better BCVA gain, a more significant reduction in central macular thickness (CMT), and less requirement for laser in DME when compared to sham [128]. However, it has been observed that Pegaptanib is less effective at improving visual outcomes than other anti-VEGF agents that target all VEGF-A isoforms [129].

4.3.2 Bevacizumab

Bevacizumab, a humanized monoclonal antibody that inhibits VEGF, was initially developed as a concomitant medication for use in combination with existing metastatic colorectal cancer regimens [130]. The FDA does not approve it for the treatment of DR or DME. However, the intravitreal Bevacizumab or laser therapy in the management of diabetic macular edema (BOLT) study examined the efficacy of Bevacizumab versus focal laser for DME and reported that Bevacizumab is superior to focal laser alone [131].

Patients in the Bevacizumab group showed significant BCVA improvement over patients in the laser group [131]. Bevacizumab costs much less than the FDA-approved intravitreal anti-VEGF drugs [132]. It is, therefore, more cost-effective in treating DME than Ranibizumab or Aflibercept [133, 134]. It is usually given as a 1.25 mg in 0.05 ml dose. The incidence of severe ocular and monocular adverse events was low for intravitreal Bevacizumab [135].

4.3.3 Ranibizumab

Ranibizumab (IVR, Lucentis®, Novartis, Basel, Switzerland) is a fully-humanized monoclonal antibody fragment that binds to VEGF-A's multiple variants [136]. The Ranibizumab for Diabetic Macular Edema (A Study of Ranibizumab Injection in Subjects With Clinically Significant Macular Edema With Center Involvement Secondary to Diabetes Mellitus (RIDE) and A Study of Ranibizumab Injection in Subjects With Clinically Significant Macular Edema With Center Involvement Secondary to Diabetes Mellitus (RISE) trials investigated the use of monthly Ranibizumab given in two doses—0.5 and 0.3 mg—for the treatment of DME [137]. The FDA approves it for the treatment of DME and DR at a dose of 0.3 mg monthly.

Port Delivery System (PDS) with Ranibizumab is a permanent refillable eye implant, approximately the size of a grain of rice, designed to deliver a customized formulation of Ranibizumab continuously over an extended duration, i.e., six months; potentially reducing the treatment burden associated with frequent eye injections [138].

The LADDER trial demonstrated that PDS with the 100 mg/mL formulation is non-inferior to monthly intravitreal injections of Ranibizumab in terms of visual and anatomical outcomes in neovascular age related macular degeneration (AMD) eyes [139]. In the ARCHWAY trial, 98.4% of PDS patients could go six months without needing additional treatment and achieved vision outcomes equivalent to in AMD patients receiving monthly Ranibizumab injections, a current standard of care [138]. Therefore, PDS could reduce the number of anti-VEGF treatments to two per year.

It is surgically implanted via a specialized tool through an incision in the sclera and pars plana. Reported adverse effects include conjunctival bleb, vitreous hemorrhage, conjunctival erosion, conjunctival retraction, endophthalmitis, rhegmatogenous retinal detachment, and hyphaema [138].

Two trials, PAGODA (will evaluate the efficacy, safety, and pharmacokinetics of the PDS With Ranibizumab in participants with DME compared with intravitreal Ranibizumab) and PAVILION (a multicenter, randomized study in participants with diabetic retinopathy without center-involved DME to evaluate the efficacy, safety, and pharmacokinetics of Ranibizumab delivered via the PDS relative to the comparator arm) are underway to study the safety and efficacy of PDS in subjects with DME and those with DR without CI-DME [140, 141].

4.3.4 Aflibercept

Aflibercept (IVA; VEGF-trap eye, Eylea, Regeneron Pharmaceuticals, NY, USA) is a recombinant chimeric fusion protein containing the second domain of VEGFR-1 and the third domain of the VEGFR-2 attached Fc portion of human IgG1 [142]. It has a dimeric structure, the molecular weight of the protein is 97kD, and the total molecule after glycosylation is 115kD [143]. Aflibercept acts as a decoy receptor binding VEGF-A, VEGF-B, and PlGF, thereby preventing their binding with their original receptors [144]. VEGF-A binds to both VEGFR-1 and VEGFR-2, but PlGF binds to only VEGFR-1. The FDA approves it for the treatment of DME and DR in patients with DME at a dose of 2 mg. It was studied in the Intravitreal Aflibercept for Diabetic Macular Edema (VISTA and VIVID) trials which compared Aflibercept with a focal laser to treat DME [145]. These studies demonstrated the superiority of Aflibercept over laser in terms of visual acuity improvement.

A comparative effectiveness randomized clinical trial compared Bevacizumab with Ranibizumab and Aflibercept for DME and found that all three agents are effective treatments at the two-year follow-up [146]. However, in eyes with visual acuity of 20/50 or worse, Aflibercept was superior to Ranibizumab and Bevacizumab at one year. In contrast, at two years, Aflibercept was no longer superior to Ranibizumab but remained superior to Bevacizumab [132, 147].

A concomitant effect of intravitreal anti-VEGF treatment for DME noticed with Ranibizumab and Aflibercept is improvement in retinopathy severity or slowing of the rate of progression of retinopathy [148]. Another concomitant effect is thinning of the choroid [149, 150].

4.3.5 Brolucizumab

Brolucizumab (IVBr, Beovu; Novartis; Basel, Switzerland), a single-chain antibody fragment, was approved for the treatment of nAMD in October 2019 and in February 2020 in the USA and the European Union [151]. The potential benefits of Brolucizumab are assumed to be related to its low molecular weight with subsequent better tissue penetration as well as higher molar concentration [152, 153]. Its use is mentioned here for completeness. It is no longer in "popular" use due to safety concerns. Brolucizumab was associated with reports of intraocular inflammation (IOI) and retinal vasculitis with or without occlusion [154, 155].

Positive 1-year results of the phase III KESTREL and KITE studies, evaluating the efficacy and safety of Beovu (Brolucizumab) 6 mg in DME were reported. Both studies met their primary endpoints of noninferiority in the change in BCVA from baseline for Beovu 6 mg versus Aflibercept 2 mg at year one [156]. However, the Beovu trials have been discontinued because Beovu was associated with higher rates of intraocular inflammation, including retinal vasculitis and retinal vascular occlusion versus Aflibercept [157].

4.3.6 Faricimab

Faricimab is a novel anti-Ang-2/anti-VEGF bispecific antibody designed explicitly for intraocular use [158, 159]. It is assembled using Roche's CrossMAb technology (Basel, Switzerland) and binds both VEGF-A and Ang-2 with high affinity and specificity [158, 160]. Faricimab is the first investigational bispecific antibody designed for the eye [161].

It targets two distinct pathways – via angiopoietin-2 (Ang-2) and vascular endothelial growth factor-A (VEGF-A) – that drive several retinal vascular diseases [161]. Ang-2 and VEGF-A contribute to vision loss by destabilizing blood vessels, causing new leaky blood vessels to form and increasing inflammation [162]. By simultaneously blocking both pathways involving Ang-2 and VEGF-A, Faricimab is designed to stabilize blood vessels, potentially improving vision outcomes for a longer duration in patients living with retinal conditions [162].

Faricimab is a promising molecule that is still undergoing investigation primarily for nAMD. The STAIRWAY Phase 2 Randomized Clinical Trial concluded that at week 52, Faricimab dosing every 16 weeks and every 12 weeks resulted in maintenance of initial vision and anatomic improvements comparable with monthly Ranibizumab [163]. TENAYA and LUCERNE phase 3 trials evaluate the efficacy, safety, and extended durability of up to 16 weekly dosing of intravitreal Faricimab in patients with nAMD [164]. YOSEMITE and RHINE are ongoing trials evaluating the efficacy, durability, and safety of Faricimab 8 weekly or a protocol-driven regimen based on treat-and-extend in DME patients [165]. Positive first-year results have been reported for Faricimab, which may emerge as an essential option if equivalent second-year results are reported with no safety flags.

4.4 Regimens

There is no consensus about the ideal treatment regimen with anti-VEGF agents [166]. Different treatment algorithms have been studied in clinical trials for AMD and applied in clinical practice, including monthly injections (ANCHOR, MARINA, CATT, HARBOR, EXCITE, IVAN, VIEW) as needed 'pro re nata' PRN (SUSTAIN, MONT BLANC, SAILOR, CABERNET, PrONTO, IVAN, CATT, HARBOR, OCTAVE), and 'treat and extend' regimen (TREND, LUCAS) [167].

Monthly maintenance dosing is a tremendous burden for both patients and the healthcare system. It has a real risk of overtreatment. The pro re nata (PRN) regimen is a treatment protocol where follow-up intervals remain fixed. At the same time, decisions to carry out an injection are based on the anatomic findings at each respective visit [168]. The PRN regiment has a risk of undertreatment or overtreatment, and patients may fail to attend. A treat-and-extend regimen (TER) is an individualized dosing scheme of titrating the injection interval based on the patient's response [169]. Therefore, if a patient shows no sign of active disease (e.g., the macula remains dry, without any leakage), intervals will be extended; if there is fluid accumulation, the next interval will be shortened. Fixed dosing lacks long-term practicability in real-world settings due to overtreatment and high costs; thus, PRNs or TERs have been suggested as feasible alternatives [169]. TERs have advantages: their cost-effectiveness due to less frequent visits and increased efficacy based on proactive treatments. However, TER involves more injections than a PRN regimen, leading to overtreatment [170].

4.5 Side effects of intravitreal injection of anti VEGFs

Endophthalmitis, intraocular inflammation (IOI), rhegmatogenous retinal detachment, intraocular pressure elevation, and ocular hemorrhage have been reported as complications of intravitreal anti-VEGF injections [171]. There are reports of ocular inflammatory events with Brolucizumab intravitreal injection [172, 173]. Recently, occlusive retinal vasculitis has been reported with the use of Brolucizumab. For this reason, the use of Brolucizumab has been discontinued. Furthermore, the experience with Brolucizumab has increased the surveillance by an ophthalmologist of drug-related IOI.

Intraocular silicone oil droplets and protein aggregates have also been reported with intravitreal anti-VEGF injections [174]. Several systemic adverse events of anti VEGFs have been reported in different studies, including systemic hypertension, cerebrovascular accidents, heart attacks, and death [175, 176].

About 40–60% of eyes that receive anti-VEGF injections show an insufficient response with recurrent and persistent macular edema, even after repeated injections [177, 178].

4.6 Intravitreal steroids

4.6.1 Corticosteroids

Corticosteroids inhibit leukostasis, adhesion, transmigration of leukocytes and downregulate the expression of prostaglandins, cytokines, and growth factors, especially VEGF [179]. They also alter the composition of the basal endothelial membrane by changing the local ratio of laminin isoforms, suppressing basement membrane dissolution, and strengthening tight junctions to limit permeability and leakage [180]. Long-term steroid use may have a neuroprotective effect on the retina [181].

Corticosteroids are now usually second-line therapy. Some of the indications for intravitreal steroids in DME include non-response to anti-VEGF, non-compliant patients, pregnancy, history of recent arterial thromboembolic events (ATEs), patients with hard exudates (HE) at the center of the fovea, pseudophakic patients (there is no risk of cataract) and vitrectomized eyes [182]. In vitrectomized eyes, corticosteroid intravitreal implants release drugs at a constant rate and provide predictable pharmacokinetics [183, 184].

In clinical trials that studied the use of intravitreal steroids in treating DME, pseudophakic eyes were shown to have better visual acuity (VA) outcomes than phakic eyes [185, 186]. The DRCRnet, protocol U concluded that pseudophakic patients with persistent DME showed better VA outcomes with combination treatment of Ranibizumab and Dexamethasone intravitreal (DEX) implant compared with Ranibizumab alone [187].

4.6.2 Dexamethasone sustained-release implants

Dexamethasone intravitreal (DEX) implant (0.7 mg) (Ozurdex, Allergan, Inc., Irvine, CA, USA) consists of micronized dexamethasone in a biodegradable copolymer of polylactic-co-glycolic acid, which slowly releases steroids into the vitreous for about 6 months [188, 189]. In 2014, based on the results of the MEAD study [190], the FDA and most European countries approved Ozurdex for the treatment of DME. DEX is a potent anti-inflammatory agent; its potency is twice that of Fluocinolone acetonide (FA) and 5-fold more than Triamcinolone Acetonide (TA) [191]. In contrast to TA, the pharmacokinetics of the DEX implant were not significantly different in vitrectomized and nonvitrectomized animal eyes [192]. There have been reports of the benefits of using DEX implant in naive DME as a first-line option [193, 194] and the advantages of early switching in patients not responding to anti-VEGF [195].

4.6.3 Fluocinolone acetonide (FA) implant

FA has a 25-fold higher anti-inflammatory potency than cortisol [196]. It has selective and potent agonist properties by binding to the cytosolic glucocorticoid receptor with high affinity; it is devoid of mineralocorticoid activity [197–199]. FA is available as an intravitreal implant. It is small (3.5 mm in length, 0.37 mm in diameter), non-biodegradable, and designed for injection using a 25-gauge injector via the pars plana into the vitreous cavity [200]. The approved implant (ILUVIEN®) contains 0.19 mg of FA initially released at 0.25 µg/day (average, 0.2 µg/day); it lasts 36 months [201]. The Fluocinolone Acetonide for Diabetic Macular Edema (FAME) studies evaluated the use of 2 different FA doses (0.2 vs. 0.5 µg/day) compared to sham injections [202, 203]. This study showed the efficacy of FA implants for chronic DME that is resistant to conventional treatment.

4.6.4 Triamcinolone Acetonide (TA)

TA has a 7.5-fold higher anti-inflammatory potency than cortisone [204]. It was the first widely used intravitreal injectable medication for DME [205]. Several clinical trials have shown the efficacy of TA in the treatment of DME [206–208]. TA Half-life in the vitreous of a nonvitrectomized eye has been reported as 18.6 days, in contrast to a much shorter duration in a vitrectomized eye, 3.2 days [209]. A single intravitreal injection of 4 mg of TA lasts approximately three months in the nonvitrectomized human eye [209, 210]. DRCR.net Protocol B investigated the efficacy and safety of 1 mg and 4 mg doses of TA compared with focal or grid laser photocoagulation and concluded that focal laser was superior to intravitreal triamcinolone [211, 212].

4.6.5 Adverse effects

Adverse effects of intravitreal steroids include ocular hypertension, cataract, infectious endophthalmitis, pseudo endophthalmitis, and sterile endophthalmitis [213]. A steroid-induced cataract is the most common adverse event of intravitreal corticosteroids [213]. Up to 50% of eyes injected with intravitreal corticosteroid will develop elevated intraocular pressure [214, 215]. Both the DEX and FA implants have been reported to migrate into the anterior chamber, potentially leading to corneal edema, corneal endothelial decompensation, and ocular hypertension [216, 217]. The DEX implant has been accidentally injected into the crystalline lens rather than into the vitreous cavity [218]. In terms of outcomes, Gillies et al. reported that the Dexamethasone implant (Ozurdex, Allergan) was as efficacious as Bevacizumab in reducing DME [219].

4.7 Macular laser photocoagulation for DME

4.7.1 Macular laser photocoagulation (MLP)

MLP was the first proven treatment for DME [220, 221]. Though its mechanism of action is not entirely understood, it improves DME through several proposed mechanisms. Photoreceptors and retinal pigment epithelium RPE cells are destroyed via a photothermal mechanism, thus reducing oxygen consumption. The reduced oxygen consumption in the outer retina is postulated to increase oxygen flux from the choroid to the inner retina, causing arteriolar constriction and decreased hydrostatic forces that drive edema [222].

Photocoagulation also induces changes to the RPE cells, causing their proliferation and releasing cytokines such as transforming growth factor-beta TGF-β, which antagonize the effects of VEGF [223].

The Early Treatment Diabetic Retinopathy Study (ETDRS) demonstrated a 50% reduction in moderate vision loss in patients with clinically significant diabetic macular edema (CSME) who underwent immediate focal laser photocoagulation [221]. MLP causes iatrogenic tissue damage, subretinal fibrosis, choroidal neovascularization, and laser scar enlargement [224, 225].

The DRCR.net re-examined this coagulation technique and reported it as a modified (m) ETDRS focal/grid photocoagulation protocol [226], but the risk of macular tissue damage remained.

The DRCR.net Protocol A reported that mETDRS laser is better than modified macular grid laser for DME while DRCR.net Protocol B noted that mETDRS focal laser is superior to intravitreal triamcinolone for DME [227]. DRCR.net Protocol K also reported that 20–60% of eyes that initially respond to focal laser might continue to improve after four months, suggesting durability of effect [228]. The macular laser had been considered the gold standard for many years [229]. According to the European Society of Retina Specialists (EURETINA) guidelines, focal/grid laser is now reserved mostly for non-center-involving DME [78].

4.7.2 Subthreshold micropulse diode (SDM) laser photocoagulation

SDM has been used in the treatment of DME [230–232]. Compared with conventional laser photocoagulation, SDM is a tissue-sparing technique: it avoids protein coagulation and prevents retinal scars, allowing retinal anatomic and functional preservation [233]. It has been hypothesized that SDM, by inducing a controlled thermal elevation of the retinal tissue, can selectively stimulate the retinal pigment epithelium (RPE) [234, 235]. Its advantages include the absence of RPE scarring, no subsequent choroidal neovascularization, and elimination of paracentral visual field scotomas [232, 236]. Its disadvantages include no visible endpoint for treatment, making it difficult to determine where treatment has and has not been applied. Furthermore, there is no standardized, consensus set of treatment parameters or guidelines for treatment within the foveal avascular zone. The reduction in macular edema after subthreshold laser photocoagulation occurs with a slower time course, and more treatments are necessary to eliminate edema [232]. Some randomized clinical trials have demonstrated that subthreshold grid laser treatment is as effective as conventional focal/grid laser photocoagulation, though slower in terms of resolution of DME, in achieving the same functional and anatomical effects [237, 238]. There have been reports of the benefits of combining SDM and intravitreal anti VEGFs in treating DME [239, 240].

4.7.3 Selective retinal therapy (SRT)

SRT is a laser procedure in which the RPE is selectively damaged without affecting the neural retina and choroid [241–243]. A microsecond pulsed laser is used to induce an instantaneous temperature rise just at the melanosomes within RPE cells, which leads to the formation of microbubbles around these melanosomes. Their temporary expansion results in a cell volume expansion and eventually mechanical cellular disruption without increasing temperature in the surrounding tissue. Studies have shown that SRT is effective in treating DME [243, 244].

4.7.4 Patterned scanned laser (PASCAL)

In PASCAL, the shorter pulse duration is used in an array of multiple burns to provide speed, better spatial localization, and reduced collateral damage by providing more precise control of the depth of the impact [245]. PASCAL is an ideal laser method to place the accurate "subthreshold" (subvisible) focal-grid laser in DME in contrast to conventional laser therapy [246, 247]. The advantages of PASCAL over conventional laser therapy include shorter treatment duration, increased safety, uniform, and precise spot placement, accurate "subthreshold" grid-pattern placement, and reduced pain and visual field defect [248]. However, the efficacy of PASCAL laser appears to be diminished compared to conventional laser therapy when the same number of laser spots were delivered [249].

4.7.5 Navigated laser (NAVILAS)

NAVILAS is a fundus imaging and laser treatment device developed by Neubauer et al. (OD-OS GmbH, Teltow, Germany) [250, 251]. The device utilizes retina navigation via computerized image capture and tracking assistance with high precision and reproducibility of <60–110 um [250]. It appears that the rate of retreatment for DME is reduced with NAVILAS when compared to the conventional mETDRS focal laser technique [251].

A 92% hit rate of microaneurysm via NAVILAS compared to 72% in conventional laser focal coagulation has been reported [252]. Focal laser therapy using NAVILAS will have more impact in the future to improve visual acuity and reduce the burden of anti-VEGF injection numbers in patients [253, 254].

4.8 Vitrectomy for DME

Optical coherence tomography has shown that vitreomacular adhesion is a risk factor for DME [255], as illustrated in **Figure 5**. Complete separation of posterior hyaloid with Posterior Vitreous Detachment (PVD) is associated with a decreased rate of DME [256]. Vitrectomy removes traction, improves macular oxygenation, removes VEGF and pro-inflammatory cytokines, and allows additional endolaser and steroids placement [257]. It was introduced for treating eyes with a taut posterior hyaloid adherent to the macula, often associated with shallow traction macular detachment, which had failed previous focal/grid laser [258, 259], as can be seen in **Figure 5**. It has also been used to treat eyes with an attached but non-thickened, non-taut posterior hyaloid or for eyes with persistent DME despite previous focal laser or intravitreal triamcinolone injection regardless of the status of the posterior hyaloid [260, 261], Illustrated in **Figures 12** and **13**.

Vitrectomy has been used as a potential primary therapy in eyes with more severe edema and greater visual acuity loss at presentation [262, 263]. Reports on the outcome of vitrectomy for DME are conflicting; some reports suggest that vitrectomy reduces macular thickening but does not improve visual acuity [264, 265]. Others have report improved visual acuities simultaneous with decreases in macular thickening or lagging behind the reduction in macular thickness by a

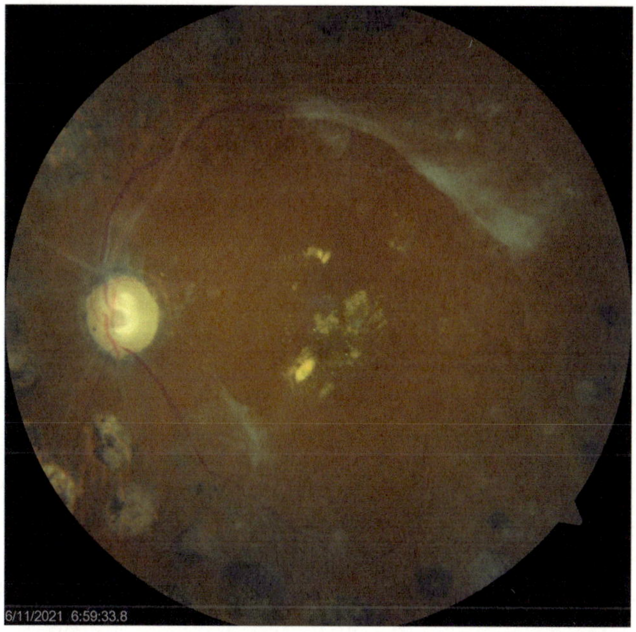

Figure 12.
This is a fundus photograph of the left eye in a patient who suffers a combination of DME and proliferative diabetic retinopathy (PDR). This eye has had vitrectomy with pan-retinal laser photocoagulation for the treatment of PDR. Notice residual fibrovascular proliferation within the superotemporal vascular arcade. Conspicuous hard exudates cluster in the foveomacula region, with few microaneurysms located inferio-nasal to the hard exudates. Retinal laser photocoagulation marks are present. There is also a pale cupped optic disc and sheathing of the retinal arteries and veins.

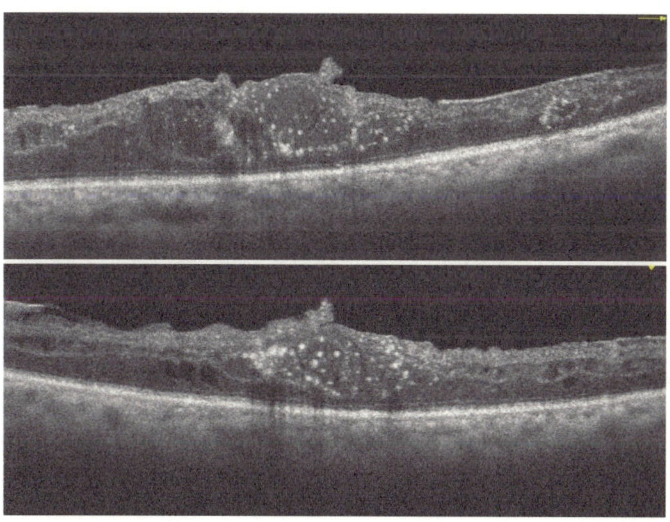

Figure 13.
*OCT of the fundus photography in **Figure 12**. This shows significant thickening of the fovea and loss of the normal foveal depression, disorganization of the intraretinal microstructure, aggregation of hard exudates, intraretinal cystoid spaces, and epiretinal membranes. This patient would have benefited from peeling of the internal limiting membrane during the vitrectomy. Post vitrectomized eyes with persistent DME can benefit from intravitreal steroid injections, e.g., Orzudex implant. Intravitreal steroids are beneficial in pseudophakic and aphakic eyes, in which the risk of cataract formation does not exist.*

few months [266, 267]. There have also been reports of improved visual acuity in cases with macular traction but no visual improvement in cases without traction [268, 269].

4.9 Plasma kallikrein inhibitors

Plasma kallikrein is highly upregulated in vitreous patients with DME [270]. It is a mediator of vascular leakage and inflammation. There is evidence that it is involved in DME pathogenesis in VEGF independent fashion and VEGF interdependent mechanisms [271]. Several small molecules and bicyclic peptides targeting the plasma kallikrein/kinin system are currently under investigation for DME treatment via intravitreal, oral, and topical administrations [271]. These include KVD001 (KalVista Pharmaceuticals) a highly potent and selective plasma kallikrein inhibitor, currently being developed as an intravitreal therapy), THR-149 (Oxurion NV), RZ402 (Rezolute Bio), and VE-3539 (Verseon Corp) [271]. Orally administered plasma kallikrein inhibitors are efficacious in reducing retinal edema and preserving retinal function in preclinical models. Plasma kallikrein inhibition is emerging as a promising new treatment modality for DME [271].

5. Clinical Studies in DME

The evidence for much of the guidelines on DME management has been gathered from clinical trials that have provided information on the safety and efficacy of different therapeutic options, investigated the systemic associations in patients diagnosed with DME, and considered newer and better therapies. This section will provide an overview of DME trials and emphasize the most important findings. Emphasis will be placed on those pharmacotherapies in current use (especially intravitreal injectable drugs).

As mentioned earlier, VEGF plays a central role in the pathogenesis of DME by increasing vascular permeability and blood flow in the setting of microvascular damage secondary to prolonged hyperglycemia. Therefore, intravitreal anti-VEGF has become the standard of care in the treatment of several forms of DME. In many cases, DME can be reversed, and this is associated with sustained improvements in vision. Several RCT have provided data and evidence for the use of intravitreal anti-VEGFs.

Ranibizumab (Lucentis, Genentech, South San Francisco, CA, USA) has been described earlier. It has a molecular weight of approximately 48 kilodaltons as it lacks an Fc region, unlike Bevacizumab. It is prepared in *Escherichia coli* with tetracycline in the nutrient medium. Due to its relatively small size, Ranibizumab penetrates the deeper layers of the retina, including the RPE and choroid.

Ranibizumab was the first anti-VEGF approved by the US Food and Drug Administration (FDA) for the treatment of DME and DR at a dose of 0.3 mg monthly. Also, the 0.5 mg dose has been used for treating DME. The 0.3 mg is as effective as the 0.5 mg. Also, the higher dose was found to confer no additional benefit compared to the 0.3 mg but was associated with more fatalities at three years (i.e., 6.4% compared to 4.4% with 0.3 mg monthly). Furthermore, at three years reported stroke rate was 4.8% and 2%; and adverse thromboembolic events (ATE) were 10.4% and 10.8% with monthly 0.5 mg and 0.3 mg Ranibizumab, respectively. Because of these systemic risks, the FDA approved the 0.3 mg dose of Ranibizumab instead of the 0.5 mg dose. However, a reduced dose is not available for other available anti-VEGF, i.e., Bevacizumab or Aflibercept. It is, however, essential to consider that the occurrence of these systemic adverse events is not uncommon after prolonged diabetes.

RISE and RIDE: These were two landmark trials. RISE was A Study of Ranibizumab Injection in Subjects With Clinically Significant Macular Edema With Center Involvement Secondary to Diabetes Mellitus. RIDE was A Study of Ranibizumab Injection in Subjects Clinically Significant Macular Edema With Center Involvement Secondary to Diabetes Mellitus [137]. These studies compared two doses of Ranibizumab with sham injections and confirmed the superiority of intravitreal Ranibizumab compared to sham injections. The study investigated using monthly Ranibizumab at two doses (0.5 and 0.3 mg) to treat DME. At month 24, the study results showed that 98% of patients-maintained vision with 0.3 mg monthly intravitreal injections, 34–45% of patients gained at least three lines (15 letters); and mean BCVA gain was 10.9 to 12.5 letters. Significantly higher numbers in the Ranibizumab arm gained >15 letters at month 24 compared to sham ie 44.8% vs. 18.1% in RISE; $P < 0.0001$, and 33.6% vs. 12.3%; $P < 0.0001$ in RIDE. Only 45–49% of patients needed macular laser compared with 91–94% in the control group. Also, there was no additional effect with the use of the higher strength 0.5 mg Ranibizumab when compared with the 0.3 mg dose.

In the RISE and RIDE extension phase, patients in the sham control group could cross over and receive monthly Ranibizumab injections in the 3rd year. The 36-month outcomes demonstrated that the rapid and sustained response of Ranibizumab in DME is further maintained for an additional 3rd year of continued monthly treatment. In addition, the group with delayed initiation of Ranibizumab therapy gained fewer letters compared to groups initially randomized to receive Ranibizumab (+4.7 vs. +10.6 letters in the 0.3 mg Ranibizumab arm). This finding suggests that chronic retinal edema (for an average of 4.5 years before Ranibizumab therapy) may result in irreversible loss of vision, and therefore prudent to initiate Ranibizumab therapy earlier. The RISE and RIDE study has become a vital landmark study against which other studies investigating more recent intravitreal pharmacotherapies have been compared.

RESOLVE: Safety and Efficacy of Ranibizumab in Diabetic Macular Edema With Center Involvement. This trial compared Ranibizumab versus sham in DME patients with BCVA of 20/40–20/160. It showed a better mean gain in letters with Ranibizumab than sham (10.3 letters gain versus a loss of 1.4 letters respectively). The patients were given three monthly injections, followed by PRN injections over a 12-month follow-up. A rescue laser could be performed if needed. CMT reduction was also more with Ranibizumab compared to sham. This study also suggested that Ranibizumab treatment was superior to laser (7.8 ETDRS letters gained versus −1.7 ETDRS letters lost).

READ-2: Ranibizumab for Edema of the mAcula in Diabetes-2). This study was A phase II, RCT to compare Ranibizumab alone (group 1), the focal laser alone (group 2), and combination of laser and Ranibizumab (group 3), i.e., randomized patients 1:1:1 to receive 0.5 mg Ranibizumab, laser, or both. Inclusion criteria were BCVA of 20/40–20/320 and CSMT of 250microns. The study demonstrated a BCVA gain of 7.4 letters in the RBZ arm at three months compared to 0.5 letters in the laser arm.

Change in mean BCVA in ETDRS letters at six months for the three groups was +7.24, −0.43, and + 3.8, respectively. However, at 24 months, it was demonstrated that Ranibizumab alone or in combination was superior to laser alone in DME.

READ-3 study (compared regular versus high dose RBZ) was a double-masked, multicenter RCT that evaluated two doses of RBZ (0.5 mg versus 2 mg). The study outcome showed that 2 mg RBZ (high dose) did not show any additional benefits over 0.5 mg dose at the primary endpoint at month 6 (+7.01 in the 2 mg group vs. +9.43 letters in the 0.5 mg group; $P = 0.161$).

RESTORE: A Twelve-Month Study to Assess the Efficacy and Safety of Ranibizumab (Intravitreal Injections) in Patients with Visual Impairment Due to Diabetic Macular Edema and a 24 month open-label extension study. It was a phase 3 RCT that was designed to compare RBZ with laser therapy. At 12 months, BCVA gain was highest in the RBZ monotherapy arm at the primary endpoint (+6.1 vs. +0.8 letters in the laser arm; $P < 0.001$).

REVEAL: A phase 3 RCT comparing Ranibizumab with laser. At the 12-month study endpoint, RBZ monotherapy was superior to laser since there was a gain of +5.9 letters in the Ranibizumab monotherapy arm vs. +1.4 letters in the laser arm;

P < 0.001. In addition, RESTORE and REVEAL studies showed that combining Ranibizumab with laser did not improve the BCVA.

LUCIDATE: Lucentis (Ranibizumab) in Diabetic Macular Oedema: Compared macular laser with Ranibizumab or combination in DME. This study further showed that in addition to improvements in BCVA and CMT, treatment of patients with center involving DME with monthly Ranibizumab was associated with an improvement in contrast threshold, retinal sensitivity on microperimetry amplitudes, and implicit times on electrophysiology.

With the use of several studies, the DRCR network answered questions relating to the effectiveness and timing of intravitreal pharmacotherapy use, combination therapy, and retinal laser photocoagulation to treat DR and DME. An example of such a study is Protocol T.

PROTOCOL-T of DRCR.net: Compared Ranibizumab, Bevacizumab and Aflibercept in DME. While the FDA had approved Ranibizumab and Aflibercept, the use of Bevacizumab was off-label. The study results revealed improvement in vision from baseline to one year with all three drugs. Improvement was most significant with Aflibercept (+13 letters) than Ranibizumab (+11 letters) or Bevacizumab (+10 letters), a statistically significant mean difference of 2–3 letters at one year. This difference appeared to be driven by baseline vision. Half of the

Name; Year of Study	Therapeutic Agents	Study Design	Study Outcome
READ -2 (2010)	RBZ / Laser	RCT	Demonstrated that Intraocular injections of Ranibizumab provided benefits for patients with DME for at least two years. When combined with focal or grid laser treatments, the amount of residual edema was reduced, as were the frequency of injections needed to control edema.
RIDE and RISE (2012)	RBZ/Sham	Two parallel Phase III RCT	Demonstrated that Ranibizumab rapidly and sustainably improved vision, reduced the risk of further vision loss, and improved macular edema in patients with DME. RISE: At 24 months, 18.1% of sham patients gained ≥15 letters versus 44.8% of 0.3-mg (P < 0.0001) RIDE: 12.3% of sham patients versus 33.6% of 0.3-mg patients (P < 0.0001).
RESTORE (2011)	RBZ/Laser	RCT	Demonstrated that Ranibizumab alone and combined with laser were superior to laser monotherapy in improving mean average change in BCVA letter score from baseline to month 1 through 12 (+6.1 and + 5.9 versus +0.8; both P < 0.0001).
RETAIN (2016)	RBZ (PRN/T&E)	RCT	Demonstrated the T&E is a feasible treatment option for patients with DME, potentially reducing the treatment burden. Slightly more injections were required versus PRN.
REVEAL (2015)	RBZ/Laser	RCT	Demonstrated that Ranibizumab monotherapy, combined with laser, showed superior BCVA improvements over laser treatment alone in Asian patients with visual impairment resulting from DME.
RESPOND (2015)	RBZ/Laser	RCT	Demonstrated that Ranibizumab as monotherapy or combined with laser resulted in significantly higher improvements in visual acuity and vision-related quality of life at month 12 than laser monotherapy.
RELATION (2018)	RBZ/Laser	RCT	Demonstrated that Ranibizumab plus laser is a valuable treatment option for the management of DME. It also showed that eyes with DME in PDR might also benefit from combined therapy compared to laser alone.

Name; Year of Study	Therapeutic Agents	Study Design	Study Outcome
DA VINCI (2011)	AFL/Laser	Phase II RCT	Demonstrated that significant gains in BCVA from baseline were achieved at week 24 and were maintained or improved at week 52 in all VEGF Trap-Eye groups.
VISTA & VIVID (2015)	AFL/Laser	Two similar Phase III RCT	Demonstrated that in both VISTA and VIVID, the 52-week visual and anatomic superiority of Aflibercept over laser control was sustained through week 100, with similar efficacy in the 2q4 and 2q8 groups.
PROTOCOL I (2011)	RBZ/Triamcinolone/ Laser	Phase III RCT	Demonstrated that anti-VEGF given by the protocol-specified prn treatment regimen was very effective for treatment of DME.
PROTOCOL T (2015)	AFL/RBZ/BEVA	RCT (Comparison of 3 Anti-VEGFs for treatment of DME)	Demonstrated that when vision was better than 20/50, the efficacy of all three intravitreal anti-VEGF medications for DME was similar. Bevacizumab thinned the retina less than Ranibizumab or Aflibercept, but the visual acuities were the same up to two years. However, when baseline vision was 20/50 or worse, Aflibercept had a superior benefit over the others with statistically significant better vision results at one year.
PROTOCOL V (2019)	AFL/Laser/ Observation	RCT	At two years, the rates of 5 or more letter vision loss were similar in all three groups (16–19%), and the mean vision in each treatment group was 20/20. Given the costs and potential adverse events associated with intravitreal injections and laser, observation is likely a reasonable initial strategy for treatment-naïve eyes with good vision despite center-involved DME as long as these eyes are followed closely and treated with anti-VEGF if vision worsens.
BOLT (2010)	BEVA/Laser	RCT	The study showed that BCVA at 12 months was 61.3+/−10.4 (range 34–79) in the Bevacizumab group and 50.0+/−16.6 (range 8–76) in the laser arm (P = 0.0006). Another finding was central macular thickness decrease from 507+/−145 microns (range 281–900 microns) at baseline to 378+/−134 microns (range 167–699 microns) (P < 0.001) in the Bevacizumab group, whereas it decreased to a lesser extent in the laser group, from 481+/−121 microns (range 279–844 microns) to 413+/−135 microns (range 170–708 microns) (P = 0.02).
BEVORDEX (2014)	BEVA/DEXA	Phase II RCT	Demonstrated that Dexamethasone implant achieves similar rates of visual acuity improvement compared with Bevacizumab for DME, with superior anatomic outcomes and fewer injections. Both treatments were associated with improvement in visual quality-of-life scores. However, more dexamethasone implant–treated eyes lost vision, mainly because of cataracts.
IBERA DME (2015)	BEVA/RBZ	RCT	This study concluded that intravitreal Bevacizumab and intravitreal Ranibizumab are associated with similar effects on central subfield thickness in patients with DME through 1 year of follow-up. Ranibizumab is associated with greater improvement in BCVA at some study visits, and the mean number of injections is higher in the Bevacizumab group.
LUCIDATE (2014)	RBZ/Laser	RCT (Single center)	Demonstrated that Ranibizumab therapy in the treatment of DME appears to improve retinal function and structure and this was demonstrated by this evaluation of different assessment methods including structural imaging and functional measures such as visual acuity, microperimetry, color contrast sensitivity, electroretinography (full field and multifocal).

Name; Year of Study	Therapeutic Agents	Study Design	Study Outcome
MEAD (2015)	DEXA/Sham	Phase III RCT	Demonstrated that DEX implant 0.7 mg and 0.35 mg met the primary efficacy endpoint for improvement in BCVA. Rates of cataract-related adverse events in phakic eyes were 67.9%, 64.1%, and 20.4% in the DEX implant 0.7 mg, DEX implant 0.35 mg, and sham groups, respectively. Only 2 patients (0.6%) in the DEX implant 0.7 mg group and 1 (0.3%) in the DEX implant 0.35 mg group required trabeculectomy.
FAME (2011)	FA/Sham	RCT	The study showed that both low- and high-dose Flucinolone Acetonide inserts significantly improved BCVA in patients with DME over 2 years, and the risk-to-benefit ratio was superior for the low-dose insert.
OZDRY (2015)	DEXA (Fixed/PRN)	RCT	Demonstrated the non-inferiority in terms of the mean change in BCVA of 5-monthly fixed dosing of Ozurdex compared to OCT-guided PRN Ozurdex therapy for refractory DME.
PLACID (2013)	DEXA/Laser	RCT	Demonstrated that though there was no difference between the groups at 12 months, significantly greater improvements in BCVA, occurred in patients with diffuse DME treated with DEX implant plus laser than in patients treated with laser alone.

AFL: Aflibercept, BEVA: Bevacizumab, DEXA: Dexamethasone, FA: Flucinolone Acetonide, RBZ: Ranibizumab, PRN: Pro re nata, T&E: Treat and Extend, RCT: Randomized Controlled Trial.

Table 1.
Summary of Anti-VEGF and Steroid for DME studies.

study participants had BCVA of 20/40 or 20/32. The mean letter score improvement in these patients was +8.3 with Ranibizumab, +8.0 with Aflibercept, and + 7.5 with Bevacizumab (each pairwise comparison $p > 0.5$).

However, when initial visual acuity was 20/50 or worse, the mean letter improvement was +18.9 with Aflibercept, +14.2 with Ranibizumab and + 11.8 with Bevacizumab (p values: Aflibercept-Bevacizumab <0.001, Aflibercept-Ranibizumab = 0.003, Ranibizumab-Bevacizumab = 0.21) (**Table 1**).

6. Variation between clinical trials and real-world outcome using intravitreal injection of pharmacotherapy

There has been a universal observation of divergence between the outcomes obtained from the use of intravitreal anti-VEGF in the real world and outcomes reported in randomized clinical trials. The visual outcomes and gains in vision observed have been much poorer. This finding has led to investigations into the reason for this difference. Some possible explanations for this observation include that participants are pre-selected using strict selection criteria and are well ahead motivated to complete the treatment schedule in clinical trials. This is not the case in real life, in which the patients have to grapple with significant challenges ranging from financial to demands on time and often have to deal with other comorbidities. These challenges could be of considerable impact on patients from low socio-economic backgrounds. It has also been shown that undertreatment is a common feature in real-world experience and that most patients do not receive the recommended number of intravitreal anti-VEGF. This real-life experience results in a mismatch between real-world visual outcomes and those of major clinical trials. The frequent clinic visits and treatment burden contributes to this discrepancy. To resolve this challenge, a host of pharmaceuticals with extended durability are at different stages of development. Hopefully, some extended durability options may make it to the bedside soon. Some of the extended durability options in the pipeline include intravitreal injections such as Faricimab, OPT-302, and KSI-301. There are implantable devices such as the Port delivery system (PDS) and Vorolanib. Gene therapy options include RGX-314, and ADVM-022. These therapeutics are currently being investigated for AMD, but could apply to DME if approved. It is expected that any therapy that will join the list of already available anti-VEGFs will be required to have the same or better safety data if compared with already available drugs.

7. Newer and emerging concepts in DME

The burden of DME and its impact on vision begs for more efficient care and better outcomes for treatment. This situation has fueled the drive for new concepts in understanding the disease process and alternative treatment.

Some of the new concepts in the understanding of DR and DME include in genetic studies, which aim to understand the variable risk diabetes poses to each person living with the disease. This risk may be affected by the individual's genetic make-up. Also, the role of epigenetics may be an essential factor in determining the response to treatment. Screening for DR and DME will take on a newer feel by introducing artificial intelligence algorithms and software, combined with the advantages of teleophthalmology. This will open up access to more persons who can benefit from screening, including persons in more remote places with limited health and eye care. Home OCT for monitoring of DME will provide information into the clinical evolution of DR and DME and answers to what happens to the eye when patients cannot attend the regular clinics. Home OCT will be an added benefit in reducing the burden of attendance to regular clinics to monitor anti-VEGF therapy. The desire for a reduction in clinic visits is a critical need.

The quest to explore alternative pathogenetic pathways outside the anti-VEGF pathway has resulted in the current progress investigating the Ang-Tie pathways and the Kallikrein pathways. In addition, pharmacotherapies are being developed based on these newer principles.

More innovation will be seen as the years unfold and will significantly benefit treatment outcomes, individualizing DME treatment, and patient satisfaction.

8. Conclusion

It is expected that the number of people living with diabetes will continue increasing, resulting in more patients diagnosed with DR and DME. There is a need to develop more efficient health systems providing holistic care for patients living with diabetes. These systems should provide for the visual needs and consider the psychological and other health needs. Medicare for such patients should ideally be with reduced treatment burden compared to the current situation and preferably fewer hospital visits.

If we succeed in creating these systems, it will positively affect the patients living with diabetes and the society. This will increase the productivity of our DR and DME patients, who then can live a happier and more fulfilling life.

Acknowledgements

Dr. Adekunle Hassan, who provided motivation and useful resources for the writing of this manuscript.

Conflict of interest

None of the authors have any relevant conflict of interest to declare.

Author details

Ogugua Ndubuisi Okonkwo[1*], Toyin Akanbi[2] and Chineze Thelma Agweye[3]

1 Eye Foundation Hospital and Eye Foundation Retina Institute, Lagos, Nigeria

2 Eye Foundation Hospital, Abuja, Nigeria

3 University of Calabar Teaching Hospital, Calabar, Nigeria

*Address all correspondence to: o_okonkwo@yahoo.com

References

[1] International Diabetes Federation. IDF Diabetes Atlas 9th Edition. 2019. Available at: www.diabetesatlas.org. Accessed: October 2020.

[2] Sarah Wild, Gojka Roglic, Anders Green, Richard Sicree, Hilary King. Global Prevalence of Diabetes. Estimates for the year 2000 and projections for 2030. Diabetes Care. 2004; 27: 1047-1053. DOI: 10.2337/diacare.27.5.1047

[3] Lightman S, Towler HM. Diabetic retinopathy. Clin Cornerstone. 2003;5:12-21. DOI: 10.1016/s1098-3597(03)90015-9. PMID: 12800477.

[4] Ling R, Ramsewak V, Taylor D, Jacob J. Longitudinal study of a cohort of people with diabetes screened by the Exeter Diabetic Retinopathy Screening Programme. Eye (Lond). 2002; 16: 140-5. DOI: 10.1038/sj.eye.6700081.

[5] Varma R, Bressler NM, Doan QV, et al. Prevalence of and risk factors for diabetic macular edema in the United States. JAMA Ophthalmol. 2014; 132(11):1334-1340. doi:10.1001/jamaophthalmol.2014.2854

[6] Ding J, Wong TY. Current epidemiology of diabetic retinopathy and diabetic macular edema. Curr Diab Rep. 2012; 12:346-54. DOI: 10.1007/s11892-012-0283-6. PMID: 22585044.

[7] Jew OM, Peyman M, Chen TC, Visvaraja S. Risk factors for clinically significant macular edema in a multi-ethnics population with type 2 diabetes. Int J Ophthalmol. 2012; 5:499-504. DOI: 10.3980/j.issn.2222-3959.2012.04.18.

[8] Klein R, Knudtson MD, Lee KE, Gangnon R, Klein BE. The Wisconsin Epidemiologic Study of Diabetic Retinopathy XXIII: the twenty-five-year incidence of macular edema in persons with type 1 diabetes. Ophthalmology. 2009; 116(3):497-503. doi:10.1016/j.ophtha.2008.10.016

[9] Do DV, Shah SM, Sung JU, Haller JA, Nguyen QD. Persistent diabetic macular edema is associated with elevated hemoglobin A1c. Am J Ophthalmol. 2005; 139:620-3. DOI: 10.1016/j.ajo.2004.10.063.

[10] Asensio-Sánchez VM, Gómez-Ramírez V, Morales-Gómez I, Rodríguez-Vaca I. Edema macular diabético clínicamente significativo: factores sistémicos de riesgo [Clinically significant diabetic macular edema: systemic risk factors]. Arch Soc Esp Oftalmol. 2008; 83:173-6.

[11] Nguyen-Khoa BA, Goehring EL, Werther W, et al. Hospitalized cardiovascular events in patients with diabetic macular edema. BMC Ophthalmol. 2012;12:11. DOI:10.1186/1471-2415-12-11

[12] Er Chen, Mark Looman, Marianne Laouri, Meghan Gallagher, Karen Van Nuys, Darius Lakdawalla & Joan Fortuny. Burden of illness of diabetic macular edema: literature review, Current Medical Research and Opinion. 2010; 26:7, 1587-1597, DOI: 10.1185/03007995.2010.482503

[13] Strain WD, Cos X, Hirst M, Vencio S, Mohan V, Vokó Z, Yabe D, Blüher M, Paldánius PM. Time to do more: addressing clinical inertia in the management of type 2 diabetes mellitus. Diabetes Res Clin Pract. 2014 Sep; 105(3):302-12. doi: 10.1016/j.diabres.2014.05.005.

[14] Yam JC, Kwok AK. Update on the treatment of diabetic retinopathy. Hong Kong Med J. 2007 Feb; 13(1):46-60.

[15] Moss SE, Klein R, Klein BE. Ten-year incidence of visual loss in a diabetic population. Ophthalmology. 1994 Jun; 101(6):1061-70. doi: 10.1016/s0161-6420(94)31217-6.

[16] WHO Europe: Diabetic Retinopathy screening: a short guide. https://www.

euro.who.int/en/publications/abstracts/diabetic-retinopathy-screening-a-short-guide-2020

[17] Liew G, Michaelides M, Bunce C. A comparison of the causes of blindness certifications in England and Wales in working age adults (16-64 years), 1999-2000 with 2009-2010. BMJ Open 2014; 4:e004015. doi: 10.1136/bmjopen-2013- 004015

[18] Jones S, Edwards RT. Diabetic retinopathy screening: a systematic review of the economic evidence. Diabet Med. 2010 Mar; 27(3):249-56. doi: 10.1111/j.1464-5491.2009.02870.x.

[19] Pearce E, Sivaprasad S. A Review of Advancements and Evidence Gaps in Diabetic Retinopathy Screening Models. Clin Ophthalmol. 2020; 14:3285-3296. Published 2020 Oct 14. doi:10.2147/OPTH.S267521

[20] Vujosevic S, Pucci P, Casciano M, Daniele A, Bini S, Berton M, Cavarzeran F, Avogaro A, Lapolla A, Midena E. A decade-long telemedicine screening program for diabetic retinopathy in the north-east of Italy. J Diabetes Complications. 2017 Aug;31(8):1348-1353. doi: 10.1016/j.jdiacomp.2017.04.010.

[21] Gunasekeran DV, Ting DSW, Tan GSW, Wong TY. Artificial intelligence for diabetic retinopathy screening, prediction and management. Curr Opin Ophthalmol. 2020 Sep; 31(5):357-365. doi: 10.1097/ICU.0000000000000693

[22] Bellemo V, Lim G, Rim TH, Tan GSW, Cheung CY, Sadda S, He MG, Tufail A, Lee ML, Hsu W, Ting DSW. Artificial Intelligence Screening for Diabetic Retinopathy: the Real-World Emerging Application. Curr Diab Rep. 2019 Jul 31; 19(9):72. doi: 10.1007/s11892-019-1189-3.

[23] Kwan CC, Fawzi AA. Imaging and Biomarkers in Diabetic Macular Edema and Diabetic Retinopathy. Curr Diab Rep. 2019 Aug 31; 19(10):95. doi: 10.1007/s11892-019-1226-2.

[24] Sim, D.A., Keane, P.A., Tufail, A. et al. Automated Retinal Image Analysis for Diabetic Retinopathy in Telemedicine. Curr Diab Rep 15, 14 (2015). https://doi.org/10.1007/s11892-015-0577-6

[25] Fuller SD, Hu J, Liu JC, Gibson E, Gregory M, Kuo J, Rajagopal R. Five-Year Cost-Effectiveness Modeling of Primary Care-Based, Nonmydriatic Automated Retinal Image Analysis Screening Among Low-Income Patients with Diabetes. J Diabetes Sci Technol. 2020 Oct 30:1932296820967011. doi: 10.1177/1932296820967011.

[26] Lois N, Cook JA, Wang A, Aldington S, Mistry H, Maredza M, McAuley D, Aslam T, Bailey C, Chong V, Ganchi F, Scanlon P, Sivaprasad S, Steel DH, Styles C, Azuara-Blanco A, Prior L, Waugh N; EMERALD Study Group. Evaluation of a New Model of Care for People with Complications of Diabetic Retinopathy: The EMERALD Study. Ophthalmology. 2021 Apr; 128(4):561-573. doi: 10.1016/j.ophtha.2020.10.030.

[27] Tiarnan D.L. Keenan, Michaella Goldstein, Dafna Goldenberg, Dinah Zur, Shiri Shulman, Anat Loewenstein. Prospective, Longitudinal Pilot Study: Daily Self-Imaging with Patient-Operated Home OCT in Neovascular Age-Related Macular Degeneration. Ophthalmology Science.2021, Volume 1, Issue 2. https://doi.org/10.1016/j.xops.2021.100034.

[28] Yu HJ, Kiernan DF, Eichenbaum D, Sheth VS, Wykoff CC. Home Monitoring of Age-Related Macular Degeneration: Utility of the ForeseeHome Device for Detection of Neovascularization. Ophthalmology. Retina. 2021 Apr;5(4):348-356. DOI: 10.1016/j.oret.2020.08.003.

[29] Tripathy K, Sharma YR, Karthikeya R, Chawla R, Gogia V, et al. Recent Advances in Management of Diabetic Macular Oedema. Current Diabetes Reviews, 2015, 11, 79-97.

[30] Romero-Aroca P. Targeting the pathophysiology of diabetic macula oedema. Diabetes care, 2010 33(11): 2484-2485.

[31] Trinh HM, Joseph M, Cholkar K, Pal D, Mitra AK. Novel strategies for the treatment of diabetic macular oedema. World J Pharmacol, 2016 March 9; 5(1): 1-14

[32] Musat O, Cernat C, Labib M, Gheorghe A, Toma O et al. Diabetic macular oedema. Romanian Journal of Ophthalmology, 2015, 59(3):133-136

[33] Powers M, Greven M, Kleinman R, Nguyen QD, Do D et al. Recent advances in the management and understanding of diabetic retinopathy. 2017, 6(2063), 1-9

[34] AbuEl-Asrar AM, Al-Mezaine HS, Ola MS. Pathophysiology and management of diabetic retinopathy. Expert Rev. Ophthalmol. 2009; 4(6): 627-647

[35] Zhang X, Zeng H, Bao S, Wang N,Gillies MC. Diabetic macular edema: new concepts in pathophysiology and treatment. Cell & Bioscience. 2014; 4(27): 1-14

[36] Maetzel A, Feener EP. Plasma Kallikrein Inhibition in Diabetic Macular Edema: Targeting a novel, VEGF-independent pathway of DME could preserve and recover vision. Retinal Physician. 2020; 17: 26-28

[37] Uriasa EA, Uriasa GA, Monickaraja F, McGuireb P, Das A. Novel therapeutic targets in diabetic macular edema: Beyond VEGF. Vision Research. 2017, 139: 221-227

[38] Akwii RG, Sajib MS, Zahra FT, Mikelis CM. Role of angiopoietin-2 in vascular physiology and pathophysiology. Cells. 2019; 8:1-19

[39] Hussain RM, Neiweem AE, Kansara V, Harris A, Ciulla TA. Tie-2/ Angiopoietin pathway modulation as a therapeutic strategy for retinal disease. Expert Opinion on Investigational Drugs. 2019:1-11

[40] Mathew C, Yunirakasiwi A, Sanjay S. Updates in the Management of Diabetic Macular oedema. Journal of Diabetes Research. 2015, 1-8

[41] Browning DJ, Stewart MW, Lee C. Diabetic macular oedema: Evidence-based management. Indian J Ophthalmol 2018; 66:1736-1750.

[42] Khan M, Aziz AA, Shafi NA, Abbas T, Khanani AM. Targeting Angiopoietin in Retinal Vascular Diseases: A Literature Review and Summary of Clinical Trials Involving Faricimab. Cells, 2020, 9 (1869): 1-14

[43] Hussain RM, Ciulla TA. Emerging vascular endothelial growth factor antagonists to treat neovascular age-related macular degeneration. Expert Opin Emerg Drugs. 2017 Sep;22(3):235-246.

[44] Elman MJ, Aiello LP, Beck RW, Bressler NM, Bressler SB et al. Randomized trial evaluating ranibizumab plus prompt or deferred laser or triamcinolone plus prompt laser for diabetic macular edema. Ophthalmology 2010, 117, 1064-1077.

[45] Elman MJ, Qin H, Aiello LP, Beck RW, Bressler NM et al. Intravitreal ranibizumab for diabetic macular edema with prompt versus deferred laser treatment: Three-year randomized trial results. Ophthalmology 2012, 119, 2312-2318

[46] Ng DS, Yip YW, Bakthavatsalam M et al. Elevated angiopoietin 2 in aqueous

of patients with neovascular age related macular degeneration correlates with disease severity at presentation. Sci Rep. 2017; 7:45081 (16)

[47] Fiedler U, Reiss Y, Scharpfenecker M et al. Angiopoietin-2 sensitizes endothelial cells to TNF-alpha and has a crucial role in the induction of inflammation. Nat Med. 2006; 12:235-239 (17)

[48] Keech A, Simes RJ, Barter P, Best J, Scott R, et al. Effects of long-term fenofibrate therapy on cardiovascular events in 9795 people with type 2 diabetes mellitus (the FIELD study): randomised controlled trial. Lancet 2005;366(9500):1849-1861.

[49] Matthews DR, Stratton IM, Aldington SJ, Holman RR, Kohner EM. Risks of progression of retinopathy and vision loss related to tight blood pressure control in type 2 diabetes mellitus: UKPDS 69. Arch Ophthalmol 2004; 122(11):1631-1640

[50] UK Prospective Diabetes Study (UKPDS) Group. Intensive blood-glucose control with sulphonylureas or insulin compared with conventional treatment and risk of complications in patients with type 2 diabetes (UKPDS 33). Lancet 1998; 352:837-853

[51] UK Prospective Diabetes Study Group. Tight blood pressure control and risk of macrovascular and microvascular complications in type 2 diabetes: UKPDS 38. BMJ 1998; 317(7160):703-713.

[52] Patel A, MacMahon S, Chalmers J, Neal B, Woodward M et al. Effects of a fixed combination of perindopril and indapamide on macrovascular and microvascular outcomes in patients with type 2 diabetes mellitus (the ADVANCE trial): a randomised controlled trial. Lancet 2007:829-840.

[53] Keenan HA, Costacou T, Sun JK, Doria A, Cavellerano J et al. Clinical factors associated with resistance to microvascular complications in diabetic patients of extreme disease duration: the 50-year medalist study. Diabetes Care 2007; 30(8):1995-1997.

[54] Wong TY, Liew G, Tapp RJ, Schmidt MI, Wang JJ et al. Relation between fasting glucose and retinopathy for diagnosis of diabetes: three population-based cross-sectional studies. Lancet 2008; 371(9614):736-743

[55] Liew G, Klein R, Wong TY. The Role of Genetics in Susceptibility to Diabetic Retinopathy. Int Ophthalmol Clin. 2009; 49(2): 35-52.

[56] Wong TY, Klein R, Islam FM, Cotch MF, Folsom AR, Klein BE, Sharrett AR, Shea S. Diabetic retinopathy in a multi-ethnic cohort in the United States. Am J Ophthalmol 2006; 141(3):446-455.

[57] Klein R, Sharrett AR, Klein BE, Moss SE, Folsom AR et al. The association of atherosclerosis, vascular risk factors, and retinopathy in adults with diabetes: the atherosclerosis risk in communities' study. Ophthalmology 2002; 109(7):1225-1234.

[58] Harris MI, Klein R, Cowie CC, Rowland M, Byrd Holt DD. Is the risk of diabetic retinopathy greater in non-Hispanic blacks and Mexican Americans than in non-Hispanic whites with type 2 diabetes? A U.S. population study. Diabetes Care 1998; 21(8):1230-1235.

[59] Bahrami B, Zhu M, Hong T, Chang A. Diabetic macular oedema: pathophysiology, management challenges and treatment resistance. Diabetologia (2016) 59:1594-1608

[60] Cabrera AP, Mankad RN, Marek L, Das R, Rangasamy S, et al. Genotypes and Phenotypes: A Search for Influential Genes in Diabetic Retinopathy. Int. J. Mol. Sci. 2020, 21(2712): 1-22

[61] Graham PS, Kaidonis G, Abhary S, Gillies MC, Daniell M et al.

Genome-wide association studies for diabetic macular edema and proliferative diabetic retinopathy. BMC Medical Genetics. 2018; 19(71): 1-8

[62] Omar AF, Silva PS, Sun JK. Genetics of diabetic retinopathy. Semin Ophthalmol 2013; 28:337-46

[63] Usman M. An Overview of Our Current Understanding of Diabetic Macular Ischemia (DMI). Cureus. 2018; 10(7):1-7

[64] Sim DA, Keane PA, Zarranz-Ventura J, et al. Predictive factors for the progression of diabetic macular ischemia. Am J Ophthalmol. 2013; 156:684-692.

[65] Garcia JM, Lima TT, Louzada RN, Rassi AT, Isaac DL, Avila M. Diabetic Macular Ischemia Diagnosis: Comparison between Optical Coherence Tomography Angiography and Fluorescein Angiography. Journal of Ophthalmology. 2016; 1-6

[66] Manousaridis K, Talks J. Macular ischaemia: a contraindication for anti-VEGF treatment in retinal vascular disease? British Journal of Ophthalmology. 2012; 96(2): 179-184.

[67] Hwang TS, Jia Y, Gao SS et al. Optical coherence tomography angiography features of diabetic retinopathy. Retina, 2015; 35 (11): 2371-2376

[68] Solomon SD, Goldberg MF. ETDRS Grading of Diabetic Retinopathy: Still the Gold Standard? Ophthalmic Res 2019; 62:190-195

[69] Jampol LM. Classifications of diabetic macular edema. European Journal of Ophthalmology 2020, Vol. 30(1) 6-7

[70] Wu L, Fernandez-Loaiza P, Sauma J, Hernandez-Bogantes E, Masis M. Classification of diabetic retinopathy and diabetic macular edema. World J Diabetes 2013, 4(6): 290-294.

[71] Early Treatment Diabetic Retinopathy Study Research Group. Grading diabetic retinopathy from stereoscopic color fundus photographs--an extension of the modified Airlie House classification. ETDRS report number 10 Ophthalmology 1991; 98: 786-806.

[72] Panozzo G, Parolini B, Gusson E, Mercanti A, Pinackatt S et al. Diabetic macular edema: an OCT-based classification. Seminars in Ophthalmology 2004, 19: 13-20

[73] Wilkinson CP, Ferris FL 3rd, Klein RE, Lee PP, Agardh CD et al. Proposed international clinical diabetic retinopathy and diabetic macular edema disease severity scales. Ophthalmology 2003; 110(9): 1677-1682

[74] Nicoară SD. Spectral Domain Optical Coherence Tomography in the Diagnosis and Monitoring of Diabetic Macular Edema. In. Intechopen. OCT-applications in ophthalmology [book on the internet].

[75] Chung Y, Kim KY, Ha SJ, Byeon H, Cho C, Kim JH, Lee K. Role of Inflammation in Classification of Diabetic Macular Edema by Optical Coherence Tomography. Journal of Diabetes Research. 2019: 1-8

[76] Alia OM, Saada MS, Hazema HAM, Dawood MN. Optical coherence tomography patterns of diabetic macular edema and their correlation with visual acuity. Journal of Current Medical Research and Practice 2020, 5:365-370

[77] Leng T, Tripathy K, Bhagat N, Lim JI. Diabetic Macular Edema. https://eyewiki.aao.org

[78] Schmidt-Erfurth U, Garcia-Arumi J, Bandello F, Berg K, Chakravarthy U, et al. Guidelines for the Management of Diabetic Macular Edema by the European Society of Retina Specialists (EURETINA). Ophthalmologica. 2017; 237:185-222.

[79] Aiello LP, Cahill MT, Wong JS: Systemic considerations in the management of diabetic retinopathy. Am J Ophthalmol. 2001; 132:760-776.

[80] Diabetes Control and Complications Trial Research Group: The effect of intensive treatment of diabetes on the development and progression of long-term complications in insulin-dependent diabetes mellitus. N Engl J Med. 1993; 329:977-986.

[81] Ciulla TA, Amador AG, Zinman B. Diabetic Retinopathy and Diabetic Macular Edema: Pathophysiology, screening, and novel therapies. Diabetes care. 2003; 2653-2664.

[82] Cole ED, Novais EA, Louzada RN, Waheed NK. Contemporary retinal imaging techniques in diabetic retinopathy: a review. Clinical and Experimental Ophthalmology 2016; 44: 289-299

[83] Cohen SR, Gardner TW. Diabetic Retinopathy and Diabetic Macular Edema. Dev Ophthalmol. 2016; 55: 137-146

[84] Fenner BJ, Wong RLM, Lam W, Tan GSW, Cheung GCM. Advances in Retinal Imaging and Applications in Diabetic Retinopathy Screening: A Review. Ophthalmol Ther. 2018 7:333-346

[85] Bresnick GH. Diabetic maculopathy. A critical review highlighting diffuse macular edema. Ophthalmology. 1983; 90:1301-1317

[86] Cheung N, Wang JJ, Klein R, Couper DJ, Sharrett AR, Wong TY. Diabetic retinopathy and the risk of coronary heart disease: the Atherosclerosis Risk in Communities Study. Diabetes Care 2007; 30: 1742-6.

[87] Kawasaki R, Cheung N, Islam FM, et al. Is diabetic retinopathy related to subclinical cardiovascular disease? Ophthalmology 2011; 118: 860-5.

[88] Alex D, Giridhar A, Gopalakrishnan M, Madan S, Indurkhya S, Haridas S, et al. Emerging retinal diseases and newer terminologies in spectral domain optical coherence tomography. Kerala JOphthalmol 2020; 32:234-43.

[89] Michl M, Fabianska M, Seeböck P, Sadeghipour A, Haj Najeeb B et al. Automated quantification of macular fluid in retinal diseases and their response to anti-VEGF therapy. Br J Ophthalmol. 2020: 317416.

[90] Lee H, Kang KE, Chung H, Kim HC. Prognostic Factors for Functional and Anatomic Outcomes in Patients with Diabetic Macular Edema Treated with Dexamethasone Implant. Korean J Ophthalmol. 2018; 32(2):116-125.

[91] Das R, Spence G, Hogg RE, Stevenson M, Chakravarthy U. Disorganization of Inner Retina and Outer Retinal Morphology in Diabetic Macular Edema. JAMA Ophthalmol. 2018; 136(2):202-208.

[92] Rasendran C, Conti TF, Hom GL, Babiuch AS, Conti FF, Singh RP. Current Understanding of the Pathophysiology of Disorganization of the Retinal Inner Layers and Relationship to Visual Acuity. Am J Ophthalmic Clin Trials 2019, 2(5) 1-10

[93] Sampani K, Abdulaal M, Peiris T, Lin MM, Pitoc C, et al. Comparison of SDOCT scan types for grading disorganization of retinal inner layers and other morphologic features of diabetic macular edema. Trans Vis Sci Tech. 2020; 9(8):45

[94] Sun JK, Lin MM, Lammer J, et al. Disorganization of the retinal inner layers as a predictor of visual acuity in eyes with center-involved diabetic macular edema. JAMA Ophthalmol. 2014; 132(11):1309-1316

[95] Sun JK, Radwan SH, Soliman AZ, et al. Neural retinal disorganization as a

robust marker of visual acuity in current and resolved diabetic macular edema. Diabetes 2015; 64(7):2560-2570

[96] Radwan SH, Soliman AZ, Tokarev J, Zhang L, van Kuijk FJ, Koozekanani DD. Association of disorganization of retinal inner layers with vision after resolution of center-involved diabetic macular edema. JAMA Ophthalmol. 2015; 133(7):820-825

[97] Salz DA, de Carlo TE, Adhi M, Moult E, Choi W, et al. Select features of diabetic retinopathy on swept-source optical coherence tomographic angiography compared with fluorescein angiography and normal eye. JAMA Ophthalmol. 2016; 134(6): 644-650.

[98] Suciu C, Suciu V, Nicoara S. Optical Coherence Tomography (Angiography) Biomarkers in the assessment and monitoring of diabetic macular edema. Journal of Diabetes Research. 2020; 20: 1-10

[99] Sousa CD, O'Keefe GD, Breda J, Tripathy K, Pinto LA, et al. Optical Coherence Tomography Angiography. https://eyewiki.aao.org.

[100] Greig EC, Duker JS, Waheed NK. A practical guide to optical coherence tomography angiography interpretation. Int J Retin Vitr. 2020; 6(55): 1-17.

[101] Moraes G, Faes L, Pal B. Optical Coherence Tomography Angiography: Principles and Application in Retinal Diseases. Delhi J Ophthalmol 2018; 29: 43-48

[102] Atta AHR, Mohamed AAM, Ali MA. Macular vessels density in diabetic retinopathy: quantitative assessment using optical coherence tomography angiography. International Ophthalmology. 2019; 39(8): 1845-1859

[103] Tang FY, Chan EO, Sun Z et al. Clinically relevant factors associated with quantitative optical coherence tomography angiography metrics in deep capillary plexus in patients with diabetes. Eye and Vision. 2020; 7 (1):1-7

[104] Sun Z, Tang F, Wong R, Lok J, Szeto SKH et al. OCT Angiography Metrics Predict Progression of Diabetic Retinopathy and Development of Diabetic Macular Edema. Ophthalmology 2019; 126:1675-1684

[105] Lee J, Moon BG, Cho AR, Yoon YH. Optical Coherence Tomography Angiography of DME and Its Association with Anti-VEGF Treatment Response. Ophthalmology. 2016; 123 (11):2368 – 2375

[106] Hsieh Y, Alam MN, Le D, Hsiao C, Yang C, Chao DL, Yao X. OCT Angiography Biomarkers for Predicting Visual Outcomes after Ranibizumab Treatment for Diabetic Macular Edema. Ophthalmol Retina. 2019; 3(10): 826-834.

[107] Russell JF, Shi Y, Hinkle JW, Scott NL, Fan KC, et al. Longitudinal Wide Field Swept Source OCT Angiography of Neovascularization in Proliferative Diabetic Retinopathy After Panretinal Photocoagulation. Ophthalmol Retina. 2019; 3(4): 350-361

[108] Bontzos G, Kabanarou SA, Garnavou-Xirou C, Kontou E, Triantafyllou D, Xirou T. Segmentation errors and motion artifacts in OCT-A associated with epiretinal membranes. Canadian Journal of Ophthalmology. 2020; 55 (4): 293 – 300

[109] Midena E, Vujosevic S. Microperimetry in diabetic retinopathy. Saudi Journal of Ophthalmology. 2011; 25:131-135.

[110] Laishram M, Srikanth K, Rajalakshmi AR, Nagarajan S, Ezhumalai G. Microperimetry – A New Tool for Assessing Retinal Sensitivity in Macular Diseases. Journal of Clinical and Diagnostic Research. 2017; 11(7): 8-11.

[111] Pereira F, Godoy BR, Maia M, Regatieri CV. Microperimetry and OCT

angiography evaluation of patients with ischemic diabetic macular edema treated with monthly intravitreal bevacizumab: a pilot study. Int J Retin Vitr. 2019; 5(24): 1-7

[112] Tehrani NM, Riazi-Esfahani H, Jafarzadehpur E, et al. Multifocal Electroretinogram in Diabetic Macular Edema; Correlation with Visual Acuity and Optical Coherence Tomography. J Ophthalmic Vis Res. 2015; 10(2):165-171.

[113] Baget-Bernaldiz M, Romero-Aroca P, Bautista-Perez A, Mercado J. Multifocal electroretinography changes at the 1-year follow up in a cohort of diabetic macular edema patients treated with ranibizumab. Doc Ophthalmol. (2017; 135:85-96.

[114] Singh R, Abhiramamurthy V, Gupta V, Gupta A, Bhansali A. Effect of multifactorial intervention on diabetic macular edema. Diabetes Care 2006; 29:463-4.

[115] Progression of retinopathy with intensive versus conventional treatment in the diabetes control and complications trial. Diabetes control and complications trial research group. Ophthalmology 1995; 102:647-61

[116] Early worsening of diabetic retinopathy in the diabetes control and complications trial. Arch Ophthalmol 1998; 116:874-86.

[117] Chew EY, Ambrosius WT, Davis MD, Danis RP, Gangaputra S, Greven CM, et al. Effects of medical therapies on retinopathy progression in type 2 diabetes. N Engl J Med 2010; 363:233-244.

[118] Klein BE, Moss SE, Klein R, Surawicz TS. The Wisconsin Epidemiologic Study of Diabetic Retinopathy. XIII. Relationship of serum cholesterol to retinopathy and hard exudate. Ophthalmology 1991; 98(8):1261-5.

[119] Chew EY, Klein ML, Ferris FL et al. Association of elevated serum lipid levels with retinal hard exudate in diabetic retinopathy. Early Treatment Diabetic Retinopathy Study (ETDRS) Report 22. Arch Ophthalmol 1996; 114(9):1079-84.

[120] Gupta A, Gupta V, Thapar S, Bhansali A. Lipid-lowering drug atorvastatin as an adjunct in the management of diabetic macular edema. Am J Ophthalmol 2004; 137(4):675-82.

[121] Baker CW, Glassman AR, Beaulieu WT, Antoszyk AN, Browning DJ, Chalam KV, et al. Effect of initial management with Aflibercept vs laser photocoagulation vs observation on vision loss among patients with diabetic macular edema involving the center of the macula and good visual acuity: a randomized clinical trial. JAMA. 2019; 321:1880-94.

[122] Nguyen, Q. D. et al. Ranibizumab for diabetic macular edema: results from 2 phase III randomized trials: RISE and RIDE. Ophthalmology 119, 789-801 (2012).

[123] The Diabetic Retinopathy Clinical Research Network. Aflibercept, bevacizumab, or ranibizumab for diabetic macular edema. N. Engl. J. Med. 372, 1193-1203 (2015).

[124] Wells, J. A. et al. Aflibercept, bevacizumab, or ranibizumab for diabetic macular edema: two-year results from a comparative effectiveness randomized clinical trial. Ophthalmology 123, 1351-1359 (2016).

[125] Heier, J. S. et al. Intravitreal aflibercept for diabetic macular edema: 148-week results from the VISTA and VIVID studies. Ophthalmology 123, 2376-2385 (2016).

[126] Brown DM, Nguyen QD, Marcus DM, Boyer DS, Patel S, Feiner L, et al. Long-term outcomes of ranibizumab therapy for diabetic macular edema: The 36-month results from two phase III trials: RISE and

RIDE. Ophthalmology. 2013; 120(10):2013-22

[127] Cunningham ET Jr., Adamis AP, Altaweel M, Aiello LP, Bressler NM, D'Amico DJ, et al. A phase II randomized double-masked trial of pegaptanib, an anti-vascular endothelial growth factor aptamer, for diabetic macular edema. Ophthalmology 2005; 112:1747-57.

[128] A Phase II Randomized Double-Masked Trial of Pegaptanib, an Anti–Vascular Endothelial Growth Factor Aptamer, for Diabetic Macular Edema. Ophthalmology 2005; 112(10):1747-57.

[129] Ahmadi MA, Lim JI (2008) Pharmacotherapy of age-related macular degeneration. Expert Opin Pharmacother 9:3045-3052

[130] J. C. Cilley, K. Barfi, A. B. Benson 3rd., and M. F. Mulcahy, "Bevacizumab in the treatment of colorectal cancer," Expert Opinion on Biological Therapy, vol. 7, no. 5, pp. 739-749, 2007.

[131] Rajendram R, Fraser-Bell S, Kaines A, Michaelides M, Hamilton RD, Esposti SD, Peto T, Egan C, Bunce C, Leslie RD, Hykin PG. A 2-year prospective randomized controlled trial of intravitreal bevacizumab or laser therapy (BOLT) in the management of diabetic macular edema: 24-month data: report 3. Arch Ophthalmol. 2012 Aug; 130(8):972-9. Doi: 10.1001/archophthalmol.2012.393. PMID: 22491395

[132] Diabetic Retinopathy Clinical Research Network, Wells JA, Glassman AR, Ayala AR, Jampol LM, Aiello LP, et al. Aflibercept, bevacizumab, or ranibizumab for diabetic macular edema. N Engl J Med 2015; 372:1193-203.

[133] Stein JD, Newman-Casey PA, Kim DD, Nwanyanwu KH, Johnson MW, Hutton DW, et al. Cost-effectiveness of various interventions for newly diagnosed diabetic macular edema. Ophthalmology 2013; 120:1835-42.

[134] Pershing S, Enns EA, Matesic B, Owens DK, Goldhaber-Fiebert JD. Cost-effectiveness of treatment of diabetic macular edema. Ann Intern Med 2014; 160:18-29.

[135] L. Wu, M. A. Mart'ınez-Castellanos, H. Quiroz-Mercado et al., "Pan American collaborative retina group (PACORES). Twelve-month safety of intravitreal injections of bevacizumab (avastin): results of the Pan-American collaborative retina study group (PACORES)," Graefe's Archive for Clinical and Experimental Ophthalmology, vol.246, no. 1, pp. 81-87, 2008.

[136] N. Ferrara, L. Damico, N. Shams, H. Lowman, and R. Kim, "Development of ranibizumab, an anti-vascular endothelial growth factor antigen binding fragment, as therapy for neovascular age-related macular degeneration," Retina, vol. 26, no. 8, pp. 859-870, 2006.

[137] Brown DM, Nguyen QD, Marcus DM, et al.: Long-term outcomes of ranibizumab therapy for diabetic macular edema: the 36-month results from two phase III trials: RISE and RIDE. Ophthalmology. 2013; 120(10): 2013-22.

[138] Campochiaro P, et al. Primary analysis results of the phase 3 Archway trial of the port delivery system with ranibizumab for patients with neovascular AMD. American Society of Retina Specialists Annual Meeting; 2020 July 24-26.

[139] Campochiaro PA, Marcus DM, Awh CC, et al. The port delivery system with Ranibizumab for neovascular age-related macular degeneration: results from the randomized Phase 2 ladder clinical trial.Ophthalmology. 2019; 126(8):1141-1154. doi:10.1016/j.ophtha.2019.03.03620.

[140] ClinicalTrials.gov. This study will evaluate the efficacy, safety, and

pharmacokinetics of the port delivery system with ranibizumab in participants with diabetic macular edema compared with intravitreal ranibizumab (PAGODA). clinicaltrials.gov/ct2/show/NCT04108156. Accessed June 9, 2021.

[141] ClinicalTrials.gov. A multicenter, randomized study in participants with diabetic retinopathy without center-involved diabetic macular edema to evaluate the efficacy, safety, and pharmacokinetics of ranibizumab delivered via the port delivery system relative to the comparator arm (PAVILION). clinicaltrials.gov/ct2/show/NCT04503551. Accessed June 9, 2021

[142] Holash J, Davis S, Papadopoulos N, et al. VEGF-Trap: a VEGF blocker with potent antitumor effects. Proc Natl Acad Sci USA 2002; 99(17):11393-8.

[143] Yog Raj Sharma, Koushik Tripathy, Pradeep Venkatesh and Varun Gogia. Aflibercept – How does it compare with other Anti–VEGF Drugs? Austin J Clin Ophthalmol 2014; 1(3):8.

[144] Chappelow AV, Kaiser PK. Neovascular age-related macular degeneration: potential therapies. Drugs 2008; 68(8):1029-36.

[145] Brown DM, Schmidt-Erfurth U, Do DV, et al.: Intravitreal Aflibercept for Diabetic Macular Edema: 100-Week Results From the VISTA and VIVID Studies. Ophthalmology. 2015; 122(10): 2044-52.

[146] Wells JA, Glassman AR, Ayala AR, et al.: Aflibercept, Bevacizumab, or Ranibizumab for Diabetic Macular Edema: Two-Year Results from a Comparative Effectiveness Randomized Clinical Trial. Ophthalmology. 2016; 123(6): 1351-9

[147] Wells JA, Glassman AR, Ayala AR, Jampol LM, Bressler NM, Bressler SB, et al. Aflibercept, bevacizumab, or ranibizumab for diabetic macular edema: Two-year results from a comparative effectiveness randomized clinical trial. Ophthalmology 2016; 123:1351-9.

[148] Brown DM, Schmidt-Erfurth U, Do DV, Holz FG, Boyer DS, Midena E, et al. Intravitreal aflibercept for diabetic macular edema: 100-week results from the VISTA and VIVID studies. Ophthalmology 2015; 122:2044-52.

[149] Kim JT, Lee DH, Joe SG, Kim JG, Yoon YH. Changes in choroidal thickness in relation to the severity of retinopathy and macular edema in type 2 diabetic patients. Invest Ophthalmol Vis Sci 2013; 54:3378-84.

[150] Lee SH, Kim J, Chung H, Kim HC. Changes of choroidal thickness after treatment for diabetic retinopathy. Curr Eye Res 2014; 39:736-44.

[151] Dugel PU, Singh RP, Koh A, et al. Hawk and harrier: Ninety-Six-Week outcomes from the phase 3 trials of Brolucizumab for neovascular age-related macular degeneration. Ophthalmology 2021; vasculitis, and retinal Occlusion-Related events with Brolucizumab: post hoc review of hawk and harrier. Ophthalmology 2020. doi:doi:10.1016/j.ophtha.2020.11.011.

[152] Dugel PU, Jaffe GJ, Sallstig P, et al. Brolucizumab versus aflibercept in participants with neovascular age-related macular degeneration: a randomized trial. Ophthalmology 2017;124:1296-304.doi:10.1016/j.ophtha.2017.03.057pmid:http://www.ncbi.nlm.nih.gov/pubmed/28551167

[153] Holz FG, Dugel PU, Weissgerber G, et al. Single-Chain antibody fragment VEGF inhibitor RTH258 for neovascular age-related macular degeneration: a randomized controlled study. Ophthalmology2016;123:10809. doi:10.1016/j.ophtha.2015.12.030pmid:http://www.ncbi.nlm.nih.gov/pubmed/26906165

[154] Baumal CR, Spaide RF, Vajzovic L, et al. Retinal vasculitis and intraocular inflammation after intravitreal injection of Brolucizumab. Ophthalmology 2020;127:1345-59.doi:10.1016/j.ophtha.2020.04.017pmid:http://www.ncbi.nlm.nih.gov/pubmed/32344075

[155] Holz FG, Heinz C, Wolf A. Intraocular inflammation with brolucizumab use: patient management, diagnosis, therapy. Ophthalmologe 2021;118:1-3.doi:10.1007/s00347-021-01321-8pmid:http://www.ncbi.nlm.nih.gov/pubmed/33007521

[156] Brown D, Wolf S, Garweg JG, et al. Brolucizumab for the treatment of visual impairment due to diabetic macular edema: 52-week results from the KESTREL & KITE studies. Presented at: The Association for Research in Vision and Ophthalmology (ARVO) 2021 Annual Meeting. May 2021.

[157] Novartis reports one year results of Phase III MERLIN study evaluating Beovu® every four week dosing and provides update on Beovu clinical program .https://www.novartis.com.

[158] Regula J.T. Lundh von Leithner P. Foxton R. et al. Targeting key angiogenic pathways with a bispecific CrossMAb optimized for neovascular eye diseases. EMBO Mol Med. 2016; 8: 1265-1288

[159] Foxton R.H. Uhles S. Gruener S. et al Evaluation of the effects of VEGF/ANG-2 neutralization on vascular, neuronal and inflammatory pathologics in a spontaneous choroidal neovascularization (CNV) mouse model.

[160] Schaefer W. Regula J.T. Bähner M. et al Immunoglobulin domain crossover as a generic approach for the production of bispecific IgG antibodies. Proc Nat Acad Sci U S A. 2011; 108: 11187-11192

[161] .Khan M, et al. Targeting Angiopoietin in retinal vascular diseases: A literature review and summary of clinical trials involving faricimab. Cells. 2020; 9:1869.

[162] Heier JS, et al. The Angiopoietin/Tie pathway in retinal vascular diseases: a review. Retina-J Ret Vit Dis. 2021; 41:1-19.

[163] Khanani AM, Patel SS, Ferrone PJ, et al. Efficacy of Every Four Monthly and Quarterly Dosing of Faricimab vs Ranibizumab in Neovascular Age-Related Macular Degeneration: The STAIRWAY Phase 2 Randomized Clinical Trial. JAMA Ophthalmol. 2020; 138(9):964-972. doi:10.1001/jamaophthalmol.2020.2699

[164] Arshad M. Khanani, Jeffrey Heier, Carlos Quezada Ruiz, Hugh Lin, David Silverman, Christopher Brittain, Jane Ives, Balakumar Swaminathan, Karen Basu, Tien Y Wong; Faricimab in Neovascular Age-Related Macular Degeneration: 1-Year Efficacy, Safety, and Durability in the Phase 3 TENAYA and LUCERNE Trials. Invest. Ophthalmol. Vis. Sci. 2021; 62(8):428.

[165] John A Wells, Charles Clifton Wykoff, Jeffrey R Willis, Zdenka Haskova, Hugh Lin, David Silverman, Anthony P Adamis, Jane Ives, Francis Abreu, Karen Basu, Ramin Tadayoni; Efficacy, durability, and safety of faricimab in diabetic macular edema (DME): one-year results from the phase 3 YOSEMITE and RHINE trials. Invest. Ophthalmol. Vis. Sci. 2021; 62(8):1037.

[166] Lalwani GA, Rosenfeld PJ, Fung AE, Dubovy SR, Michels S, Feuer W, Davis JL, Flynn HW Jr, Esquiabro M (2009) A variable-dosing regimen with intravitreal ranibizumab for neovascular age-related macular degeneration: year 2 of the PrONTO Study. Am J Ophthalmol 148(1):43-58 e41

[167] Flaxel CJ, Adelman RA, Bailey ST et al. Age-related macular degeneration preferred practice Pattern R. Ophthalmology 127(1), P1–p65 (2020).

[168] Maguire MG, Martin DF, Ying G-S, Jaffe GJ, Daniel E, Grunewald JE,

Toth CA, Ferris FL III, Fine SL, Group CoA-rMDTTR (2016) Five-year outcomes with anti–vascular endothelial growth factor treatment of neovascular age-related macular degeneration: the comparison of age-related macular degeneration treatments trials. Ophthalmology 123(8):1751-1761

[169] Spaide, R. Ranibizumab according to need: a treatment for age-related macular degeneration. Am. J. Ophthalmol. 143, 679-680 (2007).

[170] Kim, Y.C., Shin, J.P., Pak, K.Y. et al. Two-year outcomes of the treat-and-extend regimen using aflibercept for treating diabetic macular oedema. Sci Rep 10, 22030 (2020). https://doi.org/10.1038/s41598-020-78954-3

[171] Ghasemi Falavarjani, K., Nguyen, Q. Adverse events and complications associated with intravitreal injection of anti-VEGF agents: a review of literature. Eye 27, 787-794 (2013). https://doi.org/10.1038/eye.2013.107

[172] Witkin A, Hahn P, Murray T, et al. Occlusive Retinal Vasculitis Following Intravitreal Brolucizumab. Journal of VitreoRetinal Diseases 2020: 247412642093086. doi.org/10.1177/2474126420930863

[173] Kondapalli SSA. Retinal Vasculitis after Administration of Brolucizumab Resulting in Severe Loss of Visual Acuity. JAMA Ophthalmol 2020.doi: 400 10.1001/jamaophthalmol.2020.2810

[174] Schargus M, Frings A. Issues with Intravitreal Administration of Anti-VEGF Drugs. Clin Ophthalmol. 2020; 14:897-904 https://doi.org/10.2147/OPTH.S207978

[175] M. I. van der Reis, E. C. La Heij, Y. De Jong-Hesse, P. J. Ringens, F. Hendrikse, and J. S. A. G. Schouten, "A systematic review of the adverse events of intravitreal antivascular endothelial growth factor injections,"Retina,vol.31, no. 8, pp. 1449-1469, 2011.

[176] R. Nuzzi and F. Tridico, "Local and systemic complications after intravitreal administration of anti-vascular endothelial growth factor agents in the treatment of different ocular diseases: a five-year retrospective study," Seminars in Ophthalmology, vol. 30, no. 2, pp. 129-135, 2015

[177] .Das A, McGuire PG, Rangasamy S. Diabetic Macular Edema: Pathophysiology and Novel Therapeutic Targets. Ophthalmology [Internet]. 2015; 122(7):1375-94. Available from: 10.1016/ j.ophtha.2015.03.024

[178] Brown DM, Nguyen QD, Marcus DM, Boyer DS, Patel S, Feiner L, et al. Long-term outcomes of ranibizumab therapy for diabetic macular edema: The 36-month results from two phase III trials: RISE and RIDE. Ophthalmology [Internet]. 2013; 120(10):2013-22. Available from: 10.1016/ j.ophtha.2013.02.034.

[179] Antonetti DA, Wolpert EB, DeMaio L, et al: Hydrocortisone decreases retinal endothelial cell water and solute flux coincident with increased content and decreased phosphorylation of occludin. J Neurochem 2002; 80: 667-677.

[180] Silva PS, Sun JK, Aiello LP: Role of steroids in the management of diabetic macular edema and proliferative diabetic retinopathy. Semin Ophthalmol 2009;

[181] Bhisitkul RB, Winn BJ, Lee OT, et al: Neuroprotective effect of intravitreal triamcinolone acetonide against photoreceptor apoptosis in a rabbit model of subretinal haemorrhage. Invest Ophthalmol Vis Sci 2008; 49: 4071-4077.

[182] Dinah Zur, Matias Iglicki, Anat Loewenstein. The Role of Steroids in the Management of Diabetic Macular Edema. Ophthalmic Res 2019; 62: 231-236 DOI: 10.1159/000499540

[183] Pessoa B, Coelho J, Correia N, Ferreira N, Beirão M, Meireles A, et al. Fluocinolone acetonide intravitreal implant 190 μg (ILUVIEN®) in vitrectomized versus nonvitrectomized eyes for the treatment of chronic diabetic macular edema. Ophthalmic Res 2018; 59:68-75.

[184] Boyer DS, Faber D, Gupta S, Patel SS, Tabandeh H, Li XY, et al. Dexamethasone intravitreal implant for treatment of diabetic macular edema in vitrectomized patients. Retina 2011; 31:915-23

[185] Diabetic Retinopathy Clinical Research Network. A randomized trial comparing intravitreal triamcinolone acetonide and focal/grid photocoagulation for diabetic macular edema. Ophthalmology. 2008; 115:1447-9.

[186] Elman MJ, Bressler NM, Qin H, Beck RW, Ferris FL 3rd, Friedman SM, et al.; Diabetic Retinopathy Clinical Research Network. Expanded 2-year follow-up of ranibizumab plus prompt or deferred laser or triamcinolone plus prompt laser for diabetic macular edema. Ophthalmology. 2011 Apr; 118(4): 609-14

[187] Maturi RK, Glassman AR, Liu D, Beck RW, Bhavsar AR, Bressler NM, et al. Effect of adding dexamethasone to continued ranibizumab treatment in patients with persistent diabetic macular edema: a DRCR network phase 2 randomized clinical trial. JAMA Ophthalmol. 2018; 136:29-38.

[188] N. Haghjou, M. Soheilian, and M. J. Abdekhodaie, "Sustained release intraocular drug delivery devices for treatment of uveitis," Journal of Ophthalmic & Vision Research, vol. 6, no. 4, pp. 317-329, 2011.

[189] J.-E. Chang-Lin, M. Attar, A. A. Acheampong et al., "Pharmacokinetics and pharmacodynamics of a sustained release dexamethasone intravitreal implant," Investigative Ophthalmology & Visual Science, vol. 52, no. 1, pp. 80-86, 2011.

[190] D. S. Boyer, Y. H. Yoon, R. Belfort Jr. et al., "Three-year, randomized, sham-controlled trial of dexamethasone intravitreal implant in patients with diabetic macular edema," Ophthalmology, vol. 121, no. 10, pp. 1904-1914, 2014

[191] Whitcup SM, Cidlowski JA, Csaky KG, Ambati J. Pharmacology of corticosteroids for diabetic macular edema. Invest Ophthalmol Vis Sci. 2018 Jan; 59(1): 1-12.

[192] Chang-Lin JE, Burke JA, Peng Q, Lin T, Orilla WC, Ghosn CR, et al. Pharmacokinetics of a sustained-release dexamethasone intravitreal implant in vitrectomized and nonvitrectomized eyes. Invest Ophthalmol Vis Sci. 2011 Jun; 52(7): 4605-9

[193] Iglicki M, Busch C, Zur D, Okada M, Mariussi M, Chhablani JK, et al. Dexamethasone implant for diabetic macular edema in naive compared with refractory eyes: The International Retina Group Real-Life 24-Month Multicenter Study. The IRGREL-DEX Study. Retina. 2019 Jan; 39(1): 44-51

[194] Malclès A, Dot C, Voirin N, Agard É, Vié AL, Bellocq D, et al. Real-life study in diabetic macular edema treated with dexamethasone implant: The Reldex Study. Retina. 2017 Apr; 37(4): 753-60.

[195] Busch C, Zur D, Fraser-Bell S, Laíns I, Santos AR, Lupidi M, et al.; International Retina Group. Shall we stay, or shall we switch? Continued anti-VEGF therapy versus early switch to dexamethasone implant in refractory diabetic macular edema. Acta Diabetol. 2018 Aug; 55(8): 789-96.

[196] Cantrill HL, Waltman SR, Palmberg PF, Zink HA, Becker B. In vitro determination of relative corticosteroid potency. J Clin Endocrinol Metab. 1975 Jun; 40(6): 1073-7. doi: 10.1210/jcem-40-6-1073.

[197] Veritti D, Sarao V, Diplotti L, Samassa F, Lanzetta P. Fluocinolone

acetonide for the treatment of diabetic macular edema. Expert Opin Pharmacother. 2017 10; 18(14):1507-16.

[198] Syed YY. Fluocinolone Acetonide Intravitreal Implant 0.19 mg (ILUVIEN®): A Review in Diabetic Macular Edema. Drugs. 2017; 77(5):575-83.

[199] Haritoglou C, Mayer W, Wolf A. Fluocinolone acetonide for the treatment of diabetic macular edema. Expert Rev Clin Pharmacol [Internet]. 2016;9(3):367-74. Available from: 10.1080/14656566.2017.1363182

[200] Schmit-Eilenberger VK, Augustin AJ. Early experience with Iluvien for the treatment of chronic DME. Retina Today 2013: 34-37. http://retinatoday.com/2013/08/early-experience-with-iluvien-for-the-treatment-of-chronic-dme/

[201] Alimera Sciences Inc. Iluvien (fluocinolone acetonide intravitreal implant) 0.19 mg for intravitreal injection: US prescribing information. 2014.

[202] Campochiaro PA, Brown DM, Pearson A, Ciulla T, Boyer D, Holz FG, et al.; FAME Study Group. Long-term benefit of sustained-delivery fluocinolone acetonide vitreous inserts for diabetic macular edema. Ophthalmology. 2011 Apr; 118(4): 626-635.e2.

[203] Campochiaro PA, Brown DM, Pearson A, Chen S, Boyer D, Ruiz-Moreno J, et al.; FAME Study Group. Sustained delivery fluocinolone acetonide vitreous inserts provide benefit for at least 3 years in patients with diabetic macular edema. Ophthalmology. 2012 Oct; 119(10): 2125-32.

[204] Mansoor S, Kuppermann BD, Kenney MC. Intraocular sustained-release delivery systems for triamcinolone acetonide. Pharm Res 2009; 26:770-84.

[205] Jonas JB, Söfker A. Intraocular injection of crystalline cortisone as adjunctive treatment of diabetic macular edema. Am J Ophthalmol 2001; 132:425-7.

[206] Martidis A, Duker JS, Greenberg PB, Rogers AH, Puliafito CA, Reichel E, et al. Intravitreal triamcinolone for refractory diabetic macular edema. Ophthalmology. 2002 May; 109(5): 920-7.

[207] Massin P, Audren F, Haouchine B, Erginay A, Bergmann JF, Benosman R, et al. Intravitreal triamcinolone acetonide for diabetic diffuse macular edema: preliminary results of a prospective controlled trial. Ophthalmology. 2004 Feb; 111(2): 218-24.

[208] Audren F, Lecleire-Collet A, Erginay A, Haouchine B, Benosman R, Bergmann JF, et al. Intravitreal triamcinolone acetonide for diffuse diabetic macular edema: phase 2 trial comparing 4 mg vs 2 mg. Am J Ophthalmol. 2006 Nov; 142(5): 794-9.

[209] Beer PM, Bakri SJ, Singh RJ, Liu W, Peters GB 3rd, Miller M, et al. Intraocular concentration and pharmacokinetics of triamcinolone acetonide after a single intravitreal injection. Ophthalmology 2003; 110:681-6.

[210] Mason JO 3rd, Somaiya MD, Singh RJ. Intravitreal concentration and clearance of triamcinolone acetonide in nonvitrectomized human eyes. Retina 2004; 24:900-4.

[211] Elman MJ, Aiello LP, Beck RW, et al; Diabetic Retinopathy Clinical Research Network: Randomized trial evaluating ranibizumab plus prompt or deferred laser or triamcinolone plus prompt laser for diabetic macular edema. Ophthalmology 2010; 117: 1064-1077.e35

[212] Elman MJ, Bressler NM, Qin H, Beck RW, Ferris FL 3rd, Friedman SM, et al.; Diabetic Retinopathy Clinical Research Network. Expanded 2-year

follow-up of ranibizumab plus prompt or deferred laser or triamcinolone plus prompt laser for diabetic macular edema. Ophthalmology. 2011 Apr; 118(4): 609-14

[213] Chawan-Saad J, Wu M, Wu A, Wu L. Corticosteroids for diabetic macular edema. Taiwan J Ophthalmol 2019; 9:233-42. DOI: 10.4103/tjo.tjo_68_19

[214] Jones R 3rd, Rhee DJ. Corticosteroid-induced ocular hypertension and glaucoma: A brief review and update of the literature. Curr Opin Ophthalmol 2006; 17:163-7.

[215] Razeghinejad MR, Katz LJ. Steroid-induced iatrogenic glaucoma. Ophthalmic Res 2012; 47:66-80.

[216] Papastavrou VT, Zambarakji H, Dooley I, Eleftheriadis H, Jackson TL. Observation: Fluocinolone acetonide (Iluvien) implant migration into the anterior chamber. Retin Cases Brief Rep 2017; 11:44-6.

[217] Gonçalves MB, Alves BQ, Moura R, Magalhães O Jr., Maia A, Belfort R Jr., et al. Intravitreal dexamethasone implant migration into the anterior chamber: A multicenter study from the Pan-American Collaborative Retina Study Group. Retina 2019. doi: 10.1097/IAE.0000000000002475.

[218] Chalioulias K, Muqit MM. Vitreoretinal surgery for inadvertent intralenticular Ozurdex implant. Eye (Lond) 2014; 28:1523-4.

[219] Gillies MC, Lim LL, Campain A, Quin GJ, Salem W, Li J et al. A randomized clinical trial of intravitreal bevacizumab versus intravitreal dexamethasone for diabetic macular edema: The BEVORDEX Study. Ophthalmology 2014; 121 (12): 2473-2481.

[220] Meyer-Schwickerath G. History and development of photocoagulation. Am J Ophthalmol. 1967; 63:1812-4.

[221] Photocoagulation for diabetic macular edema. Early Treatment Diabetic Retinopathy Study report number 1. Early Treatment Diabetic Retinopathy Study research group. Arch Ophthalmol. 1985; 103:1796-806.

[222] Stefansson E (2006) Ocular oxygenation and the treatment of diabetic retinopathy. Surv Ophthalmol 51:364-380

[223] Matsumoto M, Yoshimura N, Honda Y (1994) Increased production of transforming growth factor-beta 2 from cultured human retinal pigment epithelial cells by photocoagulation. Invest Ophthalmol Vis Sci 35:4245-4252

[224] Schatz H, Madeira D, McDonald HR, Johnson RN. Progressive enlargement of laser scars following grid laser photocoagulation for diffuse diabetic macular edema. Arch Ophthalmol. 1991; 109:1549-51. [PubMed] [Google Scholar]

[225] Rutledge BK, Wallow IH, Poulsen GL. Sub-pigment epithelial membranes after photocoagulation for diabetic macular edema. Arch Ophthalmol. 1993; 111:608-13.

[226] Writing Committee for the Diabetic Retinopathy Clinical Research Network, Fong DS, Strauber SF, Aiello LP, Beck RW, et al. (2007) Comparison of the modified Early Treatment Diabetic Retinopathy Study and mild macular grid laser photocoagulation strategies for diabetic macular edema. Arch Ophthalmol 125: 469-480.

[227] Crosson JN, Mason L, Mason JO. The Role of Focal Laser in the Anti-Vascular Endothelial Growth Factor Era. Ophthalmol Eye Dis. 2017 Nov 21; 9:1179172117738240. doi: 10.1177/1179172117738240.

[228] Diabetic Retinopathy Clinical Research Network: The course of

response to focal/grid photocoagulation for diabetic macular edema. Retina. 2009; 29(10): 1436-43.

[229] The Diabetic Retinopathy Study Research Group, "Preliminary report on effects of photocoagulation therapy," American Journal of Ophthalmology, vol. 81, pp. 383-396, 1976.

[230] Laursen ML, Moeller F, Sander B, Sjoelie AK. Subthreshold micropulse diode laser treatment in diabetic macular oedema. Br J Ophthalmol 2004; 88:1173-9.

[231] Luttrull JK, Musch DC, Mainster MA. Subthreshold diode micropulse photocoagulation for the treatment of clinically significant diabetic macular oedema. Br J Ophthalmol 2005; 89:74-80.

[232] Akduman L, Olk RJ. Subthreshold (invisible) modified grid diode laser photocoagulation in diffuse diabetic macular edema (DDME) Ophthalmic Surg Lasers 1999; 30:706-14.

[233] Luttrull, J. K.Dorin, G. Subthreshold diode micropulse laser photocoagulation (SDM) as invisible retinal phototherapy for diabetic macular edema: a review. Curr Diabetes Rev 8, 274-284 (2012).

[234] Chhablani, J. et al. Restorative retinal laser therapy: Present state and future directions. Survey Ophthalmol 63, 307-328, https://doi.org/10.1016/j.survophthal.2017.09.008 (2018).

[235] Yu, A. K. et al. The comparative histologic effects of subthreshold 532- and 810-nm diode micropulse laser on the retina. Invest Ophthalmol Vis Sci 54, 2216-2224, https://doi.org/10.1167/iovs.12-11382 (2013).

[236] Luttrull JK, Sramek C, Palanker D, Spink CJ, Musch DC. Long-term safety, high-resolution imaging, and tissue temperature modeling of subvisible diode micropulse photocoagulation for retinovascular macular edema. Retina 2012; 32:375-86.

[237] Lavinsky D, Cardillo JA, Melo LA Jr, Dare A, Farah ME, Belfort R Jr: Randomized clinical trial evaluating mETDRS versus normal or high-density micropulse photocoagulation for diabetic macular edema. Invest Ophthalmol Vis Sci 2011; 52: 4314-4323.

[238] Figueira J, Khan J, Nunes S, Sivaprasad S, Rosa A, de Abreu JF, Cunha-Vaz JG, Chong NV: Prospective randomised controlled trial comparing sub-threshold micropulse diode laser photocoagulation. Available: 10.1016/j.ophtha.2013.02.034. and conventional green laser for clinically significant diabetic macular oedema. Br J Ophthalmol 2009; 93: 1341-1344.

[239] Abouhussein MA, Gomaa AR. Aflibercept plus micropulse laser versus aflibercept monotherapy for diabetic macular edema: 1-year results of a randomized clinical trial. Int Ophthalmol. 2020 May; 40(5):1147-1154. doi: 10.1007/s10792-019-01280-9.

[240] Furashova O, Strassburger P, Becker KA, Engelmann K. Efficacy of combining intravitreal injections of ranibizumab with micropulse diode laser versus intravitreal injections of ranibizumab alone in diabetic macular edema (ReCaLL): a single center, randomised, controlled, non-inferiority clinical trial. BMC Ophthalmol. 2020; 20(1):308. Published 2020 Jul 29. doi: 10.1186/s12886-020-01576-w

[241] Roider J, Brinkmann R, Wirbelauer C, Laqua H, Birngruber R (1999) Retinal sparing by selective retinal pigment epithelial photocoagulation. Arch Ophthalmol 117:1028-1034

[242] Brinkmann R, Roider J, Birngruber R (2006) Selective retina therapy (SRT): a review on methods, techniques,

preclinical and first clinical results. Bull Soc Belge Ophtalmol 302:51-69

[243] Roider J, Liew SH, Klatt C, Elsner H, Poerksen E, Hillenkamp J, Brinkmann R, Birngruber R (2010) Selective retina therapy (SRT) for clinically significant diabetic macular edema. Graefes's Arch Clin Exp Ophthalmol 248:1263-1272

[244] Park YG, Kim JR, Kang S, Seifert E, Theisen-Kunde D, Brinkmann R, Roh YJ (2016) Safety and efficacy of selective retina therapy (SRT) for the treatment of diabetic macular edema in Korean patients. Graefes's Arch Clin Exp Ophthalmol 254:1703-1713

[245] Jain A, Blumenkranz MS, Paulus Y, Wiltberger MW, Andersen DE, Huie P, et al. Effect of pulse duration on size and character of the lesion in retinal photocoagulation. Arch Ophthalmol. 2008; 126:78-85.

[246] Muqit MM, Gray JC, Marcellino GR, Henson DB, Young LB, Patton N, et al. In vivo laser-tissue interactions and healing responses from 20- vs 100-millisecond pulse Pascal photocoagulation burns. Arch Ophthalmol. 2010; 128:448-55.

[247] Muqit MM, Gray JC, Marcellino GR, Henson DB, Young LB, Patton N, et al. Barely visible 10-millisecond pascal laser photocoagulation for diabetic macular edema: Observations of clinical effect and burn localization. Am J Ophthalmol. 2010; 149:979-986.e2.

[248] Blumenkranz MS, Yellachich D, Andersen DE, Wiltberger MW, Mordaunt D, Marcellino GR, et al. Semiautomated patterned scanning laser for retinal photocoagulation. Retina 2006; 26:370-6

[249] Chappelow AV, Tan K, Waheed NK, Kaiser PK. Panretinal photocoagulation for proliferative diabetic retinopathy: Pattern scan laser versus argon laser. Am J Ophthalmol 2012; 153:137-42.e2.

[250] Kernt M, Cheuteu R, Vounotrypidis E, Haritoglou C, Kampik A, Ulbig MW, et al. Focal and panretinal photocoagulation with a navigated laser (NAVILAS®) Acta Ophthalmol. 2011; 89:e662-4.

[251] Neubauer AS, Langer J, Liegl R, Haritoglou C, Wolf A, Kozak I, et al. Navigated macular laser decreases retreatment rate for diabetic macular edema: A comparison with conventional macular laser. Clin Ophthalmol. 2013; 7:121-8.

[252] Kozak I, Oster SF, Cortes MA, Dowell D, Hartmann K, Kim JS, et al. Clinical evaluation and treatment accuracy in diabetic macular edema using navigated laser photocoagulator NAVILAS. Ophthalmology. 2011; 118:1119-24.

[253] Kernt M, Ulbig M, Haritoglou C. Seattle, Washington: The Association for Research in Vision and Ophthalmology; 2013. Combination of ranibizumab and navigated retinal photocoagulation vs ranibizumab mono-therapy for diabetic macular oedema: Twelve month results.

[254] Barteselli G, Kozak I, El-Emam S, Chhablani J, Cortes MA, Freeman WR. 12-month results of the standardised combination therapy for diabetic macular oedema: Intravitreal bevacizumab and navigated retinal photocoagulation. Br J Ophthalmol. 2014; 98:1036-41

[255] Gaucher D, Tadayoni R, Erginay A, Haouchine B, Gaudric A, Massin P, et al. Optical coherence tomography assessment of the vitreoretinal relationship in diabetic macular edema. Am J Ophthalmol 2005; 139:807-13.

[256] Nasrallah FP, Jalkh AE, Van Coppenolle F, et al. The role of the

vitreous in diabetic macular edema. Ophthalmology. 1988; 95(10):1335-9.

[257] Todorich, B., Mahmoud, T.H. Vitrectomy for Diabetic Macular Edema. Curr Ophthalmol Rep 2, 167-174 (2014). https://doi.org/10.1007/s40135-014-0052-6

[258] Lewis H, Abrams GW, Blumenkranz MS, Campo RV. Vitrectomy for diabetic macular traction and edema associated with posterior hyaloid traction. Ophthalmology 1992; 99:753-9.

[259] Gandorfer A, Messmer EM, Ulbig MW, Kampik A. Resolution of diabetic macular edema after surgical removal of the posterior hyaloid and the inner limiting membrane. Retina 2000; 20:126-33

[260] Hartley KL, Smiddy WE, Flynn HW Jr., Murray TG. Pars plana vitrectomy with internal limiting membrane peeling for diabetic macular edema. Retina 2008; 28:410-9.

[261] Yang CM. Surgical treatment for severe diabetic macular edema with massive hard exudates. Retina 2000; 20:121-5.

[262] Mochizuki Y, Hata Y, Enaida H, Yoshiyama K, Miyazaki M, Ueno A, et al. Evaluating adjunctive surgical procedures during vitrectomy for diabetic macular edema. Retina 2006; 26:143-8.

[263] Landers MB 3rd, Graversen VA, Stewart MW. Early vitrectomy for DME: Does it have a role? Sometimes Vitrectomy can be First-Line Treatment. Part 1 of 2. Retina Physician; 2013

[264] Patel JI, Hykin PG, Schadt M, Luong V, Fitzke F, Gregor ZJ, et al. Pars plana vitrectomy with and without peeling of the inner limiting membrane for diabetic macular edema. Retina 2006; 26:5-13.

[265] Thomas D, Bunce C, Moorman C, Laidlaw DA. A randomised controlled feasibility trial of vitrectomy versus laser for diabetic macular oedema. Br J Ophthalmol 2005; 89:81-6.

[266] Terasaki H, Kojima T, Niwa H, Piao CH, Ueno S, Kondo M, et al. Changes in focal macular electroretinograms and foveal thickness after vitrectomy for diabetic macular edema. Invest Ophthalmol Vis Sci 2003; 44:4465-72.

[267] Higuchi A, Ogata N, Jo N, Wada M, Matsumura M. Pars plana vitrectomy with removal of posterior hyaloid face in treatment of refractory diabetic macular edema resistant to triamcinolone acetonide. Jpn J Ophthalmol 2006; 50:529-31.

[268] Kadonosono K, Itoh N, Ohno S. Perifoveal microcirculation before and after vitrectomy for diabetic cystoid macular edema. Am J Ophthalmol 2000; 130:740-4.

[269] Shah SP, Laidlaw DA. Vitrectomy for diabetic macular edema. Am J Ophthalmol 2006; 141:225

[270] Kita T, Clermont AC, Murugesan N, et al. Plasma kallikrein-kinin system as a VEGF-independent mediator of diabetic macular edema. Diabetes. 2015 10; 64(10):3588-3599.

[271] Ashay D. Bhatwadekara, Viral S. Kansarab, Thomas A. Ciulla. Investigational plasma kallikrein inhibitors for the treatment of diabetic macular edema: an expert assessment. Expert Opin Investig Drugs. 2020 March; 29(3): 237-244. doi:10.1080/13543784.2020.1723078

Chapter 10

Treatment Algorithm in Proliferative Diabetic Retinopathy - From Protocols to the Real World

Jesus Hernan Gonzalez-Cortes,
Jesus Emiliano Gonzalez-Cantu, Aditya Sudhalkar,
Sergio Eustolio Hernandez-Da Mota, Alper Bilgic,
Javier Alan Garza-Chavarria and Jesus Mohamed-Hamsho

Abstract

Diabetes mellitus is a global epidemic that leads to multiple macrovascular and microvascular complications. The complex interrelated pathophysiological mechanisms triggered by hyperglycemia underlie the development of diabetic retinopathy (DR). Proliferative diabetic retinopathy (PDR) is a microvascular complication, considered the main cause of irreversible blindness in patients of productive age in the world. On the other hand, diabetic macular edema (DME) remains the clinical feature most closely associated with vision loss. In general, both manifestations are due to an increase in inflammatory factors, such as specific pro-inflammatory prostaglandins, interleukins and angiogenic substances including vascular endothelial growth factor (VEGF). Laser photocoagulation and VEGF inhibitors have been shown to be effective in the treatment of PDR and DME. Currently, randomized protocols suggest that VEGF inhibitors therapy could displace laser photocoagulation in the treatment of PDR with and without the presence of DME. The ongoing discussion still prevails about the different treatment modalities for both retinal manifestations in real-world settings.

Keywords: proliferative diabetic retinopathy, diabetic macular edema, treatment algorithm, treatment guidelines, panretinal photocoagulation, antiangiogenic therapy

1. Introduction

Diabetic retinopathy (DR) is characterized by progressive damage to retinal capillaries causing retinal ischemia. In severe cases, it leads to DR, which threatens vision induced by angiogenesis [1]. Vascular endothelial growth factor (VEGF) is an important agent in the development and progression of DR and diabetic macular edema (DME) [2, 3].

The Early Treatment of DR (ETDRS) study showed that focal photocoagulation of "clinically significant" DME reduces the risk of visual loss and increases the chances of visual improvement, decreases the frequency of persistent DME, and causes minor visual field losses [4]. Panretinal photocoagulation (PFC) has been the standard treatment for proliferative diabetic retinopathy (PDR) since the DR study (DRS) demonstrated its benefit more than 40 years ago [5]. PFC has demonstrated permanent peripheral visual field loss and decreased night vision. On the other hand, it can exacerbate existing DME or increase its incidence. Different treatment alternatives in PDR should be considered [6].

DME can affect the macular center considering it as "with center-involving" (CI-DME) or it can respect the same, considering it as "non-center-involving" (NCI-DME). Anti-angiogenic (anti-VEGF) therapy in DME, has shown superior visual acuity results and acceptable risks compared to focal, grid, or untreated laser, and has also led to the observation that DR lesions can be reversed during treatment [7–14]. Anti-VEGF therapy is currently considered the first-line treatment for DME.

The objective of this chapter is to describe an algorithm in the treatment of PDR based on current publications that could be used in real-world scenarios and different practice settings.

2. Current treatments in DME and PDR

According to the results of the DRCR.net Protocol S, at two years of follow-up, intravitreal ranibizumab (RBZ) achieved the result of non-inferiority in the change of best-corrected visual acuity (BCVA), which was no worse than in the PFC group treatment for PDR [15]. There were no statistically significant differences in BCVA between the RBZ and PFC groups, with the recognition that 53% of the PFC group received additional RBZ injections to treat DME and only 6% of the RBZ group required PFC. There was greater peripheral visual field loss (95% CI for difference, 213–531 dB) and more vitrectomies (PPV) were performed (95% CI for one difference, 4% -15%) in the PFC group compared to the RBZ group. In addition, RBZ-treated eyes were less likely to develop CI-DME causing visual impairment of 20/32 or worse, similar to the 1-year results with aflibercept (AFB) in the CLARITY randomized clinical trial [16]. In the DRCR.net Protocol S, a greater number of patients in the PFC group developed DME (28 vs. 9). At 5-year results, the mean number of injections in the PFC group was 7.9 and 19.2 in the RBZ group. The mean final BCVA in both groups was 20/25. Despite the fact that at 2 years the PFC group presented a greater visual field loss, the decrease in the peripheral visual field progressed in both groups during the following 5 years of follow-up [17].

In a post hoc analysis of the DRCR.net Protocol T [18], after 2 years of follow-up, an improvement in DR severity was demonstrated by approximately 25% for AFB, 22% for bevacizumab (BVZ) and 31% for RBZ in patients without proliferative-DR (NPDR) at baseline. This analysis also suggests a secondary benefit of DME after intravitreal AFB with respect to improvement in DR severity among patients who had PDR from baseline. Anti-VEGF therapy for DME improves the score of the DR severity scale (DRSS), evaluated in color fundus photos and can reduce the deterioration of the edema. Other randomized trials comparing anti-VEGF therapy and PFC in PDR, have demonstrated the non-inferiority of anti-VEGF over PFC in preventing PDR complications, at least during the first 2 years [19, 20]. Similar studies using ultra-wide-field (UWF) photographs and comparing them with ultra-wide-field fluorescein angiography (UWF-FAG) or wide field swept source optical coherent tomography (WF-SS-OCTA) in eyes with DR and DME [21, 22], conclude that after injections with anti-VEGF, improvement in the DRSS score can occur without vessel reperfusion or retinal capillary in UWF-FAG or WF-SS-OCTA. Therefore, the strong correlation between the number of lesions in DR and the areas of non-perfusion, established before any treatment, could no longer be relevant after anti-VEGF therapy.

These results should be taken into account in future studies, in order to demonstrate an improvement in peripheral retinal perfusion in DR after anti-VEGF therapy.

3. Changing paradigms in the treatment of PDR

Taking into account specific scenarios of PDR proposed by Sun JK et al. [23], based on the results of the DRCR.net Protocol S [15] in addition to considering the different advantages of each treatment modality, we describe a treatment algorithm that could be used in real-world scenarios and in different practice settings.

3.1 PDR without DME

Both PFC and anti-VEGF therapy are feasible therapeutic options. Anti-VEGF therapy is effective in reversing retinal neovascularization (NV) and reducing the risk of developing DME. However, it may not be cost effective overall [24].

A. If starting PFC.

- Add anti-VEGF only in case NV significantly worsens (**Table 1**) and/or DME develops (**Table 2**).

B. If starting anti-VEGF, it is suggested to perform it according to the treatment algorithm proposed by Protocol S (**Table 1**).

- If NV worsens significantly, adding PFC should be considered.
- If NV does not require further anti-VEGF and during the "sustain stability" period DME develops, add focal macular laser or anti-VEGF (**Table 2**).

The advantages and disadvantages of treatment options should be considered, as well as the individual conditions of the patient.

3.2 PDR with NCI-DME

Anti-VEGF therapy has been accepted as a first-line treatment in DME, displacing laser as a second-line therapy. Although some authors suggest the application of laser in NCI-DME [25–27], there are reports where the addition of conventional, subthreshold or micropulse laser does not add benefits to pharmacological monotherapy in any form of presentation [28–30].

1	Start with 6 monthly anti-VEGF injections (only with one exception), If the NV resolves after 4 or 5 injections, the injections may be postponed.
2	After 6 months, continue the anti-VEGF injections if NV continues to progress or continues to improve; but defer injections if NV is stable at current visit and last 2 visits ("sustained stability").
3	Resume anti-VEGF injections monthly if NV worsens after stopping injections. If "sustained stability" is achieved again, the injections can be postponed once more, but this requires at least 3 consecutive anti-VEGF injections again; one administered for the initial state of progressive NV and 2 more if the NV remains stable.

PFC is given only if NV is substantially worse despite anti-VEGF. Onset or worsening of preretinal or vitreous hemorrhage is not necessarily classified as worsening of NV, unless bleeding precludes evaluation of NV.

Table 1.
Algorithm for the treatment of PDR according to DRCR.net protocol S.

1	Start with 3 monthly ant-VEGF injections or until you achieve maximum improvement (loading phase).
2	After the loading phase, continue injecting according to reactive (Treat and Observe or Pro Re Nata) or proactive (Treat and Extend) behavior.

Table 2.
Algorithm for the treatment of DME.

A. If starting focal macular laser and PFC.

- Add anti-VEGF in case DME worsens (**Table 2**) and/or there is significant progression of NV (**Table 1**).

B. If starting anti-VEGF for DME (**Table 2**). *PFC can be deferred since the same anti-VEGF may control both (DME and PDR).*

- If DME does not require further anti-VEGF, NV status should be re-evaluated.
- If NV worsens significantly, it is suggested to decide on therapy according to Section 3.1 B (PDR without DME).
- In case of new DME activity, it is suggested to reactivate anti-VEGF therapy.

C. In the event that the DME has a poor or no response, several options should be considered (switching anti-VEGF, focal macular laser, dexamethasone implant, etc.).

Advantages and disadvantages of treatment options should be considered, as well as the individual conditions of the patient.

3.3 RDP with CI-DME

Anti-VEGF is considered first- line treatment in CI-DME. RBZ and AFB were highly effective in treating PDR [15, 16].

A. Anti-VEGF is recommended as first-line treatment in CI-DME (**Table 2**). *PFC can be deferred since the same anti-VEGF may control both (DME and PDR).*

- If DME does not require further anti-VEGF, NV status should be re-evaluated.
- If NV worsens significantly, it is suggested to decide on therapy according to Section 3.1 B (PDR without DME).
- In case of new DME activity, it is suggested to reactivate anti-VEGF therapy.

B. In the event that the DME has a poor or no response, several options should be considered (switching anti-VEGF, focal macular laser, dexamethasone implant, etc.).

Advantages and disadvantages of treatment options should be considered, as well as the individual conditions of the patient.

3.4 High-risk PDR with or without vision- impairing DME

Eyes with high-risk PDR (i.e., ≥ ETDRS level 71) face the greatest risk of severe vision loss without intervention [4, 5]. Eyes with the most advanced forms of PDR have the largest relative benefit of RBZ compared with PRP when managing PDR. Also, RBZ was superior to PRP with respect to change in visual acuity over 2 years and prevention of vision-impairing CI-DME over 2 years, regardless of baseline characteristics [31]. On the other hand, combined therapy has shown benefits in the management of high-risk PDR.

- Anti-VEGF should be considered as monotherapy (**Table 1**).
- If NV worsens significantly, it is suggested to decide on therapy according to Section 3.1 B (PDR without DME).

Although anti-VEGF may be recommended as monotherapy in eyes with high-risk PDR, complete PRP within the effective period of anti- VEGF agents might be recommended. Advantages and disadvantages of treatment options should be considered, as well as the individual conditions of the patient.

3.5 Worsening PDR

Worse baseline levels of DR severity (ETDRS scale) were associated with increased risk of worsening PDR (e.g., vitreous hemorrhage (VH), retinal detachment (RD), angle neovascularization (ANV), or neovascular glaucoma (NVG)), regardless of treatment with PRP or RBZ. There were generally fewer PDR-worsening events (e.g., VH, RD, ANV, or NVG) in eyes treated with RBZ versus PRP for PDR. Through 2-year, the cumulative probability of worsening PDR was 42% for PRP versus 34% for RBZ. The 2-year cumulative probability of VH was 39% for the PRP group and 30% for the RBZ group. The 2-year cumulative probability of RD was low in each treatment group at 11% for the PRP group and 5% for the RBZ group [20]. The fact that worsening PDR events were at higher rates in the PRP group, suggests that at least during the first two years of follow-up:

- Anti-VEGF should be considered as monotherapy (**Table 1**).
- If NV worsens significantly, it is suggested to decide on therapy according to Section 3.1 B (PDR without DME).

As in the eyes with high-risk PDR, complete PRP within the effective period of anti- VEGF agents might be recommended. Advantages and disadvantages of treatment options should be considered, as well as the individual conditions of the patient.

3.6 Vitrectomy for PDR

Eyes in both groups (RBZ or PRP) had visual loss associated with VH, being more severe in the PRP group. The protocol required investigators to wait at least 8 weeks for a nonclearing VH before proceeding to vitrectomy (in the absence of known RD, iris NV, or ANV). VH was the primary indication for most PPV, 24 (80%) procedures in the PRP group and 6 (75%) procedures in the RBZ group. Endolaser or indirect ophthalmoscopic laser during PPV were applied in 80% of procedures in the PRP group and in all procedures in the RBZ group. Only 1 eye in the RBZ group received PRP independent of PPV. Possibly for convenience, the not masked investigators, decided to continue observing VH before proceeding to PPV in the RBZ group. The authors note that because VH, only 13% (7/52) in the RBZ group compared to 42% (29/69) in the PRP group underwent PPV at the end of 2 years. Therefore, because VH was the main indication for surgery in both groups, the reduced incidence of VH in the RBZ group and the potential difference in VH severity may explain the finding that eyes in the PRP group were more likely to undergo vitrectomy [20]. Although several studies do not support the hypothesis that anti-VEGF administered to an eye with PDR, with or without high-risk features (but without macular-threatening traction at baseline), causes tractional RD (TRD) more often than eyes with PRP [7, 28, 32], we must consider the possibility of additional PPV in these patients.

4. Discussion

In clinical practice, treating PFC with one or more sessions may be sufficient to control PDR and no additional procedures are required. On the other hand, the cost of laser therapy is less expensive than anti-VEGF therapy and there is no risk of endophthalmitis or systemic adverse events [15]. The DRCR.net in a cost–benefit analysis regarding RBZ or PFC monotherapy for PDR, noted that it was more appropriate to start with PFC for patients with PDR without associated DME and RBZ for those with DME at the time of treatment detection [33]. Therefore, the relative benefits of treating PDR with anti-VEGF versus PFC could be considered in a patient presenting with DME, where anti-VEGF therapy is generally necessary, as long as the patient adheres to treatment and is able to access it. In Mexico, as in some countries, it is possible to adopt the algorithm suggested by the DRCR.net Protocol S; however, the circumstances of patients and environment could modify the scheme. Likewise, the advantages and disadvantages of treatment options should be considered, in addition to socioeconomic conditions, adherence to treatment, and access to "off-label" medications.

It is generally known that the pathogenesis and progression of DR involves changes in the vitreous structure and its relationship with the vitreoretinal interface [34–40]. A study whose objective was to evaluate the costs and usefulness of early PPV compared to PFC and intravitreal RBZ in PDR patients without DME, using a "decision analysis" based on the results of DRCR.net Protocol S at 2 years of treatment for each scenario, concluded that PPV as a treatment strategy demonstrates a similar cost utility to treatment with PFC and a more favorable cost utility compared to short-term intravitreal RBZ therapy [41]. This advantage over anti-VEGF is continuing when lifetime costs are considered. The safety of anti-VEGFs compared to primary PPV (without anti-VEGF) for persistent VH is being evaluated in the Protocol AB.

Currently, the PANORAMA study [42], a double-masked, randomized phase 3 trial, the objective of which is to evaluate the efficacy and safety of intravitreal injection of AFB compared to sham therapy in improving moderate-to-severe NPDR in the absence of CI-DME, demonstrate at week 24 that AFB improved the severity of DR in patients with moderately severe to severe NPDR and suggests that anti-VEGF can reverse disease progression in these patients.

In turn, there is interest if steroid therapy in the treatment of DME can delay the progression or even improve DR. Corticosteroids inhibit the inflammatory processes involved in DME, including the production of pro-inflammatory mediators, increased levels of VEGF, and the loss of endothelial tension-binding proteins [43, 44]. There are clinical trials that have shown some benefit of intravitreal

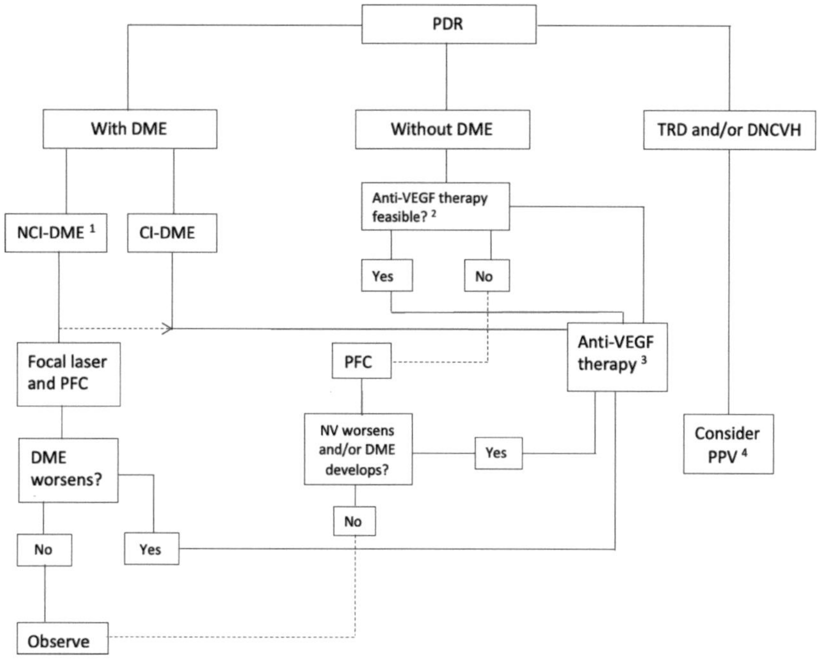

Figure 1.
Treatment flow-chart in different presenting PDR scenarios. DME: Diabetic macular edema; DNCVH: Dense non-clearing vitreous hemorrhage; CI-DME: Center-involving diabetic macular edema. NCI-DME: Non-center-involving diabetic macular edema; NV: New vessels; PDR: Proliferative diabetic retinopathy; PFC: Panretinal photocoagulation; TRD: Tractional retinal detachment threatening or involving macula; PPV: Pars plana vitrectomy. [1]If starting anti-VEGF for DME, PFC can be deferred since the same anti-VEGF may control both DME and PDR. [2]Consider factors such as risk of non-compliance, treatment cost, and treatment burden. [3]Cases with TRD should not receive only anti-VEGF therapy due to increased traction progression risk. [4]Anti-VEGF injection can be applied a few days before PPV is performed to decrease intraoperative and postoperative VH.

steroids in the progression of DR [12, 45]. The "DR-Pro-Dex" study provides the first long-term evidence that the dexamethasone implant has the potential to not only delay the progression of DR and PDR but may also improve the severity of DR in 24 months [46]. On the other hand, the results of the "TRADITION" study conclude that the implantation of dexamethasone at the end of a PPV in patients with TRD improves the severity of PDR and reduces the detachment rates [47].

In the case of DME, the little or no response of the anti-VEGF used and its relationship with persistent peripheral retinal ischemia require modifications in treatment. Alternatives should be considered such as: switching from anti-VEGF, intravitreal dexamethasone implant, additional PFC (peripheral retina), PPV or combining treatments. Although anti-VEGF monotherapy achieves stabilization of NV in PDR, adding PFC could result in a lower frequency of intravitreal applications, resulting in lower risks and costs for the patient.

In **Figure 1**, a flow-chart of treatment modalities for different presenting PDR scenarios is shown.

5. Conclusion

In general, the objective to achieve success in the treatment of PDR and DME is the inhibition of VEGF and pro-inflammatory factors, a condition that seems to be obtained more efficiently with pharmacological therapy in relation to retinal ablation. Currently the indications for laser, intravitreal drug therapy (anti-VEGF's and anti-inflammatory steroids) and PPV are increasingly clear. Based on the results previously mentioned, anti-VEGF therapy appears to be emerging as first-line therapy in PDR, as is currently suggested in the treatment of DME. Treatment regimens in patients with severe NPDR with or without DME, may be indifferent to those currently suggested in PDR patients with or without DME; including that early PPV is an alternative to prevent retinal complications of diabetic microvascular disease. This chapter suggests a treatment algorithm for PDR in different settings; however, we must not forget that both DME and PDR are different manifestations of DR and therefore must be assessed individually. Treatment decisions can be different for each manifestation and can be modified depending on its behavior. Several protocols are currently being developed to more accurately understand the behavior of PDR and DME in different settings and to provide a more solid foundation for an effective and timely treatment scheme.

6. Protocols in progress

1. **Protocol W:** Safety and efficacy of AFB vs. observation in severe NPDR and BCVA ≥20/25 without DME and without previous treatment, to assess the appearance of edema or progression of retinopathy.

2. **Protocol AA:** To evaluate lesions in the peripheral DR and their association with the progression of retinopathy in patients with NPDR, without DME or previous treatment, comparing UWF images vs. standard photographs of the seven fields (ETDRS) in order to determine if UWF photographs contribute more information than conventional ones.

3. **Protocol AB:** Treatment of early PPV versus ARB in vitreous secondary to PDR is compared by evaluating BCVA at 6 months of treatment.

4. **Protocol AD (PROMINENT):** To assess whether treatment with pemfibrate (0.2 mg / 12 h orally) compared with placebo reduces the rate of worsening of DR in patients with type 2 diabetes and NPDR.

5. **Protocol GEN:** Create a genetic material and information on the clinical phenotype, which allows evaluating genetic susceptibility or resistance in DR and determining variants on key biomarkers in the development of DME and NV.

Author details

Jesus Hernan Gonzalez-Cortes[1,2*], Jesus Emiliano Gonzalez-Cantu[1], Aditya Sudhalkar[3,4], Sergio Eustolio Hernandez-Da Mota[5], Alper Bilgic[4], Javier Alan Garza-Chavarria[2] and Jesus Mohamed-Hamsho[1]

1 Ophthalmology Department, Faculty of Medicine and University Hospital "Dr. José Eleuterio González", Universidad Autonoma de Nuevo Leon, Monterrey, Nuevo Leon, Mexico

2 Departamento de Retina y Vítreo, ISSSTE Constitucion, Universidad Nacional Autonoma de Mexico, Monterrey, Nuevo Leon, Mexico

3 MS Sudhalkar Medical Research Foundation, Baroda, India

4 Alphavision Augenarztpraxis, Bremerhaven, Germany

5 Department of Ophthalmology, Unidad Oftalmologica y Facultad de Medicina, Clinica David, Universidad Michoacana de San Nicolas de Hidalgo, Morelia, Michoacan, Mexico

*Address all correspondence to: drjesusgzz@gmail.com

References

[1] Kohner EM. Diabetic retinopathy. BMJ. *1993 Nov;307(6913):1195*-1199.

[2] Ferrara N. Molecular and biological properties of vascular endothelial growth factor. J Mol Med (Berl). 1999 Jul;77(7):527-543.

[3] Stitt AW, Curtis TM, Chen M, Medina RJ, McKay GJ, Jenkins A, et al. The progress in understanding and treatment of diabetic reti- nopathy. Prog Retin Eye Res. 2016 Mar;51: 156-186.

[4] Photocoagulation for diabetic macular edema. Early Treatment Diabetic Retinopathy Study report number 1. Early treatment diabetic retinopathy study research group. Arch Ophthalmol *1985;* 103:1796 – 1806.

[5] Diabetic Retinopathy Study Research Group. Photocoagulation treatment of proliferative diabetic retinopathy: clinical application of Diabetic Retinopathy Study (DRS) findings, DRS report number 8. Ophthalmology. 1981;88(7):583-600.

[6] Brucker AJ, Qin H, Antoszyk AN, et al; Diabetic Retinopathy Clinical Research Network. Observational study of the development of diabetic macular edema following panretinal (scatter) photocoagulation given in 1 or 4 sittings. Arch Ophthalmol. 2009;127(2):132-140.

[7] Googe J, Brucker AJ, Bressler NM, et al; Diabetic Retinopathy Clinical Research Network. Randomized trial evaluating short-term effects of intravitreal ranibizumab or triamcinolone acetonide on macular edema after focal/grid laser for diabetic macular edema in eyes also receiving panretinal photocoagulation. Retina. 2011;31(6):1009-1027.

[8] Do DV, Nguyen QD, Boyer D, Schmidt-Erfurth U, Brown DM, Vitti R, et al.; da Vinci Study Group. One-year outcomes of the da Vinci Study of VEGF Trap-Eye in eyes with diabetic macular edema. Ophthalmology. 2012 Aug;119(8):1658-1665.

[9] Heier JS, Korobelnik JF, Brown DM, Schmidt-Erfurth U, Do DV, Midena E, et al. Intravit- real Aflibercept for Diabetic Macular Edema: 148-Week Results from the VISTA and VIVID Studies. Ophthalmology. 2016 Nov; 123(11):2376-2385.

[10] Wells JA, Glassman AR, Ayala AR, Jampol LM, Bressler NM, Bressler SB, et al.; Diabetic Retinopathy Clinical Research Network. Aflibercept, Bevacizumab, or Ranibizumab for Diabetic Macular Edema: Two-Year Results from a Comparative Effectiveness Randomized Clinical Trial. Ophthalmology. 2016 Jun;123(6):1351-1359.

[11] Diabetic Retinopathy Clinical Research Network. Intravitreal Ranibizumab for Diabetic Macular Edema with Prompt versus Deferred Laser Treatment: 5-Year Randomized Trial Results. Ophthalmology. 2015;122(2): 375-381.

[12] Bressler SB, Qin H, Melia M, et al. Exploratory analysis of the effect of intravitreal ranibizumab or triamcinolone on worsening of diabetic retinopathy in a randomized clinical trial. JAMA Ophthalmol. 2013;131(8):1033-1040. [PubMed: 23807371]

[13] Brown DM, Schmidt-Erfurth U, Do DV, et al. Intravitreal aflibercept for diabetic macular edema: 100-week results from the VISTA and VIVID studies. Ophthalmology. 2015;122(10):2044-2052. [PubMed: 26198808]

[14] Nguyen QD, Brown DM, Marcus DM, et al. Ranibizumab for

diabetic macular edema: Results from 2 phase III randomized trials: RISE and RIDE. Ophthalmology. 2012;119(4):789-801. [PubMed: 22330964]

[15] Gross JG, Glassman AR, Jampol LM, Inusah S, Aiello LP, Antoszyk AN, et al.; Writing Committee for the Diabetic Retinopathy Clinical Research Network. Panretinal Photocoagulation vs Intravitreous Ranibizumab for Proliferative Diabetic Retinopathy: A Randomized Clinical Trial. *JAMA*. 2015 Nov; 314(20):2137-2146.

[16] Sivaprasad S, Prevost AT, Vasconcelos JC, et al. Clinical efficacy of intravitreal aflibercept versus panretinal photocoagulation for best corrected visual acuity in patients with proliferative diabetic retinopathy at 52 weeks (CLARITY): a multicentre, single-blinded, randomised, controlled, phase 2b, non-inferiority trial. Lancet. 2017;389(10085):2193-2203. [PubMed: 28494920].

[17] Diabetic Retinopathy Clinical Research Network. Five-Year Outcomes of Panretinal Photocoagulation vs Introus Ranibizumab for Proliferative Diabetic Retinopathy: A Randomized Clinical Trial. JAMA Ophthalmol. 2018;136(10):1138-1148.

[18] Bressler SB, Liu D, Glassman AR, Blodi BA, Castellarin AA, Jampol LM, et al.; Diabetic Retinopathy Clinical Research Network. Change in Diabetic Retinopathy Through 2 Years: Secondary Analysis of a Randomized Clinical Trial Comparing Aflibercept, Bevacizumab, and Ranibizumab. JAMA Ophthalmol. 2017 Jun;135(6):558-568.

[19] Silva PS, Dela Cruz AJ, Ledesmav MG, et al. Diabetic retinopathy severity and peripheral lesions are associated with nonperfusion on ultrawide field angiography. Ophthalmology. 2015;122:2465-2472.

[20] Bressler SB, Beaulieu WT, Glassman AR, et al. Factors associated with worsening proliferative diabetic retinopathy in eyes treated with panretinal photocoagulation or ranibizumab. Ophthalmology 2017;124:431-439.

[21] Aude Couturier, MD, PhD, Pierre-Antoine Rey, MD, Ali Erginay, MD, Carlo Lavia, MD, Sophie Bonnin, MD, Bénédicte Dupas, MD, Alain Gaudric, MD, Ramin Tadayoni, MD, PhD. Widefield OCT-Angiography and Fluorescein Angiography Assessments of Nonperfusion in Diabetic Retinopathy and Edema Treated with AntieVascular Endothelial Growth Factor. *Ophthalmology*. 2019;-:1-10 by the American Academy of Ophthalmology.

[22] Sophie Bonnin, MD, Bénédicte Dupas, MD, Carlo Lavia, MD, Ali Erginay, MD, Myriam Dhundass, MD, Aude Couturier, MD, Alain Gaudric, MD, Ramin Tadayoni, MD, PHD. Anti-vascular endothelial growth factor therapy can improve diabetic retinopathy score without change in retinal perfusion. *RETINA*. 39:426-434, 2019.

[23] Jennifer K. Sun, MD, Adam R. Glassman, MS, Wesley T. Beaulieu, PhD, Cynthia R. Stockdale, MSPH, Neil M. Bressler, MD, Christina Flaxel, MD, Jeffrey G. Gross, MD, Michel Shami, MD, Lee M. Jampol, MD for the Diabetic Retinopathy Clinical Research Network. Rationale and Application of the Protocol S Anti-Vascular Endothelial Growth Factor Algorithm for Proliferative Diabetic Retinopathy. Ophthalmology. 2019 January ; 126(1): 87-95.

[24] Ross EL, Hutton DW, Stein JD, et al. Cost-effectiveness of aflibercept, bevacizumab, and ranibizumab for diabetic macular edema treatment: Analysis from the diabetic retinopathy clinical research network comparative effectiveness trial. JAMA Ophthalmol. 2016;134(8):888-896. [PubMed: 27280850]

[25] Hooper P, Boucher MC, Colleaux K, Cruess A, Greve M, Lam WC, Shortt S, Tourville E. Contemporary management of diabetic retinopathy in Canada: from guidelines to algorithm guidance. Ophthalmologica. 2014;231(1):2-15.

[26] Bandello F, Cunha-Vaz J, Chong NV, Lang GE, Massin P, Mitchell P, Porta M, Prünte C, Schlingemann R, Schmidt-Erfurth U. New approaches for the treatment of diabetic macular oedema: recommendations by an expert panel. Eye (Lond). 2012;26(4):485-493.

[27] Mitchell P, Wong TY; Diabetic Macular Edema Treatment Guideline Working Group. Management paradigms for diabetic macular edema. Am J Ophthalmol 2014;157(3):505-513.

[28] Elman, M. J., Aiello, L. P., Beck, R. W., Bressler, N. M., Bressler, S. B., Edwards, A. R., Ferris, F. L. 3rd, Friedman, S. M., Glassman, A. R., Miller, K. M., Scott, I. U., Stockdale, C. R., & Sun, J. K. (2010). Randomized trial evaluating ranibizumab plus prompt or deferred laser or triamcinolone plus prompt laser for diabetic macular edema. *Ophthalmology*. 2010;117(6), 1064-1077.e35.

[29] Payne, J. F., Wykoff, C. C., Clark, W. L., Bruce, B. B., Boyer, D. S., & Brown, D. M. (2020). Long-term outcomes of treat-and-extend ranibizumab with and without navigated laser for diabetic macular oedema: TREX-DME 3-year results. *The British Journal of Ophthalmology*.

[30] Edgar Cuervo-Lozano, Jesús Hernán González-Cortés, Abraham Olvera-Barrios, Ezequiel Treviño- Cavazos, Josué Rodríguez-Pedraza, Karim Mohamed-Noriega, Jesús Mohamed-Hamsho. Short-term outcomes after the loading phase of intravitreal bevacizumab and subthreshold macular laser in non-center involved diabetic macular edema. *Int J Ophthalmol.* Vol. 11, No. 6, Jun.18, 2018.

[31] Bressler S, Beaulieu WT, Glassman A, et al. Photocoagulation versus ranibizumab for proliferative diabetic retinopathy: Should baseline characteristics affect choice of treatment? Retina. 2019 Sep;39(9):1646-1654.

[32] Diabetic Retinopathy Clinical Research N. Randomized clinical trial evaluating intravitreal ranibizumab or saline for vitreous hemorrhage from proliferative diabetic retinopathy. JAMA Ophthalmol. 2013;131(3):283-293. [PubMed: 23370902]

[33] Diabetic Retinopathy Clinical Research Network. Cost-effectiveness of Intravitreous Ranibizumab Compared With Panretinal Photocoagulation for Proliferative Diabetic Retinopathy Secondary Analysis From a Diabetic Retinopathy Clinical Research Network Randomized Clinical Trial. JAMA Ophthalmol. 2017;135(6):576-584.

[34] Sebag J. Anatomy and pathology of the vitreo-retinal interface. Eye. 1992;6(Pt 6):541-552.

[35] Nasrallah FP, Jalkh AE, Van Coppenolle F, et al. The role of the vitreous in diabetic macular edema. Ophthalmology. 1988;95(10): 1335-1339.

[36] Ophir A, Martinez MR, Mosqueda P, Trevino A. Vitreous traction and epiretinal membranes in diabetic macular oedema using spectral-domain optical coherence tomography. Eye (Lond). 2010;24(10):1545-1553.

[37] Ophir A, Martinez MR. Epiretinal membranes and incomplete posterior vitreous detachment in diabetic macular edema, detected by spectral-domain optical coherence tomography. Invest Ophthalmol Vis Sci. 2011;52(9): 6414-6420.

[38] Gunduz K, Bakri SJ. Management of proliferative diabetic retinopathy.

Compr Ophthalmol Update. 2007;8(5):245-256.

[39] Chu TG, Lopez P, Cano MR, et al. Posterior vitreoschisis: an echographic finding in proliferative diabetic retinopathy. Ophthalmology. 1996;103(2):315-322.

[40] Gaucher D, Tadayoni R, Erginay A, Haouchine B, Gaudric A, Massin P. Optical coherence tomography assessment of the vitreoretinal relationship in diabetic macular edema. Am J Ophthalmol. 2005;139(5): 807-813

[41] James Lin, MD, Jonathan S. Chang, MD, Nicolas A. Yannuzzi, MD, William E. Smiddy, MD. Cost Evaluation of Early Vitrectomy versus Panretinal Photocoagulation and Intravitreal Ranibizumab for Proliferative Diabetic Retinopathy. Ophthalmology. 2018 September; 125(9): 1393-1400.

[42] https://investor.regeneron.com/static-files/89add496-a979-4c71-80b5-a8aebab7d95d

[43] Nauck M, Karakiulakis G, Perruchoud AP, et al. Corticosteroids inhibit the expression of the vascular endothelial growth factor gene in human vascular smooth muscle cells. Eur J Pharmacol 1998;341:309-315.

[44] Kompella UB, Bandi N, Ayalasomayajula SP. Subconjunctival nano and microparticles sustain retinal delivery of budesonide, a corticosteroid capable of inhibiting VEGF expression. Invest Ophthalmol Vis Sci 2003;44:1192-1201.

[45] Cunha-Vaz J., Ashton P., Iezzi R., Campochiaro P., Dugel P., Holz F., et al. (2014) Sustained delivery fluocinolone acetonide vitreous implants: long-term benefit in patients with chronic diabetic macular edema. Ophthalmology 121: 1892-1903.

[46] Matias Iglicki, Dinah Zur, Catharina Busch, Mali Okada, Anat Lowenstein. Progression of diabetic retinopathy severity after treatment with dexamethasone implant: a 24-month cohort study the 'DR-Pro-DEX Study'. Acta Diabetologica 2018 Jun;55(6):541-547. doi: 10.1007/s00592-018-1117-z.

[47] Matias Iglicki, Dinah Zur, Adrian Fung, Pierre-Henry Gabrielle, Marco Lupid, Rodrigo Santos, Catharina Busch, Matus Rehak, Zafer Cebeci, Martin Charles, Dua Marsawa, Shulamit Achwarz, adiel Barak, Anat Lowenstein. International Retina group (IRG). TRActional DIabetic reTInal detachment surgery with co-adjuvant intravitreal dexamethasONe implant: the TRADITION STUDY. Acta Diabetol 2019 Oct;56(10):1141-1147. doi: 10.1007/s00592-019-01357-y.

Chapter 11

Angiopoietins as Targets for Diabetic Retinopathy Treatment

Lauren M. Ciulla, Nimesh A. Patel, Nicolas A. Yannuzzi and Rehan M. Hussain

Abstract

Diabetic eye diseases, such as diabetic retinopathy (DR) and diabetic macular edema (DME) are among the leading causes of blindness in developed countries. Anti-VEGF therapies such as, ranibizumab, aflibercept and off-label bevacizumab have become first-line treatment for DME. While randomized controlled trials show significant improvement in vision, these anti-VEGF agents have limited durability leading to a significant treatment burden, as reflected in real-world studies, which generally demonstrate under-treatment and less favorable visual acuity outcomes than observed in prospective trials. Alternative pathways, such as the Tie-2 angiopoietin pathway may address unmet needs, with potential for greater efficacy or durability when compared to anti-VEGF monotherapy. While some Tie-2 angiopoietin therapeutic agents, such as nesvacumab, ARP-1536 or AKB-9778, did not meet primary endpoints in clinical trials, other agents have shown promise. One such agent is faricimab, a bispecific antibody inhibiting both VEGF-A and Ang-2. The phase 3 DME trials (YOSEMITE and RHINE) demonstrated favorable safety, visual, and durability outcomes; patients receiving faricimab injection every 4 months achieved similar visual gains as those receiving aflibercept injection every 2 months. Another agent, AXT107 is a peptide that inhibits VEGFR2 and modifies Ang-2 to behave more similarly to Ang-1, promoting vascular stability. This drug is currently undergoing phase 1/2a trials for safety and bioactivity to be completed in May 2022.

Keywords: diabetic retinopathy, diabetic macular edema, angiopoietins, Ang-2, Ang-1, Tie2 receptor, faricimab, AXT107, nesvacumab, AKB-9778, ARP-1536

1. Introduction

The global prevalence of diabetes and its comorbidities has rapidly increased, likely due to an aging population and a high prevalence of obesity [1]. As such, DR has become one of the leading causes of blindness within the Western World [2]. Several pooled analyses have disclosed the prevalence of DR within diabetic populations is greater than 30% [3]. Previously, diabetic macular edema (DME) resulted in approximately half of affected patients losing two or more lines of visual acuity within two years [4]. Historically, laser photocoagulation was validated in clinical trials to slow visual loss in patients with DME and proliferative diabetic retinopathy (PDR), an advanced form of DR involving neovascularization, potentially complicated by vitreous hemorrhage, tractional retinal detachment, and neovascular glaucoma. However, recent and continuing medical advancements in intravitreal corticosteroids and anti-vascular endothelial growth factor (VEGF) agents have led to improvements in clinical outcomes. This chapter reviews the current treatment options and those under development for diabetic eye disease specifically in the Tie-2/Angiopoietin vascular stability pathway.

2. Diabetic retinopathy pathophysiology

Chronic hyperglycemia, hyperlipidemia, and hypertension are involved in the development of DR [5]. Specifically chronic hyperglycemia has been linked to changes within the retinal microvasculature. Chronic hyperglycemia can result in damage through multiple mechanisms including osmotic alterations due to sorbitol accumulation from the polyol pathway, increased nonenzymatic glycosylation of proteins and reactive oxygen species, and activated protein kinase C [6]. These mechanisms contribute to dysfunction of endothelial cells and pericytes, ultimately leading to DR and potentially DME. Endothelial cells support the blood-retinal barrier and pericytes regulate capillary blood flow [7]. Damage to endothelial cells results in fluid accumulation in the macula [4, 8]. Damage to pericytes causes poor regulation of blood flow and microaneurysms within these vessels [9]. Ultimately, microvascular damage of the retina culminates in vision loss due to poor retinal perfusion and ischemia, upregulation of growth factors and inflammatory cytokines, and angiogenesis [6, 10]. Among these growth factors and inflammatory cytokines, VEGF and angiopoietins play important roles and are targets of interest for therapeutic interventions [11].

3. Existing treatments: VEGF inhibitors, corticosteroids, and focal laser

VEGF proteins contribute to the regulation of vascular permeability and growth through tyrosine kinase receptors called VEGF receptors [12]. Binding of VEGF protein ligands to their VEGF receptors activates the mitogen-activating protein kinase (MAPK) signaling pathway and causes angiogenesis via increased endothelial cell growth and survival [13]. There are multiple VEGF proteins including VEGF-A, VEGF-B, VEGF-C, VEGF-D, VEGF-E, and placental growth factor (PlGF) [14]. VEGF-A primarily targets VEGF receptor 2 (VEGFR2) and increases angiogenesis, vascular permeability, and leukocyte adhesion [15, 16]. See **Figure 1** for a schematic of the relationship between the various VEGF ligands and receptors. Due to its significant role in the pathogenesis of DR/DME, many drugs inhibit the VEGF-A (referred to as simply VEGF for the remainder of this chapter) pathway to halt and decrease angiogenesis and vascular permeability within the disease [17]. Currently, two anti-VEGF medications are approved by the US Food and Drug Administration (FDA) for the treatment of DME: aflibercept (Eylea, Regeneron, Tarrytown, NY, USA) and ranibizumab (Lucentis, Genentech, South San Francisco, CA, UA). In addition, one anti-VEGF agent is frequently used off-label, bevacizumab (Avastin, Genentech, South San Francisco, CA, USA).

Ranibizumab was originally approved for the treatment of neovascular age-related macular degeneration (nAMD) in the United States in 2006, and it was approved for DME in 2012 based on the phase 3 RISE and RIDE studies [18]. It is administered intravitreally on a monthly basis. Aflibercept was approved in 2011 for nAMD and in 2014 for DME after positive results from phase 3 VIVID and VISTA studies [19]. It can be dosed in longer eight-week intervals, after 5 monthly loading doses. Bevacizumab was approved in 2004 for use in metastatic colorectal

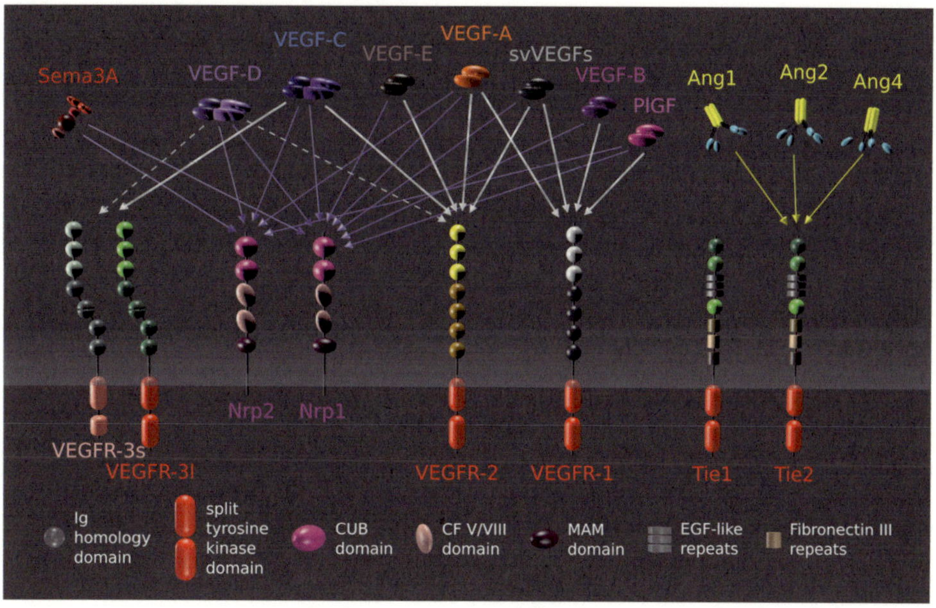

Figure 1.
Schematic depiction of the major interactions between endothelial-specific growth factors and their receptors. (Reproduced here from https://commons.m.wikimedia.org/wiki/File:Endothelial_receptors_and_growth_factors_01.png, licensed under the creative commons attribution-share alike 4.0 international license).

cancer; however, it is often used off-label for DME and is dosed intravitreally similarly to ranibizumab [20].

Intravitreal corticosteroids such as triamcinolone acetonide (Triescence, Alcon, Fort Worth, TX, USA), dexamethasone intravitreal implant (Ozurdex, Abbvie/Allergan, Irvine, CA, USA), and fluocinolone acetonide intravitreal implant (Iluvien, Alimera Sciences, Alpharetta, GA, USA) are also commonly used as a second line treatments for DME, and help reduce exudation by their broad inhibition of inflammatory cytokines. They are often used in combination with anti-VEGF therapy but have potential side effects of cataract progression and ocular hypertension [21]. Focal laser photocoagulation to leaking microaneurysms in the macula has been shown to reduce vision loss compared to no treatment, but does not provide the visual acuity gains achieved with anti-VEGF therapy [19, 22].

Although the use of anti-VEGF agents has greatly improved treatment outcomes in DR/DME patients, these agents have limited durability and require dosing as frequently as monthly, which may be required indefinitely in some cases. Additional treatment barriers include limited treatment efficacy and financial burden, particularly for the branded agents [23]. Anti-VEGF therapy has shown lower efficacy in 'real-world' studies when compared to clinical trial outcomes in DME and in nAMD patients [24–26]. This is partially due to under-treatment in clinical practice, resulting in approximately one line less of visual acuity gains compared to large randomized clinical trials. One real world database study showed that over one year U.S. DME patients received a mean of 7.5, 7.9 and 7.7 injections of aflibercept, bevacizumab and ranibizumab, respectively, which is lower than the 9.2, 9.7, and 9.4 injections received for these same drugs in the DRCR Protocol T Study [25, 27]. For the RISE and RIDE studies, DME patients received monthly ranibizumab injections (12 total), and for the VIVID and VISTA studies patients received bimonthly treatment of aflibercept after 5 monthly doses (8 total). Additionally, it has been shown that blockade of VEGF-A can lead to upregulation of other members of the VEGF family which also have pro-angiogenic effects [28]. For these reasons, there has been a heightened focus on the development of medications that target alternate pathways, such as the Tie-2/angiopoietin pathway.

4. Tie-2/angiopoietin pathway

Recently, there has been great interest in drug development within the Tie-2 transmembrane tyrosine kinase receptor pathway in exudative diseases such as DME and nAMD. This receptor is found on endothelial cells and is responsive to the opposing angiopoietins, Ang-1 and Ang-2 (see **Figure 2**) [29]. These growth factors are integral players in vessel homeostasis, permeability, and angiogenesis. Ang-1 activates the Tie-2 receptor and leads to vascular stability [30]. Ang-2 acts as a competitive antagonist to Ang-1, turning off the Tie-2 receptor, leading to abnormal vascular growth, leakage, and increased inflammatory signals within endothelial cells [31, 32]. Tumor necrosis factor α (TNFα), a central inflammation mediator, induces Ang-2 release from endothelial cells to enhance its stimulation of inflammation and vascular leakage [33]. Additionally, the enzyme vascular endothelial protein tyrosine phosphatase (VE-PTP) inactivates the Tie-2 receptor and therefore interferes with the vascular stabilizing effects of Ang-1 [34].

A number of preclinical studies have supported the importance of the Tie-2/Ang-2 pathways in DR and DME pathophysiology. Studies in the developing retina and in ischemic retinal mouse models have shown increased expression of both Ang-2 and VEGF which correlated to increased neovascularization [35, 36]. A study in double transgenic mice expressing both Ang-1 and VEGF showed that increased expression of Ang-1 led to decreased neovascularization and suppression of VEGF [37]. Additionally, high levels of Ang-2 and VEGF have been found in samples from diabetic patients following vitrectomy [38, 39]. During times of stress such as, hyperglycemia, ischemia, and oxidative stress, Ang-2 levels increase and result in aberrant vascular leakage and growth. Therapeutic interventions for exudative diseases may focus on inhibiting Ang-2 or VE-PTP therefore preventing their counterregulatory effects on the Tie-2 receptor.

4.1 Faricimab

Faricimab, previously RG7716 (Roche, Basel, Switzerland and Genentech, South San Francisco, CA, USA) is a bispecific antibody that binds to and inhibits both VEGF and Ang-2. Phase 1 and 2 trials showed promising results, supporting advancement to phase 3 trials [40, 41]. Results from four phase 3 trials from both patients with DR/DME and nAMD were released in February, 2021 from Roche [42]. All four studies demonstrated non-inferior results when administered in long-lasting dosing intervals compared to aflibercept.

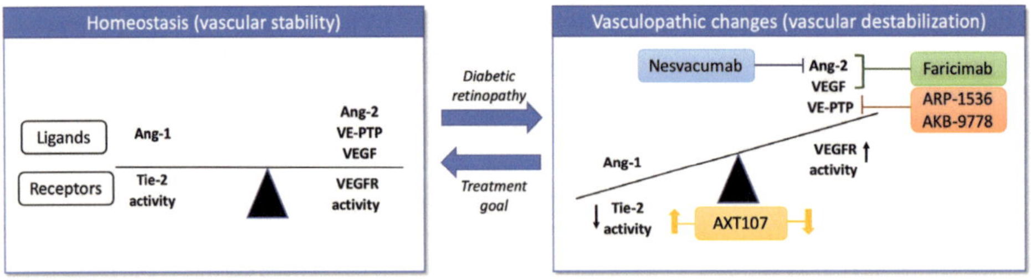

Figure 2.
Molecular targets and approaches to re-establish homeostasis in Ang–Tie-2 and VEGF–VEGFR pathways (reproduced with permission from [9]).

The YOSEMITE and RHINE studies are two identical phase 3 clinical studies that compared faricimab to aflibercept in patients with DME. The YOSEMITE and RHINE trials enrolled 940 and 951 patients respectively. These studies compared faricimab 6.0 mg given at individualized intervals (one, two, three or four months based on DR activity), faricimab 6.0 mg given at two-month intervals, and aflibercept 2.0 mg given at two-month intervals. Sham injections were given when patients within a treatment group were not scheduled to receive treatment to maintain blinding. The primary outcomes were average change in best corrected visual acuity (BCVA) at one year. Secondary outcomes were percent of individualized interval arm receiving doses at one, two, three, and four months at 52 weeks, percent of participants with a two-step or more improvement in diabetic retinopathy severity score (DRSS) from baseline, percent of participants with gain and percent without loss of 15 letters or more in BCVA, and change in central subfield thickness [43, 44].

YOSEMITE showed an average improvement of +11.6 ETDRS letters in the individualized interval faricimab arm, +10.7 ETDRS letters in the two-month interval faricimab arm, and +10.9 ETDRS letters in the aflibercept arm. Similarly, RHINE showed an average improvement of +10.8 ETDRS letters in the individualized interval faricimab arm, +11.8 ETDRS letters in the two-month interval faricimab arm, and +10.3 ETDRS letters in the aflibercept arm. Within the individualized interval faricimab arm, there were 151/286 (52.8%) participants in YOSEMITE that were dosed with a four-month interval at one year and 60/286 (21%) that were dosed with a three-month interval. Similarly, in RHINE, 157/308 (51%) participants were dosed with a four-month interval at one year and 62/308 (20.1%) achieved a three-month dosing interval. When compared to the aflibercept two-month dosing interval arm, both studies showed that the participants that achieved up to four-month dosing intervals of faricimab had larger reductions in central subfield thickness (CST) [42]. Roche has announced plan to submit a new drug application to the U.S. Food and Drug Administration and the European Medicines Agency for the treatment of DME and nAMD.

4.2 AXT107

AXT107 (Asclepix Therapeutics, Baltimore, MD, USA) is a peptide that modifies Ang-2 to function more similarly to Ang-1. This peptide is derived from the non-collagenous domain of collagen IV and ultimately activates the Tie-2 receptor and stabilizes vascular permeability [9]. In studies using confluent monolayers of endothelial cells, AXT107 attached to Ang-2 binds to the Tie-2 receptor and disrupts $\alpha5\beta1$ integrin, causing Tie-2 and $\alpha5$ to move to cell junctions. Ultimately, Ang-2 modified by AXT107 serves as an agonist of the now junctional Tie-2 receptor and acts similarly to Ang-1 even in the presence of low concentrations of Ang-1 [45]. AXT107 also suppresses TNF-α induced vascular inflammation in endothelial cells, which may provide additional benefit in treating the chronic inflammatory component of DME and other retinal vascular diseases [33]. Additionally, in animal models, AXT107 increased breakdown of VEGFR2 which ultimately decreases the effects of VEGF [46]. Studies conducted in rabbit eyes injected AXT107 into the vitreous as a clear gel depot. This gel formulation slowly releases the AXT107 and could potentially decrease the need for many repeat injections. The rabbit model studies showed that AXT107 decreased leakage by 86% and 70% at one and two months, respectively. This was compared to aflibercept which reduced leakage by 69% at one month and did not reduce leakage at two months [47].

The CONGO study is a phase 1/2a clinical trial that will evaluate the safety and bioactivity of AXT107. This is a non-randomized open label study with 18 participants with DME. Three treatment arms of low (0.1 mg), medium (0.25 mg), and high (0.5 mg) doses are included. The primary outcome is safety measured by incidence of adverse effects. Secondary outcomes are efficacy assessed by change in CST, change in BCVA, and percentage of participants improving by greater than 5, 10, 15 letters on the eye chart. This study is expected to be concluded by May 2022 [48].

4.3 Nesvacumab

Nesvacumab (Regeneron, Tarrytown, NY, USA) is a human immunoglobulin G1 (IgG1) monoclonal antibody that binds to and blocks Ang-2. Nesvacumab was coformulated with aflibercept and phase 1 trials showed promising results for nAMD and DME. The phase 2 ONYX (nAMD) and RUBY (DME) trials did not duplicate that success however; patients treated with nesvacumab-aflibercept combo did not show any significant benefit in BCVA or CST compared to aflibercept monotherapy. For the RUBY study, however, there was a significant difference in the proportion of patients with resolution of foveal edema and ≥2 step improvement in DRSS in the high dose co-formulation arm [49]. In 2017, Regeneron announced that Nesvacumab would not advance to phase 3 trials [50].

4.4 AKB-9778

AKB-9778 (Aerpio Pharmaceuticals, Cincinnati, OH, USA) is an antagonist of VE-PTP given via subcutaneous injection. The TIME-2a study was a phase 2 study that sought to determine the safety and efficacy of AKB-9778 in DME patients. There were three treatment arms within 144 participants: 15 mg AKB-9778 twice daily and monthly placebo intravitreal injections, 15 mg AKB-9778 twice daily and monthly 0.3 mg ranibizumab intravitreal injections, and placebo subcutaneous injection twice daily and monthly 0.3 mg ranibizumab injections. The primary outcome was mean change in CST at three months and secondary outcomes were BCVA, DRSS, and safety [51]. Mean change CST was significantly greater in participants receiving both AKB-9778 and ranibizumab (−164.4±24.2 μm) than in participants receiving ranibizumab alone (−110.4±17.2 μm). Regarding the secondary outcomes, the percentage of participants that gained ≥10 or ≥15 letters across the treatment arms were: 8.7% and 4.3% in the AKB-9778 alone group, 29.8% and 17.0% in the ranibizumab along group, and 35.4% and 20.8% in the combination group, respectively. The DRSS remained similar across the three groups and AKB-9778 was found to be safe [52].

The safety and efficacy of AKB-9778 in 167 patients with nonproliferative DR was studied in the Time-2b study. This study did not utilize anti-VEGF therapy in its treatment arms and instead used AKB-9778 alone. The treatment arms included: AKB-9778 15 mg once daily, AKB-9778 15 mg twice daily, and subcutaneous placebo injected twice daily [53]. The primary outcome of percentage of participants with improvement in their DRSS was not met at 48 weeks. There was a significant 20% improvement in urine albumin creatinine ratio in patients treated with AKB-9778 twice daily and there was also a significant reduction in intraocular pressure among the treatment groups versus placebo. Based on these results, Aerpio Pharmiceuticals is investigating the use of AKB-9778 in diabetic nephropathy and open angle glaucoma. AKB-9778 is also in a phase 2 study for use in hospitalized subjects with COVID-19 acute respiratory distress syndrome [54].

4.5 ARP-1536

ARP-1536 (Aerpio Pharmiceuticals, Cincinnati, OH, USA) has the same biologic activity as AKB-9778 however it is delivered by intravitreal injection rather than subcutaneously. ARP-1536 is an antagonist to VE-PTP which activates the Tie-2 receptor and provides vascular stability. It is in pre-clinical studies in combination with anti-VEGF therapy for DME and wet AMD [54].

5. Conclusion

Diabetic eye diseases are among the leading causes of blindness within the Western world. Previously, laser photocoagulation was the mainstay of treatment for DME and PDR [55]. Over the past two decades, anti-VEGF agents have become first-line treatments for DME. Although these medications have significantly improved visual outcomes for DME, limitations have been noted in 'real-world' studies [24–26]. Most notably, anti-VEGF agents require frequent injection, which acts as a treatment barrier to patients and leads to under-dosing. The investigational drugs that target the Tie-2/angiopoietin pathway may produce greater drying effect on the macula, with prolonged durability and superior visual outcomes compared to anti-VEGF monotherapy. Future trials may focus on the ability of combination anti-VEGF and Ang-2 inhibitors to treat PDR.

Author details

Lauren M. Ciulla[1], Nimesh A. Patel[2], Nicolas A. Yannuzzi[3] and Rehan M. Hussain[4]*

1 Northwestern University Feinberg School of Medicine, Chicago, IL, USA

2 Department of Ophthalmology, Massachusetts Eye and Ear Infirmary, Harvard Medical School, Boston, MA, USA

3 Department of Ophthalmology, Bascom Palmer Eye Institute, University of Miami Miller School of Medicine, Miami, FL, USA

4 Retina Associates Ltd., Elmhurst, IL, USA

*Address all correspondence to: rhussain27@gmail.com

References

[1] Danaei G, Finucane MM, Lu Y, et al. National, regional, and global trends in fasting plasma glucose and diabetes prevalence since 1980: Systematic analysis of health examination surveys and epidemiological studies with 370 country-years and 2.7 million participants. Lancet. 2011;378(9785): 31-40.

[2] Bourne RRA, Jonas JB, Bron AM, et al. Prevalence and causes of vision loss in high-income countries and in eastern and Central Europe in 2015: Magnitude, temporal trends and projections. Br J Ophthalmol. 2018;102(5):575-585.

[3] Sivaprasad S, Gupta B, Crosby-Nwaobi R, Evans J. Prevalence of diabetic retinopathy in various ethnic groups: A worldwide perspective. Surv Ophthalmol. 2012;57(4):347-370.

[4] Ferris FL, 3rd, Patz A. Macular edema. A complication of diabetic retinopathy. Surv Ophthalmol. 1984;28 Suppl:452-461.

[5] Klein R, Klein BE, Moss SE, Cruickshanks KJ. The Wisconsin epidemiologic study of diabetic retinopathy: XVII. The 14-year incidence and progression of diabetic retinopathy and associated risk factors in type 1 diabetes. Ophthalmology. 1998;105(10):1801-1815.

[6] Ciulla TA, Amador AG, Zinman B. Diabetic retinopathy and diabetic macular edema: Pathophysiology, screening, and novel therapies. Diabetes Care. 2003;26(9):2653-2664.

[7] Antcliff RJ, Marshall J. The pathogenesis of edema in diabetic maculopathy. Semin Ophthalmol. 1999;14(4):223-232.

[8] Ciulla TA, Harris A, Latkany P, et al. Ocular perfusion abnormalities in diabetes. Acta Ophthalmol Scand. 2002;80(5):468-477.

[9] Hussain RM, Neiweem AE, Kansara V, Harris A, Ciulla TA. Tie-2/ Angiopoietin pathway modulation as a therapeutic strategy for retinal disease. Expert Opin Investig Drugs. 2019; 28(10):861-869.

[10] Morello CM. Etiology and natural history of diabetic retinopathy: An overview. Am J Health Syst Pharm. 2007;64(17 Suppl 12):S3-S7.

[11] Das A, McGuire PG, Rangasamy S. Diabetic macular Edema: Pathophysiology and novel therapeutic targets. Ophthalmology. 2015;122(7): 1375-1394.

[12] Leung DW, Cachianes G, Kuang WJ, Goeddel DV, Ferrara N. Vascular endothelial growth factor is a secreted angiogenic mitogen. Science. 1989; 246(4935):1306-1309.

[13] Ferrara N, Gerber HP, LeCouter J. The biology of VEGF and its receptors. Nature medicine. 2003;9(6):669-676.

[14] Clauss M. Molecular biology of the VEGF and the VEGF receptor family. Semin Thromb Hemost. 2000;26(5): 561-569.

[15] Miller JW, Le Couter J, Strauss EC, Ferrara N. Vascular endothelial growth factor a in intraocular vascular disease. Ophthalmology. 2013;120(1):106-114.

[16] Kim I, Moon SO, Kim SH, Kim HJ, Koh YS, Koh GY. Vascular endothelial growth factor expression of intercellular adhesion molecule 1 (ICAM-1), vascular cell adhesion molecule 1 (VCAM-1), and E-selectin through nuclear factor-kappa B activation in endothelial cells. The Journal of biological chemistry. 2001;276(10):7614-7620.

[17] Boyer DS, Hopkins JJ, Sorof J, Ehrlich JS. Anti-vascular endothelial growth factor therapy for diabetic

macular edema. Ther Adv Endocrinol Metab. 2013;4(6):151-169.

[18] Nguyen QD, Brown DM, Marcus DM, et al. Ranibizumab for diabetic macular edema: Results from 2 phase III randomized trials: RISE and RIDE. Ophthalmology. 2012;119(4): 789-801.

[19] Heier JS, Korobelnik JF, Brown DM, et al. Intravitreal Aflibercept for diabetic macular Edema: 148-week results from the VISTA and VIVID studies. Ophthalmology. 2016;123(11): 2376-2385.

[20] Stefanini FR, Arevalo JF, Maia M. Bevacizumab for the management of diabetic macular edema. World journal of diabetes. 2013;4(2):19-26.

[21] Hussain RM, Ciulla TA. Treatment strategies for refractory diabetic macular edema: Switching anti-VEGF treatments, adopting corticosteroid-based treatments, and combination therapy. Expert Opin Biol Ther. 2016;16(3):365-374.

[22] Photocoagulation for diabetic macular edema. Early Treatment Diabetic Retinopathy Study report number 1. Early treatment diabetic retinopathy study research group. Archives of ophthalmology. 1985;103(12):1796-1806.

[23] Hussain RM, Ciulla TA. Emerging vascular endothelial growth factor antagonists to treat neovascular age-related macular degeneration. Expert opinion on emerging drugs. 2017;22(3): 235-246.

[24] Cohen SY, Mimoun G, Oubraham H, et al. Changes in visual acuity in patients with wet age-related macular degeneration treated with intravitreal ranibizumab in daily clinical practice: The LUMIERE study. Retina. 2013;33(3):474-481.

[25] Ciulla TA, Bracha P, Pollack J, Williams DF. Real-world outcomes of anti-vascular endothelial growth factor therapy in diabetic macular Edema in the United States. Ophthalmol Retina. 2018;2(12):1179-1187.

[26] Ciulla TA, Pollack JS, Williams DF. Visual acuity outcomes and anti-VEGF therapy intensity in diabetic macular oedema: A real-world analysis of 28 658 patient eyes. Br J Ophthalmol. 2021;105(2):216-221.

[27] Diabetic Retinopathy Clinical Research N, Wells JA, glassman AR, et al. Aflibercept, bevacizumab, or ranibizumab for diabetic macular edema. The New England journal of medicine. 2015;372(13):1193-1203.

[28] Cabral T, Lima LH, Mello LGM, et al. Bevacizumab injection in patients with Neovascular age-related macular degeneration increases Angiogenic biomarkers. Ophthalmol Retina. 2018;2(1):31-37.

[29] Asahara T, Chen D, Takahashi T, et al. Tie2 receptor ligands, angiopoietin-1 and angiopoietin-2, modulate VEGF-induced postnatal neovascularization. Circulation research. 1998;83(3): 233-240.

[30] Lee J, Park DY, Park DY, et al. Angiopoietin-1 suppresses choroidal neovascularization and vascular leakage. Invest Ophthalmol Vis Sci. 2014;55(4):2191-2199.

[31] Maisonpierre PC, Suri C, Jones PF, et al. Angiopoietin-2, a natural antagonist for Tie2 that disrupts in vivo angiogenesis. Science. 1997;277 (5322):55-60.

[32] Ziegler T, Horstkotte J, Schwab C, et al. Angiopoietin 2 mediates microvascular and hemodynamic alterations in sepsis. J Clin Invest. 2013.

[33] Mirando AC, Lima ESR, Chu Z, Campochiaro PA, Pandey NB, Popel AS.

Suppression of ocular vascular inflammation through peptide-mediated activation of Angiopoietin-Tie2 Signaling. Int J Mol Sci. 2020; 21(14).

[34] Frye M, Dierkes M, Kuppers V, et al. Interfering with VE-PTP stabilizes endothelial junctions in vivo via Tie-2 in the absence of VE-cadherin. J Exp Med. 2015;212(13):2267-2287.

[35] Oshima Y, Deering T, Oshima S, et al. Angiopoietin-2 enhances retinal vessel sensitivity to vascular endothelial growth factor. J Cell Physiol. 2004;199(3):412-417.

[36] Oshima Y, Oshima S, Nambu H, et al. Different effects of angiopoietin-2 in different vascular beds: New vessels are most sensitive. FASEB journal: official publication of the Federation of American Societies for Experimental Biology. 2005;19(8):963-965.

[37] Nambu H, Nambu R, Oshima Y, et al. Angiopoietin 1 inhibits ocular neovascularization and breakdown of the blood-retinal barrier. Gene Ther. 2004;11(10):865-873.

[38] Watanabe D, Suzuma K, Suzuma I, et al. Vitreous levels of angiopoietin 2 and vascular endothelial growth factor in patients with proliferative diabetic retinopathy. Am J Ophthalmol. 2005;139(3):476-481.

[39] Loukovaara S, Robciuc A, Holopainen JM, et al. Ang-2 upregulation correlates with increased levels of MMP-9, VEGF, EPO and TGFbeta1 in diabetic eyes undergoing vitrectomy. Acta Ophthalmol. 2013;91(6):531-539.

[40] Hussain RM, O'Leary P., Eichenbaum, D.A., Hariprasad S.M. Faricimab. Drugs of the Future. 2020;45(7):449-457.

[41] Sahni J, Patel SS, Dugel PU, et al. Simultaneous inhibition of Angiopoietin-2 and vascular endothelial growth factor-a with Faricimab in diabetic macular Edema: BOULEVARD phase 2 randomized trial. Ophthalmo logy. 2019.

[42] New phase III data show Roche's faricimab is the first investigational injectable eye medicine to extend time between treatments up to four months in two leading causes of vision loss, potentially reducting treatment burden for patients [press release]. https://roche.com, Februrary 12, 2021 2021.

[43] A Study to Evaluate the Efficacy and Safety of Faricimab (RO6867461) in Participants with Diabetic Macular Edema (YOSEMITE). https://clinicaltrials.gov/ct2/show/NCT03622580. Accessed 5-16-21.

[44] A Study to Evaluate the Efficacy and safety of faricimab (RO6867461) in participants with diabetic macular edema (RHINE). https://clinicaltrials.gov/ct2/show/NCT03622593. Accessed 5-16-21.

[45] Mirando AC, Shen J, Silva RLE, et al. A collagen IV-derived peptide disrupts alpha5beta1 integrin and potentiates Ang2/Tie2 signaling. JCI Insight. 2019;4(4).

[46] Silva RLE, Kanan Y, Mirando AC, et al. Tyrosine kinase blocking collagen IV-derived peptide suppresses ocular neovascularization and vascular leakage. Sci Transl Med. 2017;9(373).

[47] W P. Asclepix therapeutics: breakthrough next gen therapies for retinal diseases. Paper presented at: Ophthalmic Innovation Summit; 2019, 2019; Chicago (IL).

[48] AsclepiX Therapeutics, Inc. doses first patient in phase 1/2a trial of AXT107 Intravitreal self-forming gel depot peptide for diabetic macular Edema (DME) [press release]. AsclepiX Therapeutics, January 5, 2021 2021.

[49] Rodriguez M. ASRS 2018: Diabetic Retinopathy Session 1. https://retinaroundup.com/2018/07/25/asrs-2018-diabetic-retinopathy-session-1/. Updated 7-25-18. Accessed 5-22-21.

[50] Helzner J. Eylea/Ang2 combo disappoints in phase 2. Retinal Physician (Nov/Dec 2017).

[51] The TIME-2 study: a phase 2 study of AKB-9778, a novel Tie-2 activator, in patients with diabetic macular edema (TIME-2). https://clinicaltrials.gov/ct2/show/NCT02050828. Accessed 5-22-21.

[52] Campochiaro PA, Khanani A, Singer M, et al. Enhanced benefit in diabetic macular Edema from AKB-9778 Tie2 activation combined with vascular endothelial growth factor suppression. Ophthalmology. 2016;123(8):1722-1730.

[53] The Time-2b study: a study of AKB-9778, a novel Tie 2 activator, in patients with non-proliferative diabetic retinopathy (NPDR) (Time-2b). https://clinicaltrials.gov/ct2/show/NCT0 3197870. Accessed 5-22-1.

[54] Pipeline. Aerpio Pharmaceuticals https://aerpio.com. Accessed 5-22-21.

[55] Modarres M. Vitrectomy for diabetic macular edema; where are we? J Curr Ophthalmol. 2016;28(4):161-162.

Chapter 12

Diabetic Retinopathy and Stem Cell Therapy

Sevil Kestane

Abstract

This overview was evaluated by the development of diabetic retinopathy (DR) and the stem cell therapy approach. DR is a microvascular complication of diabetes mellitus, characterized by damage to the retinal blood vessels leading to progressive loss of vision. However, the pathophysiological mechanisms are complicated and not completely understood yet. The current treatment strategies have included medical, laser, intravitreal, and surgical approaches. It is known that the use of mesenchymal stem cells (MSC), which has a great potential, is promising for the treatment of many degenerative disorders, including the eye. In retinal degenerative diseases, MSCs were ameliorated retinal neurons and retinal pigmented epithelial cells in both *in vitro* and *in vivo* studies. Stem cell therapies show promise in neurodegenerative diseases. However, it is very important to know which type of stem cell will be used in which situations, the amount of stem cells to be applied, the method of application, and its physiological/neurophysiological effects. Therefore, it is of great importance to evaluate this subject physiologically. After stem cell application, its safety and efficacy should be followed for a long time. In the near future, widespread application of regenerative stem cell therapy may be a standard treatment in DR.

Keywords: diabetic retinopathy, mesenchymal stem cells, cell therapy, regenerative stem cell therapy, neurodegenerative diseases

1. Introduction

The eye is an excellent structure, both an optical and a neuronal device. There are many diseases related to the eye. Each anatomical part of this organ may show a defect and cause an eye defect. Diabetic retinopathy is one of the most common complications of type I and type II diabetes. One of the main causes of blindness worldwide is diabetic retinopathy. Although glucose controls are helpful for other diabetic complications, they cannot prevent the development of retinopathy. While many studies have been done on the physiology of the retina, there are many unknown dark spots. Studies suggest that radicals derived from reactive oxygen play an important role in the development of diabetic retinopathy. Due to high oxygen consumption, the brain and retina are very sensitive to oxidative stress. Oxidative stress has been found to cause brain and retinal damage in both diabetic humans and experimentally diabetic rats. Although various hypoglycemic drugs have been developed for the treatment of diabetes mellitus (DM), complications associated with diabetes remain major medical problems. Therefore, the development of new treatments is of great interest. The mechanisms in the development and progression of diabetic retinopathy are not yet fully understood as they are multifactorial and complex. Stem cell therapies for retinal diseases have been around for a long time. Few clinical trials are currently showing improvement [1].

The eye is the site of many acute or chronic physiopathological disorders, reversible or not, that can lead to partial or total vision loss or major changes in the quality of patients' life. The search for innovative therapeutic strategies to correct these disorders is an important current issue. Gene and cell therapies are powerful therapeutic tools, but controlling the properties and spread of the injected material is a parameter that limits its application in humans. Anatomical isolation of the eye and ease of access, on the other hand, enable the use of such treatments, which have been previously developed in tissues and whose clinical application is complex [2].

Hillard Lazarus used mesenchymal stem cell (MSC) for the first time in 1995. Today, there are more than 400 applications in a wide variety of clinical fields such as inflammatory pathologies or immunological, fibrotic, or neurological disorders [3].

The use of MSC, which has a great potential, is promising for the treatment of many degenerative disorders, including the eye. In retinal degenerative diseases, MSC ameliorated retinal neurons and retinal pigmented epithelial cells in both *in vitro* and *in vivo* studies [1]. Diabetes is among the largest medical emergencies in the world. Hyperglycemia is responsible for a wide number of complications, with the vascular ones representing the leading cause of mortality. Stem cells have the unique ability to originate any organ or tissue and are capable of self-renewal. Among stem cells, great clinical interest is reserved for MSC [4].

2. Diabetes and diabetic retinopathy

The development of modern life has brought with it an inactive life [5]. The human population is constantly increasing, and diseases are also increasing. In addition, the expectation of prolonging life, lifestyle, and dietary habits that support obesity creates possible conditions for the development of diabetes. Diabetes is shown as the third cause of death in industrialized countries after cardiovascular diseases and cancer. It is stated that about 110 million people on a global scale suffer from diabetes mellitus. This type of diabetes is also called diabetes mellitus. The main symptom of this disease is the presence of sugar in the urine. A diabetic patient occurs every 8 minutes according to the research of a health institution. DM is the inability of sugar to enter the cell and perform its function as a result of the insufficiency of pancreatic insulin secretion or the ineffectiveness of insulin or the inability of insulin to function due to structural defects in the insulin molecule. Insulin produced in the pancreas is responsible for the transition of blood glucose into cells. When insulin is deficient, the level of glucose in the blood increases and it increases the permeability of the vessel by causing defects in the inner surface and outer wall of the vessel in the vascular tissue. Diabetes damages the retina the most in the eye tissue. It is predicted that diabetes mellitus will rise sharply in the next decade. Patients with diabetes suffer from life-limiting and threatening complications and suffer from diseases such as stroke, peripheral arterial diseases, and retinopathy. [6]. Diabetic retinopathy is the most common microvascular complication of DM, resulting in blindness worldwide. Diabetic retinopathy (DR) is a global problem, affecting approximately 100 million people worldwide. Blindness is 25 times more common in diabetic patients than in non-diabetic patients. DR is the most common cause of blindness in patients aged 20–64 years in developed countries. The prevalence of the disease is related to the age of the cases and the duration of the disease. Biochemical changes detected in diabetic retinopathy increased oxidative stress, nonenzymatic glycosylation, protein kinase-C activation, polyol pathway, and increased nitric oxide [7].

Retinal neurons provide normal visual function. Vision loss in diabetes should be explained as a disorder in the function of neurons. To date, most research has generally focused on retinal vascular changes rather than the effect of diabetes on the neural retina. As a result of many studies, it has been determined that changes in neuronal function and vitality are effective in the pathological mechanism of diabetic retinopathy that starts in the early stage of diabetes. Neurophysiological changes have been observed immediately after the onset of diabetes in both humans and experimental animals [8].

The most common cause of retinopathy is diabetes. Retinopathy is responsible for about a third of vision loss and blindness in children. Microaneurysms, non-perfusion capillaries, hemorrhages and/or lipoprotein exudates, which are the onset of DR, indicate that DR is primarily a microvascular disease [9]. There is ample evidence of early retinal neurodegenerations in diabetes. Neuronal degenerations and early retinal disorders were observed in some animal models and studies in humans before the onset of diabetic vasculopathy [10]. Neurodegeneration, which causes thinning of the retina layer in animal studies, is not only limited to cell death and tissue loss but also causes functional disorders in neurotransmitters [11]. The most prominent feature of neurodegenerative diseases is increased neuronal loss with apoptosis. Increasing neuron frequency is accepted as an important component of pathology in diabetic retinopathy. Early studies characterized vascular lesions in postmortem specimens of human retinas [12–14].

Indeed, neurophysiological changes have been observed immediately after the onset of diabetes in both humans and experimental animals. It has been reported that vascular changes such as permeability changes during diabetes occur 8 days after the onset of diabetes in rats. Capillary dilation and increased blood flow are the earliest signs of diabetes in both humans and animals. Capillaries begin to close within a few years in dogs whereas in about 1 year of diabetes in rats. Typical retinopathy begins to develop in humans at 5–10 years, with microaneurysm, hemorrhage, macular edema, and neovascularization. The neural retina is transparent and invisible, so it is not visible on clinical examination. Vascular changes provide information about the course of the disease and the possibility of blindness. Apart from insulin therapy, the only proven treatment is laser photocoagulation, which destroys retinal regions with overt vascular disorders. This manipulation reduces macular edema and can improve visual acuity, but it cannot restore normal vision and prevent neuronal loss. If neurodegeneration begins shortly after the onset of diabetes, irreversible neuron damage occurs during laser therapy. Early neurophysiological and neurodegenerative changes should be considered as targets for current DR treatments. Psychophysical measurements also showed changes in vision in the early stage of diabetes onset. Contrast sensitivity decreases especially at mid and low spatial frequencies [1, 15].

Obesity is a major health problem in the world that is responsible for type II diabetes mellitus (DM) and its serious complications, such as retinopathy, cardiovascular disease, and nephropathy. In diabetic eyes, neovascularization results in blindness through a vitreous hemorrhage, retinal detachment, or glaucoma. Retinal hypoxia is the crucial factor for these complications [16]. Diabetic retinopathy is one of the most common complications of type I and type II diabetes. One of the main causes of blindness worldwide is diabetic retinopathy. Although glucose controls are helpful for other diabetic complications, they cannot prevent the development of retinopathy. The pathology of retinopathy is due to the deterioration of the vessels of the eye, which occurs due to various metabolic disorders in diabetic patients. These metabolic disturbances range from the level of vascular endothelial growth factor (VEGF) to the accumulation of end products of its glycosylation. The primarily tissue-damaging effects of chronic hyperglycemia cause a complex interplay of multiple mechanisms, which cause abnormal permeability within the retinal vessels, and occlusion with ischemia and subsequent neovascularization. Current treatments include laser photocoagulation and vitreotomy, but these treatments are not curative and do not target the pathological mechanism of the disease. Various studies have been conducted in diabetic rats and human models. Immunohistochemical studies were able to show that intravitreally injected stem cells were localized to the inner retina and it has been stated that this increases visual function. Human clinical trials are ongoing to evaluate the safety, success, and utility of hematopoietic stem cell (HSC) injection in treating retinal vascular diseases. Two patients with diabetic retinopathy injected with HCC showed improvement in visual acuity and ophthalmic measurements even 12 weeks after treatment. The mechanism of the behavior of HSC is unclear, but is thought to be dependent on paracrine signaling. In animal models, intravitreal HSC has been shown to improve retinal damage caused by light, ischemia, and diabetes. Apart from HSC, other stem cells such as mesenchymal stem cell (MSC), endothelial progenitor cell (EPC), and adipose stromal cell are also being investigated for their use in the treatment of diabetic retinopathy. Diabetes mellitus causes both functional and structural deficiencies by affecting both the peripheral and central nervous systems. Peripheral disorders develop within a few weeks after the onset of diabetes, while central disorders take months to develop [17]. Diabetic retinopathy is a major complication of diabetes. However, the effect of a prediabetic condition on the retina has not been clarified. Prediabetes refers to a metabolic disorder defined by glycemic variables lower than diabetes but higher than normoglycemia and considered a high-risk condition for the development of diabetes. It has been stated that the majority of prediabetic patients will eventually develop diabetes [18, 19]. Current treatments for DR as laser photocoagulation, intravitreal anti-VEGF agents, intravitreal corticosteroids, and vitreoretinal surgery are applicable only at advanced stages of the DR and are associated with significant adverse effects [20]. Therefore, new treatments for the early stages of the DR are needed. Retinal diseases are the leading cause of vision loss in the world. Because of the ability of stem cells to self-renewal and differentiation to various types of cells, stem cells are becoming an attractive source of cell therapy in repairing damaged cells as retina pigment epithelium or photoreceptors. Consequently, retinal stem cell therapy is one of the promising therapeutic alternatives to recover vision [21].

3. Stem cells

The organism begins to form from a cell and then develops into a complete organism with more than 200 cell types. This phylogenetic trend, the tendency to switch from pluripotent cells to mature cells is an integral part of human development. This process, in which cells differentiate and turn into cells without plasticity, is necessary to form all special tissues of the human and to minimize the risk of tumor proliferation. Basically, for a cell to be accepted as a stem cell, this cell should first be able to renew itself without losing its plasticity, and then lose its plasticity and differentiate into different sub-cell types [22]. A stem cell is an undifferentiated cell with the capacity to self-renewal and differentiate. These cells have also the capacity to differentiate into special cells that make up tissues and organs. Self-renewal is the capacity for a cell to reproduce indefinitely by maintaining its undifferentiated state. Differentiation potential is the capacity for a cell to differentiate into one or more types of mature cells.

In addition, stem cells are also characterized by maintaining a certain calm-stagnant state, apart from their capacity for self-renewal and differentiation. This quiescent phase is the G_0 phase of the cell cycle, in which cells enter in the absence of mitotic factors. With this calm phase, stem cells can protect themselves against possible "attacks" and maintain their vitality. However, none of these features are sufficient to define the 'root' character of the cell. In fact, it should have the potential to rebuild the tissue's excellent function in the long run. This means a large number of cellular divisions and differentiation *in vivo*. These properties also play a vital role in organogenesis and adult tissue regeneration. There are many stem cells used and studied in research. Particularly, some researchers can find new stem cell sources today [23–25].

The two largest types of stem cells in mammals are embryonic stem cells isolated from the inner cell mass of the blastocyst and adult stem cells found in most adult tissues.

3.1 Embryonic stem cells (ESC)

They are the first discovered and studied stem cells. They are cells that can renew themselves and have the capacity to differentiate into all cell types that can form a whole organism.

3.2 Adult stem cells

With the development of the embryo, embryonic pluripotent stem cells are replaced by stem cells with a more limited capacity, which will provide organ and tissue formation. Cells of different tissues are now specialized. Organs need a mechanism to regenerate cells by replacing cells lost by apoptosis or lesion, thus maintaining their homeostasis. An adult loses about 20 billion cells in a day. This requires a permanent restructuring system [26]. Some organs such as the brain, heart, and kidney are less regenerated [27]. On the other hand, tissues such as bone marrow, skin, and intestines are constantly renewed. To ensure the regeneration prosess, organs have a cell reservoir; adult stem cells which serve throughout life. Their stocks are provided by the balance between self-renewal and differentiation capacities. Adult stem cells are also known as somatic stem cells. It is assumed that all organs of the body have mature stem cells, and in most organs, they are active throughout life. They constantly form new cells to ensure tissue regeneration (skin, cornea, bone marrow, intestine) [28–30]. In some organs, these cells become active after birth and then go into dormancy. We see them in organs with slow or almost no cellular regeneration; it is seen only in organs such as the brain and liver, where stem cells divide only during serious injuries or rarely [31, 32]. Hematopoietic stem cells, stromal stem cells, and stem cells in organs are adult stem cells.

Bone marrow contains two types of cells: hematopoietic stem cells (HSC) and stromal mesenchymal stem cells (MSC). HSC can form all mature hematopoietic cells such as myeloid and lymphoid. MSC plays a supportive role in hematopoiesis. Bone marrow also contains other types of cells. Progenitor endothelial cells (PEC) are found in the marrow as well as adult multipotent progenitor cells [33]. When necessary, PEH enters the circulation and plays a role in angiogenesis. In addition, some studies refer to bone marrow stem cells (F-MSCs), which represent a heterogeneous stem cell population. These cells can differentiate into many different types of cells, such as hepatocytes, endothelial cells, epithelial cells, cardiac or skeletal muscle cells, neuronal cells, or astrocytes. This indicates that bone marrow cells have the potential to differentiate into cells of another tissue [34]. Stem cells are ubiquitous. Some niches are yet to be discovered. Although bone marrow-derived stem cells have been cited as a potential resource for regenerative therapy, their potential and usefulness are still open to debate [35, 36].

Deterioration in tissues or organ functions for any reason constitutes a very important problem in terms of seriously affecting an individual's quality of life. For this reason, regenerative medicine is concerned with repairing the damage and restoring normal body functions through stem cell therapies. Advances in stem cell research have shown cell-based therapy as a useful option to treat medically incurable diseases [36]. Stem cells can migrate to damaged tissue. The effect and cellular mechanisms of stem cells vary according to their environment. They have excellent plasticity that allows these cells to adapt to their environment and act appropriately [33].

"Plasticity" is the ability of a stem cell to acquire different differentiation programs under certain microenvironmental conditions. Endogenous MSC or exogenously administered MSC can migrate to the injured tissue and participate in its healing. The therapeutic effects of MSC can be attributed to its ability to secrete a wide variety of paracrine factors. These mechanisms are likely independent, but they can also act together. In many cases, a combination of these protective mechanisms can work together to heal the damage [37]. However, the mechanism of the therapeutic effect of stem cell is still open to debate. There are two basic explanations; these are cell differentiation and the paracrine effect of stem cells. The combination of these two mechanisms seems to be a third theory [38].

4. Mesenchymal stem cells and retinal degenerations

Retinal degenerations are pathologies that affect the light-sensitive cells of the retina, photoreceptors, cones, and rods. Cell therapy is accepted as an interesting alternative for retinal degenerations. A mouse model of retinal degeneration has been shown to improve visual function after transplantation of photoreceptors [39]. Other cells, including MSC, also show great potential by altering photoreceptors or protecting against degenerations due to their paracrine effects [40]. Some researchers also emphasize that MSC can differentiate into retinal cells, especially photoreceptor-like cells. This plasticity feature of MSC has been observed *in vitro* [41]. It has also been observed *in vivo* by subretinal injection in a rat model with retinal degeneration [42]. These results reveal the possibility of regenerative therapy in pathologies involving photoreceptor losses.

In general, cellular therapy works in two ways: to replace dead cells in the tissue to restore tissue function or to prevent/attenuate/slow tissue degeneration by reducing inflammatory infiltration or reduce apoptosis and cell death phenomena.

5. Stem cell and eye

The eye is a small organ, and the number of stem cells required therapeutically is theoretically less than in larger organs. Compared to other internal organs, the retinal environment is easily accessible with small-gauge vitrectomy needles, greatly increasing the potential for stem cell-based therapy for the treatment of retinal degenerative diseases. The retina is layered and thin. It depends on the preservation of cells, nerve anatomy, and synaptic networks to maintain vision. Retinal neuron connectivity is an important therapeutic goal to alleviate blindness in millions of people worldwide for the preservation or restoration of the original neural structure of the retina and photoreceptor [43]. The emergence of studies shows the possibility of cell regeneration in the adult central nervous system, which makes it possible to envision the implantation of stem cells or progenitor cells as an approach to cell therapy. The restorative approach offers strong hope, given that key questions about the biology of development need to be explored. The transplantation of differentiated or undifferentiated retinal tissue (embryonic, newborn) in the subretinal position of the graft poses the problem of its structural and functional organization.

It is seen that different types of stem cells are used considering transplantation studies. When we look at transplantation studies, in studies using different types of stem cells (retina progenitor cell, neural stem cell, bone marrow-derived stem cell, and embryonic stem cell), although they settle in the retina, they are not able to express retinal-specific markers and cannot establish synaptic connections are encountered [44].

The discovery of stem cells has caused great excitement in the hopes of using such treatments to restore vision. Already, stem cells in the anterior segment of the eye have a remarkable clinical effect. Stem cell therapy provides re-epithelialization of the cornea and improves vision. The trabecular meshwork, located on the inner side of the junction of the sclera and the cornea, can also be regenerated with stem cells [38]. However, the most interesting studies have been done in the posterior segment of the eye. Most retinal degenerations begin with the loss of a neuron or damage to a neuron. Therefore, these cells should be replaced with a cell layer that is differentiated and functional in the appropriate medium. Sometimes pathology develops and destroys many cells. In this case, a graft consisting of several layers is required. To perform a transplant treatment for blindness, progenitor neuronal cells are isolated and transferred to different cells of the retina.

Studies on neuronal cell cultures that can differentiate are done. Today, very few of these differentiation mechanisms have been fully elucidated. Therefore, the use of cell transplantation in the retina seems distant [45].

Considering that stem cell therapy is promising in retinal diseases, studies were started with embryonic stem cells, and induced pluripotent stem cells were obtained. Many retinal cells such as retinal pigment epithelium, photoreceptors, and ganglion cells were obtained from induced pluripotent stem cells [46].

It is stated that the neuroretina, which is attached to the pigment epithelium (RPE), has a complex structure. Therefore, it has been stated that there are three different cells that can be considered in cell therapy: neuroretina (photoreceptors, bipolar cells, ganglion cells, and glial cells), RPEs, and vascular endothelial cells. Depending on retinal diseases, strategies to place different cells need to be developed [47].

6. Conclusion

Diabetic retinopathy (DR) is one of the largest causes of vision loss worldwide. The use of autologous stem cells for organ reconstruction offers a potential solution for the replacement of tissue or whole organs mechanisms in the development and progression of DR are not fully understood yet. Although many studies have been done about retinal physiology, many unknown dark spots are available about it. Stem cell therapy appears to be a possible option both to prevent neurovascular damage and to repair the damaged retina. Mesenchymal stem cell attracts great attention in retinal degenerations due to their ability to differentiate into neurons. However, the way and amount of stem cell administration will create different effects, it is important to know the effect of cell therapy on body after administration in relation to its use in the clinical practice.

To date, no treatment has been developed for the regeneration of retinal vasculature damage resulting from prolonged hyperglycemia. Cell therapy seems to be a possible option both to prevent neurovascular damage and to repair damaged retina [48]. Although clinical evaluations and retinal autopsies of diabetic patients provide information about the progression and features of diabetic retinopathy, its pathophysiological mechanism is not yet understood. Studies on animal models continue in order to better understand the development of diabetic retinopathy at the molecular and cellular level [49]. Retina, in the nervous system, provides a suitable environment to study the functions and distribution of stem cells. It is stated that intravenously administered mesenchymal stem cell transplantation can inhibit retinal apoptotic cells, reduce inflammatory responses, and limit the spread of damage [50].

In a study in which intravitreal mesenchymal stem cell application was performed, some physiological parameters were examined and it was seen that although there were decreases in body weight in diabetics, there was no change in body weight in the group administered intravitreal stem cells. These findings were interesting for us. While it was reported that body weight increased significantly in the mouse model in which the human adipose tissue-derived mesenchymal stem cell was transplanted *via* the tail. It has been stated that intravitreal stem cell application also reduces intraocular pressure and provides a better cognitive function in the diabetic model [51].

As a result, more clinical trials should evaluate the application methods, the timing of the practice, using cell count and repetition dose of stem cell and their results. In the near future, the regenerative stem cell therapy may be a standard treatment in many degenerative eye disorders.

Author details

Sevil Kestane
Medical Faculty, Department of Physiology, Basic Medical Science, Kirşehir Ahi Evran University, Turkey

*Address all correspondence to: kestanesevil@gmail.com

References

[1] Sevil K. The Effect of Mesenchymal Stem Cell Applications on Diabetes and Tamoxifen Retinopathy in Diabetic Rats. Kayseri, Turkey: Erciyes University; 2020

[2] Trapani I, Puppo A, Auricchio A. Vector platforms for gene therapy of inherited retinopathies. Progress in Retinal and Eye Research. 2014;**43**:108-128. DOI: 10.1016/j.preteyeres.2014.08.001

[3] Galderisi U, Peluso G, Di Bernardo G. Clinical trials based on mesenchymal stromal cells are exponentially increasing: Where are we in recent years? Stem Cell Reviews and Reports. 2021;**17**(4):1-14. DOI: 10.1007/s12015-021- 10231-w

[4] Bassi R, Trevisani A, Tezza S, Ben Nasr M, Gatti F, Vergani A, et al. Regenerative therapies for diabetic microangiopathy. Experimental Diabetes Research. 2012;**2012**:916560. DOI: 10.1155/2012/916560

[5] Mutlu S. The Effect of Exercise on Physical Profile and Some Physiological Parameters in Pregnant Women. Kayseri, Turkey: Erciyes University; 2019

[6] Duh EJ, Sun JK, Stitt AW. Diabetic retinopathy: Current understanding, mechanisms, and treatment strategies. JCI Insight. 2017;**2**(14):e93751. DOI: 10.1172/jci. insight.93751

[7] Berkit İ. The Effect of Intravitreal Triamcinalone Acetonide on Retinal Vascular Endothelial Growth Factor Release in Diabetic Rats. Aydın, Turkey: Adnan Menderes University; 2008

[8] Lieth E, Gardner TW, Barber AJ, Antonetti DA, Penn State Retina Research Group. Retinal neurodegeneration: Early pathology in diabetes. Clinical & Experimental Ophthalmology. 2000;**28**(1):3-8. DOI: 10.1046/j.1442-9071.2000.00222.x.(2000)

[9] Lecleire-Collet A, Audo I, Aout M, Girmens JF, Sofroni R, Erginay A, et al. Evaluation of retinal function and flicker light-induced retinal vascular response in normotensive patients with diabetes without retinopathy. Investigative Ophthalmology & Visual Science. 2011;**52**(6):2861-2867. DOI: 10.1167/iovs.10-5960

[10] Lasta M, Pemp B, Schmidl D, Boltz A, Kaya S, Palkovits S, et al. Neurovascular dysfunction precedes neural dysfunction in the retina of patients with type 1 diabetes. Investigative Ophthalmology & Visual Science. 2013;**54**(1):842-847. DOI: 10.1167/iovs.12-10873

[11] Barber AJ, Baccouche B. Neurodegeneration in diabetic retinopathy: Potential for novel therapies. Vision Research. 2017;**139**:82-92. DOI: 10.1016/j.visres.2017.06.014

[12] Bloodworth JM Jr. Diabetic microangiopathy. Diabetes. 1963;**12**:99-114. DOI: 10.2337/diab.12.2.99

[13] Bloodworth JM Jr, Molitor DL. Ultrastructural aspects of human and canine diabetic retinopathy. Investigative Ophthalmology. 1965 Dec;**4**(6):1037-1048

[14] Cunha-Vaz JG. Pathophysiology of diabetic retinopathy. The British Journal of Ophthalmology. 1978;**62**(6):351-355. DOI: 10.1136/bjo.62.6.351

[15] Chihara E, Matsuoka T, Ogura Y, Matsumura M. Retinal nerve fiber layer defect as an early manifestation of diabetic retinopathy. Ophthalmology. 1993;**100**(8):1147-1151. DOI: 10.1016/s0161-6420(93)31513-7

[16] Arjamaa O, Nikinmaa M. Oxygen-dependent diseases in the retina: role of hypoxia-inducible factors. Experimental Eye Research. 2006;**83**(3):473-483. DOI: 10.1016/j.exer.2006.01.016

[17] Biessels GJ, Cristino NA, Rutten GJ, Hamers FP, Erkelens DW, Gispen WH. Neurophysiological changes in the central and peripheral nervous system of streptozotocin-diabetic rats. Course of development and effects of insulin treatment. Brain. 1999;**122**(Pt 4):757-768. DOI: 10.1093/brain/122.4.757

[18] Alves MRP, Boia R, Campos EJ, Martins J, Nunes S, Madeira MH, et al. Subtle thinning of retinal layers without overt vascular and inflammatory alterations in a rat model of prediabetes. Molecular Vision. 2018;**24**:353-366

[19] Cai J, Boulton M. The pathogenesis of diabetic retinopathy: Old concepts and new questions. Eye (London, England). 2002;**16**(3):242-260. DOI: 10.1038/sj.eye.6700133

[20] Simó-Servat O, Hernández C, Simó R. Usefulness of the vitreous fluid analysis in the translational research of diabetic retinopathy. Mediators of Inflammation. 2012;**2012**:872978. DOI: 10.1155/2012/872978

[21] Feng X, Chen P, Zhao X, Wang J, Wang H. Transplanted embryonic retinal stem cells have the potential to repair the injured retina in mice. BMC Ophthalmology. 2021;**21**(1):26. DOI: 10.1186/s12886-020-01795-1

[22] Dominici M, Le Blanc K, Mueller I, Slaper-Cortenbach I, Marini F, Krause D, et al. Minimal criteria for defining multipotent mesenchymal stromal cells. The International Society for Cellular Therapy position statement. Cytotherapy. 2006;**8**(4):315-317. DOI: 10.1080/14653240600855905

[23] Meng X, Ichim TE, Zhong J, Rogers A, Yin Z, Jackson J, et al. Endometrial regenerative cells: A novel stem cell population. Journal of Translational Medicine. 2007;**5**:57. DOI: 10.1186/1479-5876-5-57

[24] Reinisch A, Hofmann NA, Obenauf AC, Kashofer K, Rohde E, Schallmoser K, et al. Humanized large-scale expanded endothelial colony-forming cells function in vitro and in vivo. Blood. 2009;**113**(26):6716-6725. DOI: 10.1182/blood-2008-09-181362

[25] Humphries A, Graham TA, McDonald SA. Stem cells and inflammation in the intestine. Recent Results in Cancer Research. 2011;**185**:51-63. DOI: 10.1007/978-3-642-03503-6_3

[26] Fuchs E. The tortoise and the hair: Slow-cycling cells in the stem cell race. Cell. 2009;**137**(5):811-819. DOI: 10.1016/j.cell.2009.05.002

[27] Bergmann O, Bhardwaj RD, Bernard S, Zdunek S, Barnabé-Heider F, Walsh S, et al. Evidence for cardiomyocyte renewal in humans. Science. 2009;**324**(5923):98-102. DOI: 10.1126/science.1164680

[28] Barker N, van Es JH, Kuipers J, Kujala P, van den Born M, Cozijnsen M, et al. Identification of stem cells in small intestine and colon by marker gene Lgr5. Nature. 2007;**449**(7165):1003-1007. DOI: 10.1038/nature06196

[29] Greco V, Chen T, Rendl M, Schober M, Pasolli HA, Stokes N, et al. A two-step mechanism for stem cell activation during hair regeneration. Cell Stem Cell. 2009;**4**(2):155-169. DOI: 10.1016/j.stem.2008.12.009

[30] Takizawa H, Regoes RR, Boddupalli CS, Bonhoeffer S, Manz MG. Dynamic variation in cycling of hematopoietic stem cells in steady state and inflammation. The Journal of Experimental Medicine.

2011;**208**(2):273-284. DOI: 10.1084/jem.20101643

[31] Lugert S, Basak O, Knuckles P, Haussler U, Fabel K, Götz M, et al. Quiescent and active hippocampal neural stem cells with distinct morphologies respond selectively to physiological and pathological stimuli and aging. Cell Stem Cell. 2010;**6**(5): 445-456. DOI: 10.1016/j.stem.2010.03.017

[32] Furuyama K, Kawaguchi Y, Akiyama H, Horiguchi M, Kodama S, Kuhara T, et al. Continuous cell supply from a Sox9-expressing progenitor zone in adult liver, exocrine pancreas and intestine. Nature Genetics. 2011;**43**(1):34-41. DOI: 10.1038/ng.722

[33] van Haaften T, Thébaud B. Adult bone marrow-derived stem cells for the lung: Implications for pediatric lung diseases. Pediatric Research. 2006;**59** (4 Pt 2):94R-99R. DOI: 10.1203/01.pdr.0000203550.50258.5a

[34] Tomita M, Adachi Y, Yamada H, Takahashi K, Kiuchi K, Oyaizu H, et al. Bone marrow-derived stem cells can differentiate into retinal cells in injured rat retina. Stem Cells. 2002;**20**(4):279-283. DOI: 10.1634/stemcells.20-4-279

[35] Machalińska A, Baumert B, Kuprjanowicz L, Wiszniewska B, Karczewicz D, Machaliński B. Potential application of adult stem cells in retinal repair--challenge for regenerative medicine. Current Eye Research. 2009;**34**(9):748-760. DOI: 10.1080/02713680903050592

[36] Enzmann V, Yolcu E, Kaplan HJ, Ildstad ST. Stem cells as tools in regenerative therapy for retinal degeneration. Archives of Ophthalmology. 2009;**127**(4):563-571. DOI: 10.1001/archophthalmol.2009.65

[37] Li H, Fu X. Mechanisms of action of mesenchymal stem cells in cutaneous wound repair and regeneration. Cell and Tissue Research. 2012;**348**(3):371-377. DOI: 10.1007/s00441-012-1393-9

[38] Marchetti V, Krohne TU, Friedlander DF, Friedlander M. Stemming vision loss with stem cells. The Journal of Clinical Investigation. 2010;**120**(9):3012-3021. DOI: 10.1172/JCI42951

[39] Pearson RA, Barber AC, Rizzi M, Hippert C, Xue T, West EL, et al. Restoration of vision after transplantation of photoreceptors. Nature. 2012;**485**(7396):99-103. DOI: 10.1038/nature10997

[40] Ng TK, Fortino VR, Pelaez D, Cheung HS. Progress of mesenchymal stem cell therapy for neural and retinal diseases. World Journal of Stem Cells. 2014;**6**(2):111-119. DOI: 10.4252/wjsc.v6.i2.111

[41] Nadri S, Yazdani S, Arefian E, Gohari Z, Eslaminejad MB, Kazemi B, et al. Mesenchymal stem cells from trabecular meshwork become photoreceptor-like cells on amniotic membrane. Neuroscience Letters; **541**:43-48. DOI: 10.1016/j.neulet.2012.12.055

[42] Huo DM, Dong FT, Yu WH, Gao F. Differentiation of mesenchymal stem cell in the microenviroment of retinitis pigmentosa. International Journal of Ophthalmology. 2010;**3**(3):216-219. DOI: 10.3980/j.issn.2222-3959.2010.03.08

[43] Singh R, Cuzzani O, Binette F, Sternberg H, West MD, Nasonkin IO. Pluripotent stem cells for retinal tissue engineering: Current status and future prospects. Stem Cell Reviews and Reports. 2018;**14**(4):463-483. DOI: 10.1007/s12015-018-9802-4

[44] Goureau O, Sahel JA. Cellules souches rétiniennes: mécanisme de différenciation et potentiel

thérapeutique [Retinal stem cells: Mechanism of differentiation and therapeutic application]. Pathologie Biologie (Paris). 2006;**54**(2):64-71. French. DOİ: 10.1016/j.patbio.2005.02.002.

[45] Limb GA, Daniels JT, Cambrey AD, Secker GA, Shortt AJ, Lawrence JM, et al. Current prospects for adult stem cell-based therapies in ocular repair and regeneration. Current Eye Research. 2006;**31**(5):381-390. DOI: 10.1080/02713680600681210

[46] Garg A, Yang J, Lee W, Tsang SH. Stem cell therapies in retinal disorders. Cells. 2017;**6**(1):4. DOI: 10.3390/cells6010004

[47] Siqueira RC. Stem cell therapy in retinal diseases? Revista Brasileira de Hematologia e Hemoterapia. 2012;**34**(3):222-226. DOI: 10.5581/1516-8484.20120054

[48] Kramerov AA, Ljubimov AV. Stem cell therapies in the treatment of diabetic retinopathy and keratopathy. Experimental Biology and Medicine (Maywood, N.J.). 2016;**241**(6):559-568. DOI: 10.1177/1535370215609692

[49] Lai AK, Lo AC. Animal models of diabetic retinopathy: Summary and comparison. Journal Diabetes Research. 2013;**2013**:106594. DOI: 10.1155/2013/106594

[50] Jiang Y, Zhang Y, Zhang L, Wang M, Zhang X, Li X. Therapeutic effect of bone marrow mesenchymal stem cells on laser-induced retinal injury in mice. International Journal of Molecular Sciences. 2014;**15**(6):9372-9385. DOI: 10.3390/ijms15069372

[51] Sevil K, Bekir C. Effect of mesenchymal stem cell on vep in dıabetıc rat. International Journal of Advances in Science, Engineering and Technology (IJASEAT). 2009, 2019;**7**(3):5-11 DOIONLINE NO - IJASEAT-IRAJ-DOIONLINE-16111

Chapter 13

Vitrectomy in Diabetic Retinopathy

Payal Naresh Shah, Mahesh P. Shanmugam and Divyansh K. Mishra

Abstract

Diabetic vitrectomy is a complicated vitreoretinal surgery due to the complex interaction of various factors. Indications of vitrectomy in diabetes patients would comprise of non-resolving vitreous haemorrhage, taut posterior hyaloid causing vitreo-papillary traction, vitreomacular traction, non-resolving macular edema due to epiretinal membrane, posterior pole tractional retinal detachment or combined retinal detachment. Pre-operative systemic evaluation, a thorough clinical evaluation with ancillary investigations like ultrasound and optical coherence tomography are important for planning the surgery. In this chapter, we would be discussing the basic principles of PVD induction, surgical steps and techniques involved in diabetic vitrectomy. Complications associated can be intraoperative or post-operative. Intra-operative complications would include corneal edema, cataract, bleeding and iatrogenic breaks. Post-operative complications can be divided into early and late, which include vitreous cavity bleeding, raised intraocular pressure, reproliferation, epiretinal membrane, cataract, glaucoma and hypotony.

Keywords: diabetic vitrectomy, proliferative diabetic retinopathy, fibrovascular membrane dissection, delamination, diabetic retinal detachment

1. Introduction

Diabetic retinopathy is one of the leading causes of blindness across the world. The estimated global prevalence of proliferative diabetic retinopathy amongst diabetic patients is 7.5%, and it is higher in type 1 compared to type 2 diabetes [1].

The first pars plana vitrectomy was performed for persistent vitreous haemorrhage in a diabetes patient by Robert Machemer in 1970 using a single port instrument called vitrectomy infusion suction cutter (VISC) [2, 3]. There has been a drastic evolutionary change in the technique of diabetic vitrectomy since then. In this chapter, we would be discussing the current indications of vitrectomy in diabetes patients, various surgical techniques and complications.

1.1 Indications of vitrectomy in diabetic retinopathy

1. Non-resolving vitreous haemorrhage (VH)

2. Dense subhyaloid haemorrhage (SHH) over the macula

3. Tractional retinal detachment (TRD) threatening or involving the fovea

4. Combined retinal detachment (CRD)

5. Vitreomacular traction (VMT) or epiretinal membrane (ERM) causing non-resolving macular edema

6. Taut posterior hyaloid causing vitreopapillary traction [4].

Surgery for extramacular TRDs is generally not advocated as vision is preserved in most cases. Patients who become symptomatic with visual complaints or metamorphopsia or if there is a progression of extramacular TRD to threaten the macula would benefit from surgery [5].

2. Pre-operative assessment

Thorough anterior segment evaluation with special attention to health of corneal epithelium, anterior and posterior synechiae, neovascularisation of angles and iris, and cataract need to performed. Vitreous haemorrhage with dense anterior opacities in the Berger's space or significant cataracts can hinder the view behind. Thus a combined cataract surgery along with vitrectomy can be planned in these cases.

2.1 What to look for, while examining the fundus?

1. Assess the posterior hyaloid separation clinically and assess the areas of dense attachments and planes of separation in order to plan the surgery and site of initiation.

2. FVP-flat or elevated—A flat fibrovascular proliferation without hyaloid separation may be much more surgically challenging compared to an elevated proliferation with separated hyaloid.

3. Configuration of detachment—A tractional detachment is usually concave, while a convex or bullous configuration suggests a combined rhegmatogenous component.

4. Extent of TRD/CRD with FVP membranes beyond the equator and extending anteriorly—indicate that the dissection of these peripheral membranes would be difficult and if its inferior quadrants may warrant external support with a belt buckle (BB)/segmental buckle (SB) based on the extent.

5. Presence of any abnormal vitreoretinal attachments (lattice degenerations/ FVP membranes/breaks) in the periphery and midperiphery—so as to plan for an external tamponade—BB/SB.

6. Associated lesions like macular schisis (implies long standing traction) or macular hole (to plan for inverse flap ILM peeling).

7. Looking at the vascularity of the membranes—more vascular—better to consider pre-operative anti-VEGF injection to reduce the risk of bleeding.

8. Presence of sclerosed vessels would suggest thin retina with higher chances of iatrogenic damage, which one needs to be cautious about.

9. Sometimes, a subretinal bleed or subretinal gliotic (SRG) bands may be noted which also point towards a combined detachment.

10. Long standing traction over disc, papillomacular bundle or fovea—can have a guarded visual prognosis.

2.2 Ancillary investigations

2.2.1 Role of OCT

In patients with media clarity, an optical coherence tomography (OCT) scan can be of utmost value to assess the vitreomacular anatomy, extent of macular detachment, status of fovea, vitreopapillary traction, vitreomacular traction, tractional schisis, epiretinal membrane and macular edema. It can also help in identifying progression of detachment on follow-up. Patients with ERM or macular edema can also be benefited with ERM and internal limiting membrane (ILM) peeling.

Figure 1 shows pre-operative and post-operative OCT and fundus photo comparison. This is a patient with PDR with florid NVD and NVE with VMT and CME with vitreoschisis with vitreopapillary traction pre-operatively. Post-operative OCT shows resolution of all traction and edema with temporal retinal thinning.

A widefield OCT helps in better understanding of the vitreomacular anatomy in the centre as well as mid periphery. It can also help in identifying the plane of dissection and thus help planning the site of initiation [6].

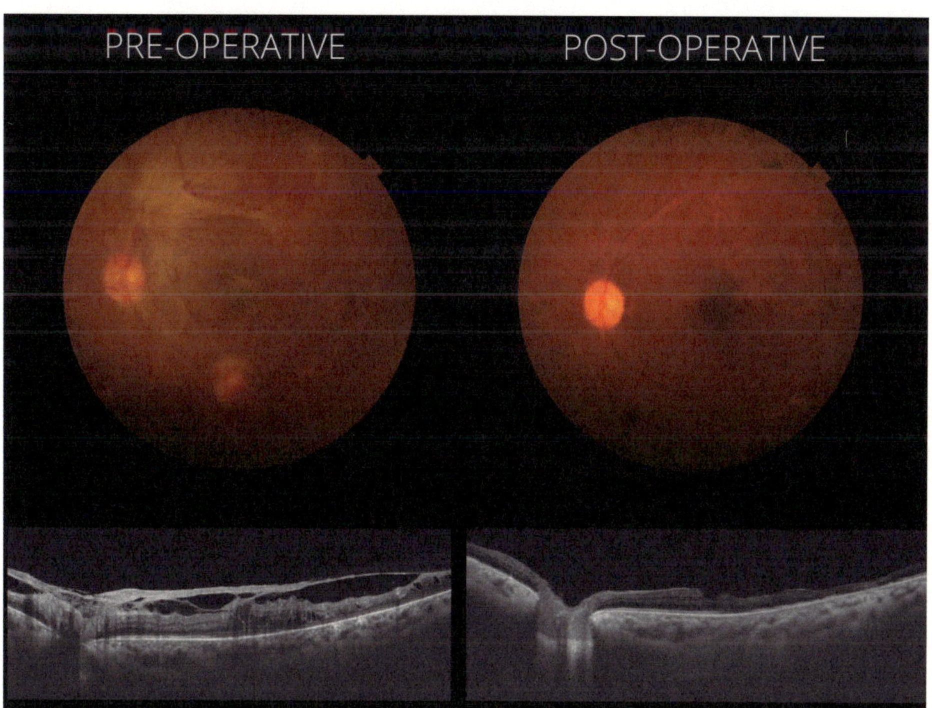

Figure 1.
Preoperative and postoperative colour fundus photograph and OCT scans of a patient with PDR with florid NVD and NVE with VMT and CME with vitreoschisis and vitreopapillary traction.

2.2.2 Role of ultrasound

In patients with dense media opacities like cataract or vitreous haemorrhage, a pre-operative ultrasound evaluation is warranted. This will help to understand the status of posterior hyaloid, location of focal attachments of posterior hyaloid onto the retina, any traction on retina, and co-existing retinal detachment. **Figure 2** shows ultrasound image of a patient with vitreous haemorrhage with subhyaloid haemorrhage with thickened and incomplete hyaloid separation.

Systemic evaluation and stabilisation of the patient is important before taking up for surgery. In patients who are on haemodialysis, a pre-operative heparin-free dialysis should be recommended in order to reduce the chances of intraoperative and post-operative bleeding.

2.2.3 Patient counselling

Besides advocating for surgery, it is very important to counsel the patient about the visual potential since despite good anatomical outcomes, in patients with long standing detachments and macular ischemia, functional outcomes may not be very satisfying. The chances of multiple surgeries due to recurrent vitreous cavity bleeds or redetachments due to reproliferations should be explained. Need for subsequent cataract surgery or silicon oil removal surgery should be explained clearly beforehand. Importance of good systemic control should be re-emphasised.

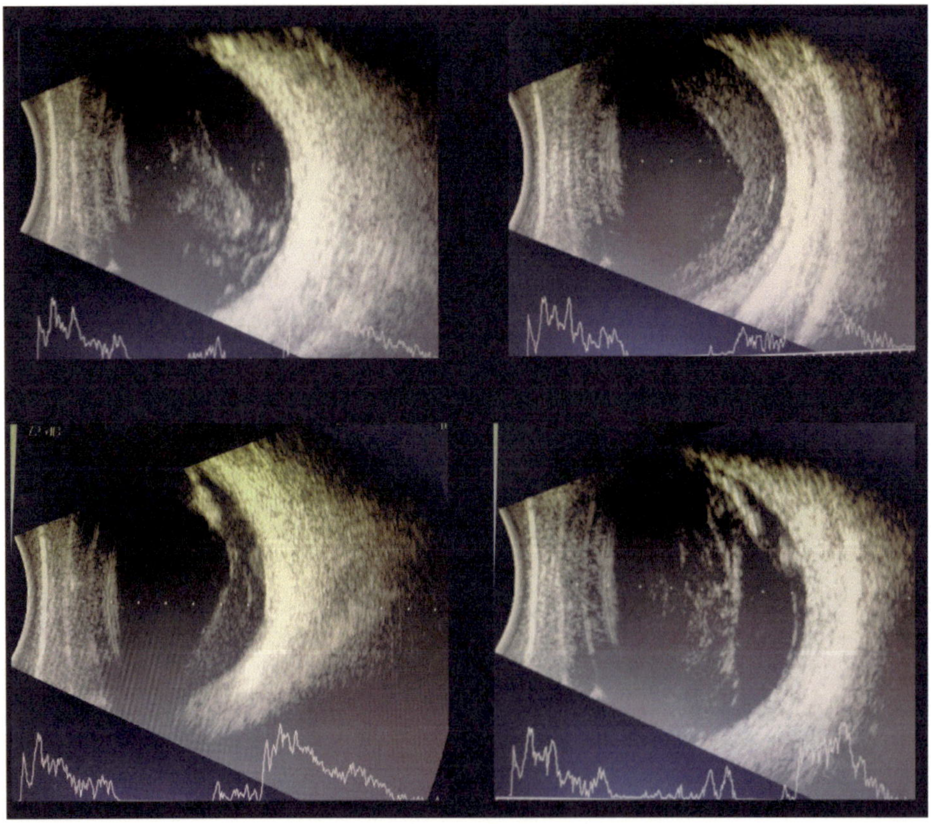

Figure 2.
Ultrasound images of a patient with vitreous haemorrhage with subhyaloid haemorrhage with thickened and incomplete hyaloid separation.

Various studies have shown that a pre-operative intravitreal anti-VEGF injection 3–14 days prior to surgery can help in controlling intra-operative bleeding [7, 8]. Nonetheless, one has to keep in mind that bleeding may occur despite an anti-VEGF injection. Some patients can develop *Crunch syndrome* after anti-VEGF injection. In these cases, TRD worsens due to development of denser fibrotic connections between the retina and overlying tissue, thus making it harder to identify tissue planes. In a retrospective review of TRD following intravitreal bevacizumab, anti-VEGF crunch developed at 5 days or more after initial IVB injection in nearly 80% of cases [9].

3. Timing of vitrectomy in diabetic vitreous haemorrhage

At the time of diabetic retinopathy vitrectomy study (DRVS), vitrectomy was performed in patients who had non-resolving vitreous haemorrhage for more than 12 months. The results of DRVS showed that eyes undergoing early vitrectomy for severe vitreous haemorrhage were more likely to have VA ≥ 20/40 at 2 years and greatest benefit was seen in patients with type 1 diabetes [10]. With the evolution of better surgical techniques and instruments (MIVS), early vitrectomy is more effective in achieving better visual outcomes [11]. Usually, patients with type 1 or type 2 diabetics with VH and no underlying traction, can be observed for 1 month [12]. In the meantime, if haemorrhage improves, visible panretinal photocoagulation (PRP) or intravitreal anti-VEGF injection can be given to allow for neovascularisation to regress. In patients with visually demanding jobs, an early vitrectomy can be performed.

In patients with persistent VH, especially aphakic and pseudophakic patients with posterior capsular defect, there is an increased risk of ghost cell glaucoma and neovascular glaucoma. In these patients, anti-VEGF can be considered prior to surgery and an early vitrectomy is warranted to control IOP.

Vitreous haemorrhage can sometimes develop after panretinal photocoagulation due to contraction of the fibrous component as the vascular component of the fibrovascular membrane regresses or due to posterior vitreous detachment (PVD).

4. Surgical technique

Use of wide-angle non-contact systems would be preferred in diabetic vitrectomy as this would reduce the chances of corneal epithelial defects (since wound healing is delayed in these patients), give a better understanding of vitreous attachments and reduce the chances of iatrogenic breaks.

4.1 Diabetic vitreous haemorrhage

If the ultrasound does not show any co-existing traction or detachment, pars plana vitrectomy along with panretinal photocoagulation would suffice. Pars plana ports are made using biplanar incisions using 23/25G trocar cannula. After clearing the anterior hyaloids, a thorough core vitrectomy should be performed. Care should be taken while clearing the peripheral vitreous, as it may be difficult to distinguish between retina and blood stained vitreous. In case of dense VH, a burr hole vitrectomy can be performed in the superonasal quadrant until the retina is visualised and then further truncation of cone can performed. If the posterior hyaloid is separated at the disc, then the PVD induction is completed if there are no focal areas of traction. If the posterior hyaloid is not separated completely or not moving freely or causes a fluttering movement, suspect an underlying FVP. Thus the truncation of cone should be gentle and graded with a watch on underlying retina/FVP/dense vitreoretinal adhesions.

In some cases, PVD separation may not be complete and there may be subhyaloid haemorrhage (SHH). In such cases, an opening can be made in the taut hyaloid overlying the SHH using the cutter or rarely 26G needle to incise the hyaloid if it is very close to retina and the blood can be drained using cutter aspiration or flute.

Once the blood is cleared and underlying retina visualised, PVD can be completed as far anteriorly as safely possible. The aim should be to segment peripheral base of the vitreous from the any posterior hyaloid to prevent reproliferation and rebleeds. It is not mandatory to shave the vitreous base in these cases. One has to be very careful while performing vitreous base shaving in cases of VH, as the peripheral vitreous base would be harbouring the haemorrhage within itself, sometimes difficult to distinguish from the underlying retina. Also, the blood can leach from the uncut vitreous into the fluid filled vitreous cavity and can cause post-operative dispersed haemorrhage.

It is important look for any sites of blood ooze as this can give rise to post-operative rebleeds. Transient lowering of intraocular pressure (IOP) can help to identify the bleeders. Small oozes can be allowed to clot and then trimmed off with cutter, while large bleeders need immediate attention. Clots should not be pulled as they can cause rebleed. Peripheral examination by indentation to look for breaks or sites of bleeding is crucial. A 360° panretinal photocoagulation using endolaser is performed. While performing endolaser, a straight or a curved laser probe can be used. In case a straight endolaser probe is being used, care has to be taken while performing anterior laser to move away from the retina as the curvature of the globe need to be kept in mind to avoid inadvertent retinal touch. Also, exchanging instruments in both hands while performing anterior laser rather than crossing over instruments will help to avoid inadvertent lens touch. A partial or complete fluid air exchange is performed. It is important to ensure that the sclerotomy sites are not leaking and eye is not hypotonous at the end of surgery as these can also lead to dispersed vitreous cavity haemorrhage post-operatively.

In patients with coexisting macular edema or epiretinal membrane, an ERM with ILM peeling after injecting brilliant blue dye should be performed. Anti-VEGF or steroid injection [13] can also be planned at the end of surgery in such cases after partial or complete fluid air-exchange.

4.2 Diabetic retinal detachment

4.2.1 Understanding the anatomy

The fibrovascular proliferation (FVP) in a diabetic patient grows along the posterior hyaloid and causes tangential traction leading to pleatlike folds on the retina. As the posterior hyaloid starts separating from the retina, it causes an anteroposterior traction over the retina causing tractional retinal detachment. Thus the PVD creates a cone of vitreous extending from the vitreous base to the posterior pole in diabetic eyes [14]. Thus the goal of surgery would be to initially relieve the anteroposterior traction by truncating the cone and then relieve the tangential traction by dissecting the membranes. Once the detachment becomes long standing, the underlying retina becomes then and atrophic creating breaks, leading to combined retinal detachment. Sometimes, one may also notice subretinal gliotic bands (SRGs) due to long standing CRD. It may not always be possible to identify the breaks preoperatively in CRD. Bullous configuration of detachment, SRG or subretinal bleeds may be indirect indicators of CRD.

4.2.2 Principles of surgery

Thus induction of PVD in diabetics is not similar to that performed regularly. In these patients, the primary step is truncation of cone. It is important to identify an area with hyaloid separation, and this leading edge can be held as a bucket handle and go circumferentially to truncate the cone (Video 1; https://cdn.intechopen.com/public/chapter_videos/241965/VIDEO_1.mov). In areas with dense adhesions, switching the site and going forth can help. At sites where the vitreous is very densely adherent and the above technique fails, viscodissection can be utilised to help induce separation. Once the anteroposterior traction is relieved, the membranes need to be carefully dissected out using a combination of various techniques described below to relieve the tangential traction caused by the FVP.

Two basic approaches to handle the membrane dissection are *outside-in* and *inside-out* approaches. Depending on where the hyaloid is maximally separated, one would decide the approach. Although outside-in is a safer and commonly practised approach since the macula is spared, in some cases with flat and densely adherent membranes and/or where there is no PVD, an inside-out approach may be more helpful. However, it is not uncommon to encounter situations where one will require to use a combination of both these approaches depending on the hyaloid adherence. Sometimes, pockets of hyaloid separation can be noted adjacent to NVE and can be used as an initiating site.

Various techniques can be employed in the dissection of membranes as follows:

1. Segmentation: Involves sharp dissection of membranes using scissors or even sometimes cutter. One blade of scissors is inserted beneath the membrane after finding a cleavage plane, while the other blade lies above the membrane. One must be careful not to pinch retina in between the blades to avoid iatrogenic breaks. Initially, this technique was described using a vertical scissors, but these are no longer used after the introduction of curved scissors as they occupy lesser space. Segmentation basically isolates the membranes and does not essentially require complete removal of membranes (Video 2; https://cdn.intechopen.com/public/chapter_videos/241965/VIDEO_2.mov).

2. Delamination: Developed subsequently to address the issue of residual membranes after segmentation causing redetachment. Delamination involves complete removal of membranes rather than just isolating them and identifying the right plane is very important for delamination. This is the most commonly used technique to remove the proliferative membranes. Delamination can be performed using a scissors or a cutter.

In scissors delamination, after identifying the cleavage plane, both the blades are placed beneath the membrane to severe them from underlying vascular attachments. Although initially described using horizontal scissors, these are now replaced by curved scissors (Video 3; https://cdn.intechopen.com/public/chapter_videos/241965/VIDEO_3.mov).

Cutter delamination is now more commonly performed with the advent of smaller guage instruments, where the port is much closer to the tip and thus helps in better delamination. Various techniques of cutter delamination have been described [15]:

a. *Conformal cutter delamination:* Used for rigid membranes, where the port opening is placed at the outer margin of the membrane (Video 2; https://cdn.intechopen.com/public/chapter_videos/241965/VIDEO_2.mov).

b. *Foldback technique:* In this technique, cutter is placed on the anterior surface of the membrane and the vaccum is used to separate the membrane and fold into the cutter, thus protecting the retinal surface. One should allow the membrane to fold up and fall back into the mouth of cutter rather than chasing the membrane into the cutter (Video 3; https://cdn.intechopen.com/public/chapter_videos/241965/VIDEO_3.mov).

c. *Lift and shave:* With the advent of smaller guage (25 and 27G) instruments, it now enables the surgeon to complete the membrane dissection with the cutter alone. A cleavage plane is identified and then using the cutter, membranes are lifted using aspiration and cutting is used once resistance is encountered. This alternate aspiration and cutting the membranes is used to shave them off the surface [16]. Here the cutter is initially used as a pic forceps to lift the membrane and then cutting is applied to shave it off. The advantage of the smaller probes is the higher cutting rates (7000–10,000 cuts/min), which allows controlled movements with minimal movement of the retina underneath and also the port location being closer to tip enables better grasp (Video 1; https://cdn.intechopen.com/public/chapter_videos/241965/VIDEO_1.mov).

d. *Lawnmower technique:* In this technique cutter is used for lifting and blunt dissection, once an opening within the membranes is identified [17]. Here an opening can be made using smaller guage instruments, in the peripapillary area where there is a potential space. Although, the disadvantage would be that, if one encounters bleeding during this manoeuvre, it would be difficult to achieve haemostasis over the disc.

3. En bloc dissection: Although originally described as a technique where the posterior hyaloid was used to lift the membranes and remove as a single unit, there was a high risk of posterior breaks [18]. This technique is no longer used with the advent of minimally invasive vitreoretinal surgery (MIVS) due to higher chances of retinal breaks.

4. Bimanual dissection: In this technique, various illuminated instruments/sources are used, so that the surgeon can use both his hands for membrane peeling. From illuminated infusion cannulas to illuminated picks [19] or chandelier assisted light source, surgeon can use forceps in the non-dominant hand to lift the membrane and scissors or picks in the dominant hand to peel the membranes. This technique is usually reserved for densely adherent diffuse/broad FVP which are usually difficult to dissect otherwise. Care should be taken not to apply undue traction while lifting the membrane by the non-dominant hand, as it can pull the retina and make the detachment more bullous/cause iatrogenic breaks. While using a chandelier light source, an additional sclerotomy can be planned at 12 or 6 o clock position based on the surgeons' preference (Video 4; https://cdn.intechopen.com/public/chapter_videos/241965/VIDEO_4.mov).

5. Viscodissection: In this technique, viscoelastic substance is injected initially into the potential space between the membranes and the retina, in cases where there are densely adherent membranes to aid in the cleavage of the plane. This technique has the risk of creating retinal breaks [20].

6. Perfluoro carbon liquid (PFCL) dissection: In this technique, an opening is made in posterior hyaloid and PFCL is injected to separate the posterior hyaloid from the retina [21]. PFCL can be used as a third hand to stabilise the posterior pole in cases of CRDs or TRDs. It also helps to salvage the macula from surrounding haemorrhage and provides a counter force during membrane

peeling. One has to be cautious while using PFCL in cases of posterior breaks, where traction is not relieved as there can be a chance of subretinal PFCL migration. Also forceful jet while injecting in cases with thin atrophic retinas can cause iatrogenic breaks during injection.

4.3 Vitreoschisis or second membrane identification

Often the posterior vitreous gel splits into an anterior and a posterior leaflet [22]. One may be easily mistaken by looking at the posterior leaflet as the edge of the hyaloid near the FVP and start pulling it. It is important to identify the anterior leaflet that extends beyond the FVP sometimes as thin flimsy glistening membrane onto the surface of TRD/adjacent retina and start separating it from the retina. Once this is identified using a pic or a needle and separated, it is easier to get the right plane for further dissection. If not correctly identified, one can have multiple iatrogenic breaks, since the anterior leaflet of posterior hyaloid (also known as second membrane) is still adherent to underlying retina. Though the aetiology is uncertain, some authors believe that the split may be caused due to the bleeding from the vascular epicentres (Video 3; https://cdn.intechopen.com/public/chapter_videos/241965/VIDEO_3.mov).

In rare circumstances, where the hyaloid is very densely adherent extending till periphery, with flat broad and dense fibrovascular proliferations, one of the authors (Dr. MPS) have tried intravitreal autologous serum injection 24 hours prior to the surgery for induction of PVD with a successful outcome. In the event of any iatrogenic break in the periphery or near the vitreous base better, one can also support with BB/SB to avoid transmitted tractions from the vitreous base.

Hybrid vitrectomy: Some surgeons prefer hybrid vitrectomy using 23G trocar cannulas and 25G or 27G cutters for better membrane delamination. This has the advantage of higher cut-rate and the port site being closer to the tip of cutter helps in easier grasp of membranes [23]. Newer cutters (27G) with very high cutting rates with low vaccum can allow precise cutting in close proximity to the retina with reduced risk of breaks [24].

4.4 Special considerations in CRD

Most often, one may not be able to identify a break pre-operatively. Convex configuration of detachment, SRG, subretinal haemorrhage are indirect clues towards CRD.

1. It is important to keep in mind not to drain the surbretinal fluid (SRF) from the break in case of CRD before completing the membrane dissection, as it helps to keep the retina taut. Once the SRF is drained, retina starts becoming bullous and further membrane dissection becomes very difficult.

2. Use of valved cannulas can help in cases of bullous detachments to reduce the continuous egress of fluid which increases the fluid currents inside and aggravates the bullosity.

3. It is important to finish membrane peeling before retina starts becoming bullous.

4. All attempts should be made to keep the break free from any surrounding membrane or significant blood clot to avoid late lifting of the break and recurrence.

5. Rarely, one can also support with an external segmental buckle if further dissection of membranes is not possible and the posterior traction is relieved as a last resort.

6. Once the membrane dissection is completed and clots are managed, SRF needs to be drained initially by fluid-fluid exchange to dilute the thick SRF and drain better before switching to fluid-air exchange (Video 1 ending; https://cdn.intechopen.com/public/chapter_videos/241965/VIDEO_1.mov).

7. In presence of SRGs not allowing retina to settle, a drainage retinotomy can be made to remove the SRG (Video 1 ending; https://cdn.intechopen.com/public/chapter_videos/241965/VIDEO_1.mov).

Apart from truncating the cone, identifying the right plane and second membranes, dissection of fibrovascular proliferation, another major challenge in diabetic vitrectomy is controlling the haemorrhage or clot management. Bleeding can occur from multiple sources, i.e., vascular nails during FVP dissection, edges of FVP during dissection, optic nerve head due to dense adhesion of posterior hyaloid or FVP at the disc, arcade vessels due to iatrogenic damage, edges of retinal breaks or trimmed NVEs. Despite multiple techniques to arrest the bleeding, it may sometimes be very difficult to handle these blood clots as they get densely adherent to the underlying thin retina.

4.5 Management of haemorrhage

This is one of the crucial and sometimes most challenging step during diabetic vitrectomy. Clot management should always be preferred in the fluid filled cavity, as the air would cause the clot to diffusely get adhered to the retina and will be more catastrophic. Once all the bleeders are managed, before switching to air, one can decrease the IOP to look for any residual oozing and manage accordingly. This would help to reduce post-operative bleeding.

In case of an active visible bleeder as seen from either the edge of FVP or NVEs, one can immediately cauterise them using endodiathermy. In cases where the bleeding is from a major arcade vessel, one has to be cautious to use diathermy as it may cause vascular occlusion subsequently. Light burns using endolaser probe (Power: 150–200 mW and shorter duration—100 ms) can be attempted instead. Rarely, one can also try pinching of the vessel gently using forceps as a last resort.

In case of bleeding from the disc, we cannot use diathermy or endolaser over the disc. Hence either increasing the bottle height of infusion (in case of gravity assisted infusion) or temporarily increasing the intraocular pressure may help to arrest the bleed. If nothing works, a fluid air exchange can also be tried to use air as a temporary tamponade and wait for few minutes to arrest the active bleeding. One has to be patient and may need to make repeated attempts of the above manoeuvres to achieve haemostasis. One does not have to always peel the membrane over disc, as it may bleed unstoppably if it is densely adherent and vascular. This can be circumcised or trimmed and left behind.

Not always, every blood clot needs immediate attention. Sometimes if it has clotted and is not hampering further membrane dissection, then the clot may be left alone and addressed at the end once all membranes are dissected. Small clots can be removed using flute, while larger clots may need cutter. Clots not covering the macula can be left alone if there is no surrounding break or traction if they cannot be safely removed.

4.6 Vitrectomy in tractional versus non-tractional DME

Patients with tractional macular edema in diabetes are known to benefit with vitrectomy and ERM with ILM peeling [25]. In non-tractional DME, role of vitrectomy has been controversial. While some studies show that patients with refractory DME would benefit with vitrectomy [26], other studies have shown no significant visual improvement with ILM peeling although there may be anatomical improvement [27, 28]. Addition of intravitreal steroid along with ILM peeling in some cases of refractory DME, has shown to improve visual outcome in long-term [29].

In patients with long standing macular ischemia or FVP causing traction over fovea, sometimes a macular hole may be noted. Visual prognosis in such cases is guarded despite ILM peeling in contrast to idiopathic macular holes [30].

4.7 Choice of tamponade

In patients with vitreous or subhyaloid haemorrhage or tractional macular edema with no retinal breaks, a simple fluid air exchange would suffice in most cases. In TRD with no iatrogenic breaks, it is not required to drain the SRF using drainage retinotomy. A gas tamponade may suffice in such cases, as the SRF gets absorbed over a period of time gradually. In CRD or TRD with iatrogenic breaks, a gas or a silicon oil tamponade would be required.

5. To summarise

Step 1: After placing sclerotomy ports using valved cannulas, perform anterior and core vitrectomy.

Step 2: Relieve antero-posterior traction—identify areas of posterior hyaloid separation and complete the truncation of cone. If unable to identify, can inject triamcinolone acetonide for better identification. The leading edge of the posterior hyaloid should be held as a bucket handle and the separation should be continued circumferentially, thus separating the posterior hyaloid from the peripheral vitreous base.

Step 3: Relieve tangential traction—identify the site of initiating membrane dissection by identifying the cleavage plane and second membrane. Membranes can be dissected using segmentation or one of the delamination techniques mentioned above.

Step 4: Achieve haemostasis—vascular nails during membrane dissection can be severed using one of the above techniques. Smaller oozes can be dealt later at the end of membrane dissection, while large bleeders which would hamper visualisation should be dealt immediately during membrane dissection.

Step 5: Complete peripheral vitreous clearing.

Step 6: BBG assisted ILM peeling if planned.

Step 7: Endolaser photocoagulation—panretinal and surrounding the retinal breaks.

Step 8: Fluid air exchange and injection of endotamponade.

Step 9: Injection of anti-VEGF or steroid implant.

Step 10: Removal of ports with or without suturing the sclerotomies.

6. Complications

6.1 Intraoperative complications

1. Corneal edema: Can happen due to prolonged surgical time or raised intraocular pressure. Viscoelastic lubrication of cornea intraoperatively and optimal IOP control can help to have better view of fundus. Sometimes, corneal

epithelial debridement may be needed although slow healing in diabetic patients need to be kept in mind.

2. Cataract: This can occur preoperative/intraoperative/postoperative. Diabetic patients are known to have a higher risk and vitrectomy would further increase the risk of cataract. Sometimes intraocular lens touch or hydration of lens can further aggravate the process. With the advent of minimally invasive cataract surgery (MICS), combining cataract surgery along with vitrectomy would be a better choice in older patients with lens changes.

3. Bleeding: This is one of the most dreadful complication encountered intra-operatively in diabetic vitrectomies. Preoperative anti-VEGF injection may help to mitigate this to some extent. Use of valved cannulas also helps to some extent. Lesser exchange of instruments causes lesser IOP fluctuations. Finally, the most important cause is bleeding during dissection of FVP which has been explained above.

4. Iatrogenic breaks: These can occur usually during dissection of FVPs. If the edge of break is oozing blood, it is important to cauterise immediately to achieve haemostasis. It is important to ensure that all the posterior hyaloid and traction has been relieved from surrounding the break, as it can lead to reproliferations or recurrent detachment. Also, it is not a good idea to drain the SRF from the break before completely removing the membranes, as the retina would then start becoming bullous and make further dissection difficult. It is important to indent the periphery at the end to look for any peripheral breaks especially near the active port site.

6.2 Post-operative complications

These can be further classified as early and late post-operative complications.

6.2.1 Early

1. Vitreous cavity bleeding: Dispersed bleeding in the vitreous cavity can be noted either immediately in the post-operative period most often, or sometimes as a delayed complication. Causes in the immediate post-operative period would be inadequate haemostasis intra-operatively or continuous ooze from the sites of vascular nails, or sometimes from peripheral vitreous or sclerotomy sites and hypotony. Sometimes lowering the IOP before closing intraoperatively, can help to locate the possible sites of rebleed/ooze and can be managed appropriately [31]. Pre-operative anti-VEGF can also help to some extent. These bleeds usually resolve by themselves within 2–4 weeks and if persist for long may need a vitreous lavage.

2. Late causes of vitreous cavity bleeding can be reproliferations or inadequately lasered ischemic retina, neovascularisation of retina/iris, or rarely anterior hyaloid fibrovascular proliferation (AHF). An indirect clue to AHF proliferation can be to look for a dilated episcleral vessel. An ultrasound biomicroscopy (UBM) can help to rule out AHF proliferation. These complications can be prevented by doing an aggressive panretinal laser photocoagulation involving the anterior retina, although not always. Rarely, a patient may develop neovascular glaucoma, which may require an anti-VEGF injection along with vitreous lavage and intense laser photocoagulation involving anterior retina.

3. Raised intraocular pressure: In the early post-operative period, clogging of erythrocytes or cellular debris in the trabecular meshwork can cause raised IOP, which can be managed by topical anti-glaucoma medications or oral acetazolamide in most cases [32]. In patients with silicon oil tamponade, sometimes over-filling can cause increased IOP. In such cases, an oil tap using a 23G trocar cannula at 12 o clock can help to reduce the IOP. Pupillary block or anterior chamber migration of oil can be other causes especially in aphakic patients. An inferior peripheral iridectomy (PI) intraoperatively before performing fluid air exchange would help to prevent pupillary block. Steroid induced ocular hypertension or worsening of pre-existing glaucoma can be other causes. Identifying the right cause and treating the underlying problem is the key to successful management. Topical aqueous suppressants would be the first line of choice, since prostaglandin analogues can aggravate cystoid macular edema and/or promote inflammation [33].

4. Suboil haemorrhage: This can happen sometimes due to persistent ooze from the vascular nails of FVP or dense attachments at disc. In most cases, they resolve by themselves and are mobile. One can wait upto 2–4 weeks for the blood to resolve.

6.2.2 Late

1. Reproliferations/redetachments: Reproliferations can develop due to residual FVP or sequestrated growth factors and VEGF in the peripheral vitreous or from the edges of large retinectomies or rarely across the vitreous base as anterior hyaloid fibrovascular proliferations. Reproliferations not causing traction or detachment can be observed. Sometimes they can be managed during silicon oil removal or can be peeled under silicon oil.

2. Epiretinal Membrane: Incidence of ERM after diabetic vitrectomy is 20–50% [34]. Several studies have reported that ILM peeling during vitrectomy can help to reduce the incidence of post-operative ERM [35]. Removal of ERM can be planned along with silicon oil removal in patients with oil tamponade. ERM removal is indicated only if it causes a traction or decrease in visual acuity has been recorded which can be attributed to presence of ERM.

3. Cataract: Diabetes per se, vitrectomy, gas and oil tamponade all are known to be risk factors for faster progression of cataract. Although some surgeons prefer to perform combined cataract and vitrectomy surgery in elderly patients irrespective of lens status, doing a staged procedure can help to reduce post-operative inflammation if the view is adequate to enable vitrectomy [36].

4. Glaucoma: Causes of late glaucoma can be synechial angle closure or emulsified silicon oil blocking the trabecular meshwork or neovascular glaucoma secondary to long standing ischemia [37]. A blocked PI can cause late-onset pupillary block glaucoma. Reopening of PI by Yag laser iridotomy can help in most cases. Some patients may require multiple PIs.

Hypotony: Extensive AHF proliferation or cyclitic membranes over the ciliary body or ciliary body shutdown due to cyclophotocoagulation or anterior segment ischemia can cause persistent hypotony in some patients.

7. Poor prognostic factors

Presence of macular detachment, vitreopapillary traction, thinned out retina, sclerosed vessels, pale disc, neovascularisation of iris or NVG, macular ischemia, poor initial VA (<5/200) and loss of photoreceptor layers, ELM and ellipsoid zone on OCT are poor visual prognostic factors despite a successful anatomical outcome [27].

For a successful anatomic outcome, it is very important to understand the anatomy and surgical principles in a case of diabetic vitrectomy. One has to counsel the patient that visual outcomes may not always correlate with anatomical outcomes. Importance of good systemic control should always be emphasised.

Video links

1. https://cdn.intechopen.com/public/chapter_videos/241965/VIDEO_1.mov
2. https://cdn.intechopen.com/public/chapter_videos/241965/VIDEO_2.mov
3. https://cdn.intechopen.com/public/chapter_videos/241965/VIDEO_3.mov
4. https://cdn.intechopen.com/public/chapter_videos/241965/VIDEO_4.mov

Author details

Payal Naresh Shah*, Mahesh P. Shanmugam and Divyansh K. Mishra
Department of Vitreoretinal and Ocular Oncology Services, Sankara Eye Hospital, Bangalore, India

*Address all correspondence to: n.payalshah@gmail.com

References

[1] Yau JW, Rogers SL, Kawasaki R, Lamoureux EL, Kowalski JW, Bek T, et al. Meta-analysis for eye disease (META-EYE) study group. Diabetes Care. 2012;**35**(3):556-564

[2] Machemer R, Buettner H, Norton EW, Parel JM. Vitrectomy: A pars plana approach. Transactions - American Academy of Ophthalmology and Otolaryngology. 1971;**75**(4):813-820

[3] Machemer R, Parel JM, Buettner H. A new concept for vitreous surgery. 1. Instrumentation. American Journal of Ophthalmology. 1972;**73**:1

[4] De Maria M, Panchal B, Coassin M. Update on indications for diabetic vitrectomy and management of complications. Annals of Eye Science. 2018;**3**(9):51

[5] Stewart MW, Browning DJ, Landers MB. Current management of diabetic tractional retinal detachments. Indian Journal of Ophthalmology. 2018;**66**(12):1751-1762. DOI: 10.4103/ijo.IJO_1217_18

[6] Mishra DK, Shanmugam MP, Ramanjulu R, Sagar P. Comparison of standard and "innovative wide-field" optical coherence tomography images in assessment of vitreoretinal interface in proliferative diabetic retinopathy. Indian Journal of Ophthalmology. 2021;**69**(1):99-102

[7] Zhao XY, Xia S, Chen YX. Antivascular endothelial growth factor agents pretreatment before vitrectomy for complicated proliferative diabetic retinopathy: A meta-analysis of randomised controlled trials. The British Journal of Ophthalmology. 2018;**102**(8):1077-1085. DOI: 10.1136/bjophthalmol-2017-311344

[8] Wang DY, Zhao XY, Zhang WF, et al. Perioperative anti-vascular endothelial growth factor agents treatment in patients undergoing vitrectomy for complicated proliferative diabetic retinopathy: A network meta-analysis. Scientific Reports. 2020;**10**:18880. DOI: 10.1038/s41598-020-75896-8

[9] Arevalo JF, Maia M, Flynn HW Jr, Saravia M, Avery RL, Wu L, Eid Farah M, Pieramici DJ, Berrocal MH, Sanchez JG. Tractional retinal detachment following intravitreal bevacizumab (Avastin) in patients with severe proliferative diabetic retinopathy. The British Journal of Ophthalmology. 2008;**92**(2):213-216

[10] Early vitrectomy for severe vitreous hemorrhage in diabetic retinopathy. Two-year results of a randomized trial. Diabetic Retinopathy Vitrectomy Study Reports 2. The Diabetic Retinopathy Vitrectomy Study Research Group. Archives of Ophthalmology. 1985; **103**:1644-1652

[11] Lin L, Chen Y, Wang L, Shen L. Timing of optimal surgical intervention for vitreous hemorrhage in patients with proliferative diabetic retinopathy. 11 March 2020, PREPRINT (Version 1). DOI: 10.21203/rs.3.rs-16666/v1

[12] El Annan J, Carvounis PE. Current management of vitreous hemorrhage due to proliferative diabetic retinopathy. International Ophthalmology Clinics. 2014;**54**(2):141-153

[13] Kulkarni M, Mishra DK, Shanmugam MP. Slow-release technique of dexamethasone implant. Acta Scientific Ophthalmology. 2021;**4**(5): 87-89

[14] Meredith TA, Kaplan HJ, Aaberg TM. Pars plana vitrectomy techniques for relief of epiretinal traction by membrane segmentation. American Journal of Ophthalmology. 1980;**89**(3):408-413

[15] Charles S. Vitreous Microsurgery. Baltimore: Williams and Wilkins; 1981. pp. 107-120

[16] Berrocal MH. All-probe vitrectomy dissection techniques for diabetic tractional retinal detachments: Lift and shave. Retina. 2018;**38**(Suppl. 1):S2-S4

[17] Berrocal M. A minimalist approach to surgery for diabetic retinal detachment. Retina Today. 2014;**9**(3): 65-69

[18] Abrams GW, Williams GA. "En bloc" excision of diabetic membranes. American Journal of Ophthalmology. 1987;**103**:302-308

[19] Williams GA, Abrams GW, Mieler WF. Illuminated retinal picks for vitreous surgery. Archives of Ophthalmology. 1989;**107**(7):1086

[20] Grigorian RA, Castellarin A, Bhagat N, et al. Use of viscodissection and silicone oil in vitrectomy for severe diabetic retinopathy. Seminars in Ophthalmology. 2003;**18**:121-126

[21] Arevalo JF. En bloc perfluorodissection for tractional retinal detachment in proliferative diabetic retinopathy. Ophthalmology. 2008;**115**:e21-e25

[22] Schwatz SD, Alexander R, Hiscott P, Gregor ZJ. Recognition of vitreoschisis in proliferative diabetic retinopathy. A useful landmark in vitrectomy for diabetic traction retinal detachment. Ophthalmology. 1996;**103**(2): 323-328

[23] Khan MA, Samara WA, Hsu J, Garg S. Short-term outcomes of hybrid 23-, 25-, and 27-gauge vitrectomy for complex diabetic tractional retinal detachment repair. Retinal Cases and Brief Reports. 2019;**13**(3):244-247

[24] Oellers P, Mahmoud TH. Surgery for proliferative diabetic retinopathy: New tips and tricks. J. Ophthalmic Vis. Res. 2016;**11**(1):93-99

[25] Committee Diabetic Retinopathy Clinical Research Network Writing. Vitrectomy outcomes in eyes with diabetic macular edema and vitreomacular traction. Ophthalmology. 2010;**117**(6):1087-1093.e3

[26] Hu XY, Liu H, Wang LN, Ding YZ, Luan J. Efficacy and safety of vitrectomy with internal limiting membrane peeling for diabetic macular edema: A meta-analysis. International Journal of Ophthalmology. 2018;**11**(11):1848-1855

[27] Modarres M. Vitrectomy for diabetic macular edema; where are we? Journal of Current Ophthalmology. 2016;**28**(4): 161-162

[28] Simunovic MP, Hunyor AP, Ho IV. Vitrectomy for diabetic macular edema: A systematic review and meta-analysis. Canadian Journal of Ophthalmology. 2014;**49**(2):188-195

[29] Hwang S, Kang SW, Kim KT, et al. Three-year outcomes of vitrectomy combined with intraoperative dexamethasone implantation for non-tractional refractory diabetic macular edema. Scientific Reports. 2021;**11**:1292

[30] Sharma T, Fong A, Lai TY, Lee V, Das S, Lam D. Surgical treatment for diabetic vitreoretinal diseases: A review. Clinical and Experimental Ophthalmology. 2016;**44**:340-354

[31] Tan SZ, Dell' Aversana Orabona G, Robins JJ, Kumaran N, Wong R. "Delamination Plus": A Technique to Reduce Immediate Postoperative Diabetic Cavity Hemorrhage. Retina. 2020 May 13. DOI: 10.1097/IAE.0000000000002833

[32] Machemer R, Norton EWD. A new concept for vitreous surgery: III. Indications and results. American

Journal of Ophthalmology. 1972; **74**:1034-1056

[33] Alm A, Grierson I, Shields MB. Side effects associated with prostaglandin analog therapy. Survey of Ophthalmology. 2008;53(Suppl. 1): S93-105

[34] Mehta A, Rana-Rahman R, Klaassen I, Rees J, Steel DH. The effect of internal limiting membrane cleaning on epiretinal membrane formation after vitrectomy for proliferative diabetic retinopathy. Ophthalmologica. 2020; **243**:426-435

[35] Michalewska Z, Bednarski M, Michalewski J, Jerzy N. The role of ILM peeling in vitreous surgery for proliferative diabetic retinopathy complications. Ophthalmic Surgery, Lasers & Imaging Retina. 2013; **44**(3):238-242

[36] Ogawa LS, Ozawa Y, Nagasaki K, Inoue M, Katsura H. Posterior synechia of the iris after combined pars plana vitrectomy, phacoemulsification, and intraocular lens implantation. Japanese Journal of Ophthalmology. 2001; **45**:276-280

[37] Branisteanu DC, Moraru AD, Maranduca MA, Branisteanu DE, Stoleriu G, Branisteanu CI, Balta F. Intraocular pressure changes during and after silicone oil endotamponade (Review). Experimental and Therapeutic Medicine. 2020;**20**(6):204